BANISH
your
Belly, Butt & Thighs
forever!

The <u>Real</u> Woman's Guide
to Body Shaping & Weight Loss

By the Editors of
PREVENTION
Health Books
for **Women**™

Foreword by Michele Stanten
Fitness Editor, Prevention *Magazine*

RODALE

Library of Congress Cataloging-in-Publication Data

Banish your belly, butt & thighs forever! : the real woman's guide to body shaping & weight loss / by the editors of Prevention Health Books for Women ; foreword by Michele Stanten
    p.   cm.
Includes index.
ISBN 1–57954–036–8   hardcover
ISBN 1–57954–037–6   paperback
1. Reducing exercises.   2. Exercise for women.
3. Weight loss.   I. Title: Banish your belly, butt, and thighs forever!.   II. Prevention Health Books for Women.
RA781.6.B36   1999
613.7'045—dc21   99–045686

Distributed to the book trade by St. Martin's Press

      6 8 10 9 7   hardcover
2 4 6 8 10 9 7 5 3   paperback

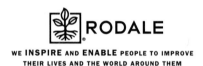

RODALE

WE **INSPIRE** AND **ENABLE** PEOPLE TO IMPROVE
THEIR LIVES AND THE WORLD AROUND THEM

About *Prevention* Health Books for Women

The editors of *Prevention* Health Books for Women are dedicated to providing you with authoritative, trustworthy, and innovative advice for a healthy active lifestyle. In all of our books, our goal is to keep you thoroughly informed about the latest breakthroughs in natural healing, medical research, alternative health, herbs, nutrition, fitness, and weight loss. We cut through the confusion of today's conflicting health reports to deliver clear, concise, and definitive health information that you can trust. And we explain in practical terms what each new breakthrough means to you, so you can take immediate, practical steps to improve your health and well-being.

Every recommendation in *Prevention* Health Books for Women is based upon interviews with highly qualified health authorities, including medical doctors and practitioners of alternative medicine. In addition, we consult with the *Prevention* Health Books Board of Advisors to ensure that all of the health information is safe, practical, and up-to-date. *Prevention* Health Books for Women are thoroughly factchecked for accuracy, and we make every effort to verify recommendations, dosages, and cautions.

The advice in this book will help keep you well-informed about your personal choices in health care—to help you lead a happier, healthier, and longer life.

Banish Your Belly, Butt, and Thighs Forever! Staff

EDITOR: Sharon Faelten

CONTRIBUTING WRITERS: Donna Raskin; Kristine Napier, R.D.; Kim Galeaz, R.D.; Roberta Duyff, R.D.; Elizabeth Ward, R.D.; Betsy Bates; Judith Lin Eftekhar; Susan Huxley; Larry Keller

ART DIRECTOR: Darlene Schneck

COVER AND INTERIOR DESIGNER: Carol Angstadt

PHOTO EDITOR: James A. Gallucci

COVER PHOTOGRAPHER: Mitch Mandel

ILLUSTRATOR: Karen Kuchar

ASSISTANT RESEARCH MANAGER: Anita C. Small

BOOK PROJECT RESEARCHER: Teresa A. Yeykal

EDITORIAL RESEARCHERS: Molly Donaldson Brown, Lori Davis, Christine Dreisbach, Bella Hebrew, Mary Kittel, Elizabeth B. Price, Staci Sander, Elizabeth Shimer, Lucille Uhlman, Nancy Zelko

SENIOR COPY EDITOR: Amy K. Kovalski

PRODUCTION EDITOR: Cindy Updegrove

LAYOUT DESIGNER: Keith Biery

ASSOCIATE STUDIO MANAGER: Thomas P. Aczel

MANUFACTURING COORDINATORS: Brenda Miller, Jodi Schaffer, Patrick T. Smith

Rodale Healthy Living Books

VICE PRESIDENT AND PUBLISHER: Brian Carnahan

VICE PRESIDENT AND EDITORIAL DIRECTOR: Debora T. Yost

EDITORIAL DIRECTOR: Michael Ward

VICE PRESIDENT AND MARKETING DIRECTOR: Karen Arbegast

PRODUCT MARKETING MANAGER: Tania Attanasio

BOOK MANUFACTURING DIRECTOR: Helen Clogston

MANUFACTURING MANAGERS: Eileen Bauder, Mark Krahforst

RESEARCH MANAGER: Ann Gossy Yermish

COPY MANAGER: Lisa D. Andruscavage

PRODUCTION MANAGER: Robert V. Anderson Jr.

OFFICE MANAGER: Jacqueline Dornblaser

OFFICE STAFF: Suzanne Lynch Holderman, Julie Kehs, Mary Lou Stephen, Catherine E. Strouse

To get in the best shape of your life...

...start with your index finger!

BANISH**BBT**.COM

👆

It's an exclusive Web site created just for you!

Congratulations! You are joining an innovative program guaranteed to get you in the best shape of your life. *Banish Your Belly, Butt, and Thighs Forever!* has a companion Web site that functions as your training buddy, confidante, and supportive friend. Go to **banishbbt.com**, go to the "Members Only" area, enter your special password (yours is below), and discover how to customize this revolutionary program to meet your individual needs.

Web site: `http://www.banishbbt.com`
Password: `slender`

For the support you need 24 hours a day!

Need support at 3:00 P.M. or 3:00 A.M? We're there for you at banishbbt.com! Log on anytime day or night to:

Buddy up for better results. Get inspired by other women who are also following the program, through the interactive message center on the site.

Ask the experts. Get answers you can trust from the exercise experts and dietitians who contributed to the book, plus editors from *Prevention* magazine.

Get inspired by success stories. Meet women just like you who have already successfully completed the program and reached their body-shaping goals. You'll see their "before" and "after" photos and learn from their challenges and successes.

Inspire others. Share your own success story online on the site's interactive message center.

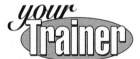   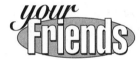

THE BANISHBBT.COM "TOOL KIT"

Click here to find all the tools you need to tailor the program to fit your needs, including how to:

Enhance your workout with tips from "Your Trainer." Learn expert techniques and strategies for getting even more out of every workout.

Trim your trouble spots. Do you have an apple-shaped, pear-shaped, or classic baby-making physique? A quick and easy quiz helps you decide, then shows you which activities will give you the shape you've always wanted.

Make every move count. Step-by-step animated exercise demonstrations will show you how to do exercises correctly the first time, and every time.

Chart your progress. Keep track of your accomplishments with weekly log printouts, including words of encouragement and inspiration. Stick a new printout on your fridge each week to keep yourself motivated!

Customize the burn. Break down your calorie-burning potential based on your weight and the length and intensity of your activity. Want to see faster results? You'll know exactly what to do!

Eat your way lean. Decide what to have for breakfast, lunch, dinner, or just a snack. Find delicious low-fat meals custom-made for this program!

Plus, you'll get updates on cellulite remedies, diet pills, and other weight-loss news!

And we'll even link you up to the best sites for workout gear, exercise equipment, fitness activities, and more!

Getting in shape has never been so much fun!
To get started, just log on to **banishbbt.com**.

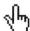

Contents

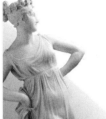

Part One
The Art of Body Shaping

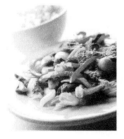

Part Two
Eating Lean

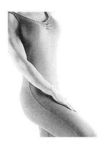

Part Three
Body-Shaping Workouts

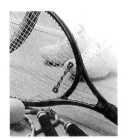

Part Four
Aerobics for Overall Slimness

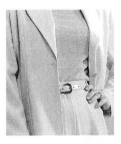

Part Five
Self-Coaching the New You

Foreword

Throw away those dowdy overblouses and sweatpants. *Banish Your Belly, Butt, and Thighs Forever!* offers a comprehensive program that shows you how to flatten your belly, trim your thighs, and firm your butt so you can stop hiding behind layers of baggy clothes—forever.

As fitness editor of *Prevention* magazine, every day I hear from women who, like you, want to target these trouble spots. Even women who aren't overweight want to get rid of that paunch around their middles or tone jiggly thighs or sagging butts. Now you can! The authors talked to leading weight-loss, nutrition, fitness, psychology, and fashion experts to develop a plan that will take you from your first walk down the block to your final walk through the mall for a new wardrobe in a smaller size. Whether this is your 1st or 50th attempt at losing inches, *Banish Your Belly, Butt, and Thighs Forever!* tells you everything you need to know to go from fat to fabulous.

Here are some comments from real women who tried this program and loved it.

- "I can't believe what a difference such a simple program has made. And I never felt like I was on a diet!" says Janine Slaughter, age 37.

- "I have tons of energy! And my husband keeps commenting on how skinny I'm getting," says Laura Kaplus, age 32.

- "The exercises are straightforward and simple to do thanks to the photos, and they work," says Brooke Myers, age 31.

What makes this program so successful is that you can customize it to meet your needs. If the most exercise you're used to getting is lapping the grocery store aisle, you can start with the low-intensity, beginner workouts. That way, you'll avoid one of the most common beginner mistakes—doing too much too soon—which can sideline you with injuries or leave you hating exercise. If you're exercising regularly now but aren't satisfied with your progress, start with the high-intensity workouts for experienced exercisers.

Plus, you'll discover 25 fun ways to exercise—everything from bicycling and cross-country skiing to walking and water aerobics—that target your specific trouble spots.

No weight-loss program would be complete without a healthy diet. But this book does more than just give you a "one-size-fits-all" meal plan. The Best and Worst Body-Shaping Foods chapter can help you develop a shopping list of low-fat, flavorful foods that will help you to shed pounds. Stock up on the best ones, and you'll never feel hungry again. Best of all, you have the freedom to indulge. Even chocoholics can indulge their pleasure. What's more, you can dine out without blowing your diet. Expert dietitians show you how.

Most important, you'll feel good while you lose weight—you'll learn how to set the right goals for success; how to dress to look two sizes smaller, even before you drop a pound; and how to incorporate strategies to help you stick with your exercise program. After years of coaching women, I know that you can't slim down if you don't feel good about yourself.

Finally, you won't be doing this alone. Research has shown that online support groups can help you lose more pounds—and keep them off. Just log on to the companion Web site for this book, at www.banishbbt.com, to hear from other women using the program and experts quoted in the book.

Turn the page and watch your trouble spots disappear.

Michele Stanten

Michele Stanten
Fitness Editor
Prevention magazine

Acknowledgments

Special thanks to **Marjorie Albohm**, an exercise physiologist, certified athletic trainer, and director of sports medicine at Kendrick Memorial Hospital in Mooresville, Indiana, for developing the Body-Shaping Workouts for this program.

Thanks also to the following registered dietitians for creating and writing the Eating Lean portion of this program.

Kristine Napier, R.D., a registered dietitian and nutrition consultant in Mayfield Village, Ohio; consultant director of the Nutrition Enhancement Project at the Cleveland Clinic Heart Center, Preventive Cardiology Program; and author of *Power Nutrition for Chronic Illness*.

Kim Galeaz, R.D., a registered dietitian and food and nutrition consultant in Indianapolis.

Roberta Duyff, R.D., a registered dietitian and food and nutrition consultant in St. Louis, Missouri, and author of *The American Dietetic Association's Complete Food and Nutrition Guide*, among other books.

Elizabeth Ward, R.D., a registered dietitian and nutrition consultant in Stoneham, Massachusetts, spokesperson for the American Dietetic Association, and author of *Pregnancy Nutrition: Good Health for You and Your Baby*, among other publications.

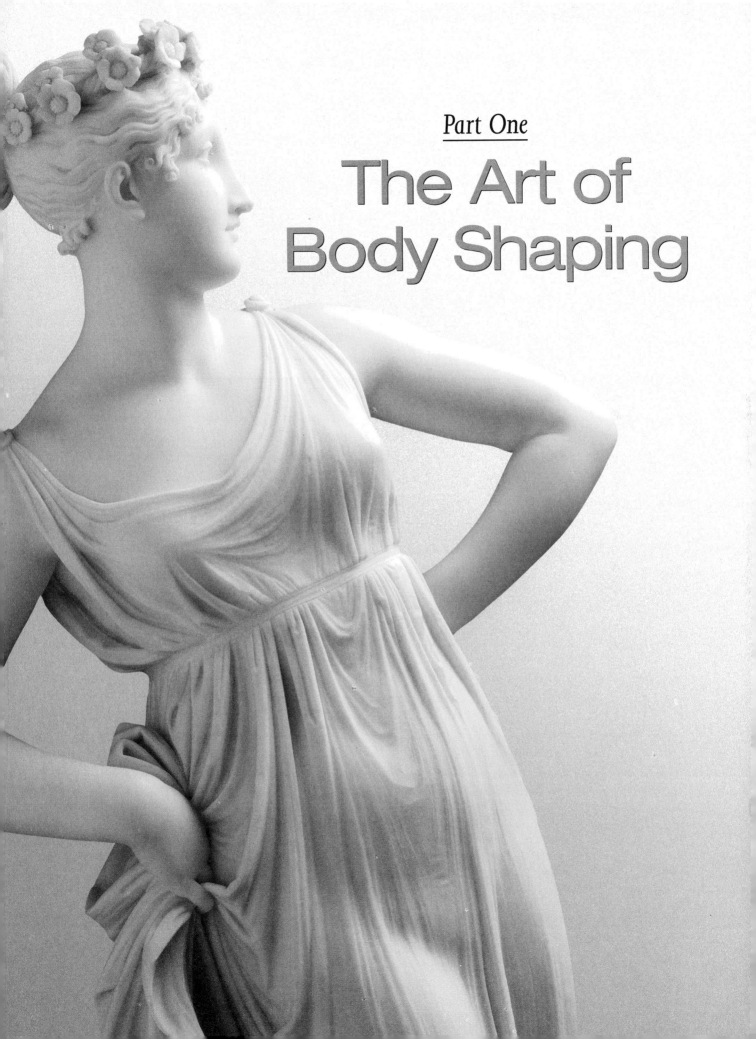

Part One

The Art of Body Shaping

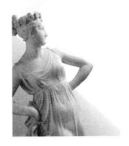

It's a Lifestyle, Not a Diet

It's an all too familiar experience: You take your favorite jeans out of the clothes dryer, and you can't zip them. You figure the dryer shrunk them. The next morning, you get dressed for work, and you can't button your skirt. That night, you pull your favorite dress out of the closet, and it pulls across your backside.

You've gained weight. Again. The last diet you tried worked, but you regained all the weight. Worse, it settled just where you least want the extra curves—in your belly, butt, and thighs.

If you're unhappy with your physique, you have lots of company. No doubt you've read the headlines proclaiming that more than half of all Americans over the age of 20 are overweight, and that nearly one out of every four people is clinically obese.

Despite our national obsession with getting thinner, more women (and men) are overweight.

Fad diets don't seem to be helping. Americans spend as much as $40 billion a year on weight-loss treatments, primarily diets and dietary foods. We buy diet books that claim to be the next miracle or revolution with the zeal of a chocoholic attacking a hot fudge sundae. We try high-protein diets, cabbage soup diets—even chewing gum diets.

Still we've become a country of pudgy people with chubby children; one-fourth of our kids are overweight or obese. As other nations inexorably follow our example, their people likewise are gaining in girth. Information is sketchy, but data suggest that the number of obese people in the United Kingdom, Brazil, Canada, and Thailand (among others) is rising.

These trends seem to suggest that we will see a worldwide expansion of waistlines, hips, and thighs rivaling global warming in scope.

It's Not Your Fault

It's not hard to figure out where all this extra weight comes from: supersize portions and mega meals. Everything from candy bars to breakfast cereals comes in bigger packages than in the past. Food portions in many restaurants have mushroomed to the point of becoming gargantuan. The average "serving" per order could feed a family of five.

"There is enormous commercial pressure for people to eat more," says Marion Nestle, Ph.D., professor in the department of nutrition and food studies at New York University. "Food companies are competing for the American food dollar in two ways. They want you to eat their product instead of somebody else's. And they want you to eat more. In every possible way, this society is going to conspire to get you to eat more. It's good for business."

The obvious solution? "Eat less," says Dr. Nestle. "Train yourself to stop eating when you feel full. You need to be vigilant."

Granted, this is easier said than done. But it is doable. Dr. Nestle and several colleagues have begun practicing what they preach by eating smaller portions at meals. "The pounds just fall off," she says. "We're astounded."

Developing a general knowledge of the fat and calorie content of foods is useful for planning what to eat, but don't measure and weigh your food to the point of obsession.

If you eat out, calorie counting is impossible because you don't see how the food is prepared, explains Dr. Nestle. She cites an experiment in which she and several other nutritionists were taken to lunch by a newspaper reporter who asked them to estimate the number of calories and grams of fat in what they ate.

"We couldn't do it," she says. "We didn't even come close. It was inconceivable to me that the food we were eating had as much fat and calories as it turned out to have."

Why Dieting Doesn't Work

There are lots of things you can—and should—do, however, in the fight against fat. In part 2, Eating Lean, you'll learn how to shop for the right kind of food prepared in weight-friendly ways and substitute foods that are kind to your waistline and hips. Add new, healthier foods to your repertoire. Keep a food diary. Eat more fiber. Eat small meals throughout the day. You'll find out that you don't need to deny yourself the occasional brownie or slice of pie—just set limits for yourself and stick to them.

In fact, you don't have to limit yourself to cabbage soup or other unusual foods to lose weight.

There is no hard evidence that anybody benefits from dieting per se. In fact, 90 to 95 percent of women who attempt to lose weight via dieting fail. Emerging data suggest that when women diet and then begin to lose and regain weight over and over again, the process may be driving their bodies' normal natural set point for weight upward. Also, this so-called yo-yo dieting can lead to frustration and overeating.

The real weight-loss experts are women just like you who figured out how to pare pounds and pinch inches painlessly. Take Cindi Arvanites, who along with her husband changed the way she cooked meals—and improved her figure in the process. (See page 119.) By substituting lower-fat ingredients for fatty ones or using less of the latter and eating smaller portions, Cindi

has eaten healthier and lost weight at the same time. Yet the couple still adds some "caloric luxuries," such as butter, to their recipes—just less of it. You'll find out how Cindi did it and learn some cooking techniques that will help you shape up, too.

Being Active Made Easy

Monitoring what you place in your mouth is half the equation. It will work only if you also burn more calories. Some of you are thinking, "Not me." You feel silly flouncing about in a step aerobics class with young, leotard-clad women who look like they leaped from the pages of a *Victoria's Secret* catalog. Or the idea of hard exercise appeals to you about as much as 10 hours of labor pains.

But as you'll learn in this book, you don't have to become G.I. Jane in order to become more active. In fact, exercising can be fun. Really.

And you don't have to follow a strict regimen—unless you want to. Experts say that your chances for success are higher if you incorporate aerobic activities into your lifestyle. Take a 30-minute walk during your lunch hour, for example. Like many women, you probably associate the term *aerobic* with calisthenics done to music in a class. But technically, any sustained activity that gets your heart pumping can contribute to weight loss. And you don't have to huff and puff for hours: 30 minutes of aerobic activity most days of the week may do the trick, says Laurie L. Tis, Ph.D., associate professor in the department of kinesiology and health at Georgia State University in Atlanta.

What's more, there are dozens of ways to work exercise into your lifestyle, including but not limited to aerobics classes.

- If you're a homebody, you can garden or work around the house or yard.

- If you have teenage kids, you can bicycle, skate, or cross-country ski with them.

- If you're competitive, you can play table tennis, badminton, tennis, or racquetball.

- If you like to dance, you can take up dancing. (What better way to work your abs than belly dancing?)
- If you like to work out in the privacy of your own home, or you can't get to a gym, you can skip rope or use a step machine or rowing machine.
- If you have knee or back problems, you can swim.
- If you love to vacation in the tropics, you can snorkel. If you vacation in the mountains, you can hike.

The list goes on.

"When we talk about healthy lifestyle and quality of life issues, we're finding that it's less about that '20-minute, 75 percent of maximum heart rate three times a week,' and more about just being generally active," says Dr. Tis. The idea is to get a minimum of 30 total minutes of moderate activity throughout the day.

On page 229, you will meet Kate Flynn, whose story shows how a change in lifestyle can improve physique. A single mother of two, she enjoyed aerobics classes, but found it hard to make the time or shell out the money for them. Interested in keeping fit, Kate also tried running, but it hurt her knees. She didn't give up, though. Instead, she became an avid gardener who has maintained a firm body and a youthful appearance by weeding, raking, and the like.

Kate illustrates what more and more exercise and weight-loss experts are recommending: Experiment with various forms of physical activity until you find one or more that you like. The advantage of doing so is that you are more likely to keep at it consistently, says Charles Corbin, Ph.D., professor in the department of exercise science and physical education at Arizona State University in Tempe. "The activity doesn't have to be vigorous," he adds. If you work out about as hard as brisk walking, you can exercise for a fair amount of time without getting tired.

"When you were a kid, you enjoyed being active," notes Dr. Corbin. "If you can find that enjoyment again, you may be much better off than

if you are a member of four different health clubs, getting on treadmills all the time and doing calisthenics. It's best to find things you really enjoy."

A Little Goes a Long Way

Still skeptical about exercise? There's a wealth of research suggesting that even modest increases in physical activity pay off.

In one study, for example, a group of 40 women who were each 33 pounds or more overweight was divided into two groups. One group participated in structured aerobic exercise for 16 weeks and ate a daily diet of 1,200 calories, while the other group increased their moderate-intensity physical activity by 30 minutes a day, most days of the week, while also eating a 1,200-calorie diet for 16 weeks.

The first group participated in a step aerobics class, reaching a peak of 45 minutes of stepping by the eighth week. The second group was encouraged to walk rather than drive short distances, take the stairs instead of elevators, and the like. After 16 weeks, women in both groups had lost weight, but there were not significant differences between them.

In another, two-year study, 235 sedentary, overweight men and women were divided into groups similar to those in the above study. When it was over, the group that had simply begun living a more physically active lifestyle had lost slightly more weight and a greater percentage of body fat than the group that was in a structured exercise program.

In a third study, Mayo Clinic researchers fed 16 women and men of average weight food containing 1,000 calories per day above what was required to maintain their weight, and limited them to low levels of exercise. Then they measured which participants stored the most and the least amounts of the additional calories as fat.

The study volunteers gained an average of 10 pounds in two months. But those who were most active without actually exercising—they fidgeted, moved around, adjusted their posture, and so forth—gained the least weight. One volunteer burned up an average of 692 calories per day through such mundane movements. Conversely, those participants who moved around the least gained the most weight.

Finally, in yet another study, more than 1,000 women and men who were trying to maintain their weights were monitored for a year. Researchers found that those who spent the most time watching television gained the most weight. Among high-income women, each hour of TV viewed per day equated to an extra half-pound of weight gained over the year.

Television per se is not to blame, of course. But it's a sedentary activity. Getting up during commercial breaks to load the dishwasher, fold clothes, or take a brief exercise break by doing jumping jacks or jogging in place are among the things you can do to break the lethargy cycle, says Dr. Nestle.

Maybe you think vanity is a poor reason to lose weight. Fine, but your appearance isn't the only reason to shake a tail feather. Think about your health. Physically active women have less risk of dying from coronary heart disease and developing high blood pressure, colon cancer, and diabetes. And all that movin' and groovin' may enhance the effect of estrogen-replacement therapy in decreasing bone loss after menopause.

Certainly most of us could improve on this score. More than three out of five women in the United States don't engage in the recommended amount of physical activity. The Surgeon General defines moderate physical activity as activity that uses 150 calories per day, or 1,000 calories per week. You can achieve this rate by gardening or playing table tennis for 30 to 45 minutes six days a week.

While a common stereotype is that of a pot-bellied guy slumped in front of the television, experts report that women are more apt to be physically inactive than men. True, you may be running around all day and up until all hours taking care of your job and family. But that isn't necessarily the kind of activity that improves your figure.

"But I don't have time to exercise," you might say. Or, "I don't have time to shop for special food—I have to eat what my family eats."

No problem. On page 308, you'll learn how any woman, no matter how busy, can work exercise into her schedule. And in part 2, you'll discover innovative advice from dietitians who specialize in teaching women how to shop for and prepare foods that the whole family will enjoy.

You won't even know you're on a diet. Because you're not. You're living a lifestyle that puts you in control, once and for all.

For stories of how real women lost weight and shaped up using the exercises and eating plan in this book, visit our Web site at www.banishbbt.com.

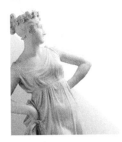

Your Unique Body

Three women get together for lunch. One of them, a harried woman whose life is filled with young children and a full-time job, orders a turkey sandwich, hold the mayo, and don't forget the dessert menu. The oldest woman, who works part-time when not tending house, asks for the diet plate—fruit salad and cottage cheese. The youngest woman, who is single, active, and loving it, hasn't eaten anything yet today, and she's starving. She orders a taco salad in a shell.

All three of these women think they are on a diet.

We'd like to introduce you to Margie, Sarah, and Ann, three completely different women who have one big thing in common: They each want to lose weight.

• Margie, at age 40, wants to lose 20 pounds from her hips and backside, which is the extra weight that she has put on since having two children.

• Sarah, 52, is a career dieter. She has 30 pounds to lose—weight that she's lost and regained (plus a little more) over and over again.

• And finally there is Ann, 29 and single. She only has 10 pounds to lose, but it's 10 pounds that have settled mostly on her thighs and backside within the last few years.

Do these women sound like you or your friends? They should. You see, Margie, Sarah, and Ann are composites, based on what surveys reveal—and weight-loss experts confirm—to be the most common types of women dieters. Margie is the stressed-out career woman who blames her weight gain on having children. Sarah is the nurturing, sedentary, plump mother who spends an inordinate amount of time in the kitchen. Ann is the life-at-full-speed single who hardly thinks about her health. Margie, Sarah, and Ann are

familiar to all of us, as are their weight-loss concerns.

In fact, you probably already recognize yourself—or parts of yourself—in one or more of them. And that's good, because in this chapter, you're going to get to know Margie, Sarah, and Ann intimately—their bodies, their eating habits, their exercise needs, their goals, their struggles. More important, you'll discover expert advice for how each can sculpt a weight-loss and body-shaping program that is absolutely best for her. You'll learn how they can eat well, live active lives, and feel better. Using Margie, Sarah, and Ann as examples, you'll be able to take advice experts offer these women and apply it to your own weight-loss and body-shaping efforts. If they can do it, so can you.

The Common Theme: Uniqueness

Why go through this exercise? Simple: While the major themes of weight loss are universal—eat smarter, be more active—each person needs to apply these maxims in her own way, based on the special needs of her body and circumstance.

"One of the most important considerations in weight loss is to remember that we each have a unique biochemistry, just as we each have unique fingerprints," says Michael Steelman, M.D., a weight-loss specialist in Oklahoma City, Oklahoma. "While there are absolute dietary and lifestyle changes we all need to make, we also have to remember that each of these changes will be unique and individual to every person."

That means that what works for Margie isn't going to work for Ann and what works for Ann isn't going to work for Sarah. Take breakfast, for example. Margie could add a piece of fruit to her meal and replace her high-sugar cereal for one low in sugar and high in fiber. Sarah might try having a poached egg and turkey bacon, rather than the fried eggs and sausage that her husband demands. And Ann should try to start eating a real breakfast instead of going without food until lunch.

"The basics of weight loss are really the same across the board," says Dr. Steelman. "The 'recipe' includes nutritious food, exercise, an active lifestyle, and stress management. But to lose weight, each woman has to add specific ingredients in the right percentages in order to create the recipe that tastes just right to her palate."

So where do you begin in building the right program for you? By learning why you've gained weight. Like many women, Margie, Sarah, and Ann have all spent a lot of time trying to figure out how to shed their extra pounds, but they haven't spent any time trying to understand why they have weight problems in the first place.

To formulate a weight-loss and body-shaping plan that works for you, listen carefully to these women's stories. If you're typical of women who struggle in frustration with their weight, certain elements will mirror your experience. Do you attribute your weight gain to hormones, as Margie does? Have you been dieting your whole life and now worry about your health like Sarah? Do you skip meals and then binge at night like Ann? Perhaps you're a combination of all three, or just two. Whatever your situation, you're likely to find some underlying truths to why you, too, might be struggling with weight loss.

Margie: Wants to Lose Her "Baby Fat"

At 40, Margie has two wonderful kids, a demanding job, a great husband, and 20 extra pounds on her body. Her hips are wider than they used to be, and she hates to see her rear end in the mirror.

Margie attributes her weight gain to the hormonal changes that come with having children—along with certain lifestyle changes that come with raising children. For example, she often ends up at fast-food restaurants as she shuttles her kids between activities after school or on weekends. In order to stick to her "diet," she tries to minimize the caloric damage by ordering small—a hamburger, small fries, and a diet soda. Small or not, the food she orders still contributes more fat and calories than a carefully planned home-cooked meal would.

Like so many office workers, Margie also faces a constant barrage of cakes and cookies at work—the going-away chocolate cake, the happy birthday carrot cake, and the weekly-meeting doughnuts. Margie thinks that she does a pretty good job of limiting the damage, helping herself to just a cookie or two or a small piece of cake.

The problem is, that isn't the only time Margie eats sweets. She would never tell anyone, but when she fights with her husband or gets upset at work, she'll stop at a convenience store to get something sweet. Sometimes it's candy, sometimes it's a packaged dessert, but it's always high in fat and calories. When life isn't going right for Margie, food is her best friend.

Margie thinks she's dieting, but she's just kidding herself. A menu that focuses on tiny this and tiny that—fast food and sweets included—is not a diet, no matter how small the portions.

Is Having Babies Really to Blame?

Childbearing is only an excuse for being overweight. It is possible for a woman to have children without having to sacrifice her physique.

But like a lot of women, Margie is sure that having children caused her to gain weight. "It's not true," says Blenda Eckert, R.D., a registered dietitian in Clarksville, Maryland. "Mother Nature has it set up so that if we watch our calories before and during pregnancy, during lactation, and after lactation, then our weight should return to the pre-pregnancy weight."

Margie should recognize that if she had just paid attention to the amount and types of food she ate as well as her level of physical activity, then her weight wouldn't have gotten out of hand, Eckert says. The weight came on because she eats high-fat, high-calorie, non-nutritious fast food with her kids and because she doesn't get any exercise. Ultimately, Margie will need to deal with the underlying causes of her emotional eating, learn healthier eating patterns, and become more physically active.

Sarah: The Veteran Dieter

Her four adult children are out of the house and Sarah, at 52, works three days a week in a doctor's office. Her life is quiet, finally. She and her husband are happy to watch a little TV at night and see their friends and grandchildren on the weekends.

Sarah has been on every diet under the sun. She has lost and regained the same 30 pounds with each of them. Of course, she never stopped cooking proper meals for her husband and kids during any of these phases. They always had eggs and bacon for breakfast and meat and potatoes for dinner. Sarah's husband likes it that way. In fact, he still likes it that way, even though he needs to lose 30 pounds, too. She hates to say it, but she even overfeeds the dog, as the vet recently pointed out.

At this point in their lives, Sarah is actually beginning to worry about how the extra weight is affecting her and her husband's health. He, at least, gets some exercise at his weekly bowling game, but Sarah's hobbies are sedentary, even fattening. She likes to sew—and cook! She'll try any new recipe as long as she thinks her husband will like it.

The Problem with Yo-Yo Thinking

Sarah's idea of a diet is to buy the latest weight-loss gimmicks, including shakes, pills, and formulas. When she was younger, they worked—for a while. She knew that whenever she needed to lose weight, she could try the latest over-the-counter weight-loss aid and shed a few pounds quickly.

Now, it seems harder to lose weight, no matter what weight-loss aid she tries. After years of losing and regaining the weight, Sarah is convinced that she has permanently broken her fat thermostat. She's sure the extra weight she has kept on since her last diet is here to stay. But here's the good news: It isn't years of yo-yo dieting that have led to Sarah's weight gain. You can't break your metabolism. "Yes,

your body composition probably changes each time you lose and regain weight," says Eckert. "But that doesn't mean the situation is hopeless."

Sarah's biggest problem, says Eckert, is that she thinks of weight loss as a light switch—it's either on or off. "This is a sure road to failure," Eckert says. "Sarah needs to realize that she needs to eat properly and be active for the rest of her life. Period."

Nevertheless, Eckert doesn't minimize the effect Sarah's husband is having on her. "Not getting support is hard; it's a real issue," she says. "Sarah is really going to have to take steps to deal with that."

Ann: A Question of Genetics?

Ah, to be 29 and single again, Margie and Sarah think, looking longingly at Ann's slim waist and torso. What they don't realize is that when Ann gets out of the shower and looks in the mirror, she focuses on her thighs. And when she thinks about what to order for lunch, she's thinking about her thighs. And her mother's thighs. And her sister's thighs. Ann is pretty convinced that genetics is a curse. Sure, she has beautiful jet black hair and a lovely complexion—inherited as well from her mother—but she's also 10 pounds heavier than she was five years ago. Hidden under a sarong skirt, Ann's thighs may not be obvious to Margie and Sarah. But Ann thinks about them enough to keep them hidden.

Ann always skips breakfast and often skimps at lunch. By dinnertime, she's ravenous. And most nights she's out, hitting a new restaurant with her friends. She eats pretty sensibly then, she thinks: broiled fish, pasta with pesto, or sweet-and-sour shrimp and broccoli with a vegetable (not pork) egg roll. Plus, she limits herself to a glass or two of wine—or a light beer.

Ann used to run regularly, but her job keeps her too busy to jog on weekdays anymore. Her gym membership lapsed about three months ago, and she can't remember the last time she lifted a weight. She tries to get out for a run on Sundays, though. And she often works in a game of tennis or some inline skating on Saturdays, if the weather is good.

Ann's 3,000-Calorie Meal

How can someone gain weight when she's only eating one big meal a day? Pretty easily, says Eckert.

"First of all, Ann is eating more fat and calories than she realizes," Eckert explains. Pesto and even fish (if it is broiled in butter) are brimming with fat. And restaurant portions routinely run double or triple the size of a "regular," healthy serving. Add it up, and what Ann considers to be a sensible meal is landing her a full day's quota of calories—and then some.

"Plus, Ann is slowing down her metabolism by starving herself the rest of the day," says Eckert. "This mindset of starvation-binge, starvation-binge is a big problem." Indeed, Ann is breaking most every principle of sound eating. She must learn to eat reasonable portions of less fatty food, spread throughout the day. She doesn't have the discipline—yet—of a grown-up eater.

Finally, Ann's exercise doesn't do her much good. She may burn a few extra calories, but not nearly enough to compensate for the extra calories she consumes during the week.

The Hidden Problem (and the Real Solution)

Even though Margie, Sarah, and Ann think they have nothing in common, they do. They all see their extra weight as a problem caused by some external force—the kids or a husband, the failure of diets, or the legacy of genetics. The reality, however, is that they are each fully responsible for the extra weight they carry on their bones. It's their own habits that have created the problem. And it's changing their habits that will save them.

"All three of these women need to take the focus off what they think caused the weight gain and begin to look at realistic ways to change their daily lives in order to lose weight and live healthier lives," says Terry Passano, R.D., a registered dietitian in Columbia, Maryland.

For example, Margie is going to have to keep low-calorie snacks on hand for herself and her kids while they're driving to soccer games. Or she's going to have to order chili or grilled chicken and a salad, skip the fries, and hold the dessert at the drive-up window.

"Each of these women has options and lots of things going for her that will help make her weight loss successful," Passano says. "It's great, for instance, that Sarah loves to cook. Now she just has to get used to experimenting with healthier recipes and making subtle changes in her old ones, such as switching to low-fat cheese. The whole family may actually enjoy the new, healthier meals."

Learning by Example

How much weight do *you* want to lose? 10 pounds? 30? 100? Do you carry your extra weight on your belly? Your backside? Your hips and thighs? Or all over?

Do you credit (or blame) heredity for your figure? Childbearing? Menopause? Do you realize all too well that you need to exercise, but hate the idea of getting all sweaty? Or just can't imagine where you'd find the time?

Do you feel that buying and preparing meals for others—your husband or kids—limits your food choices to what they're willing to eat?

Even if you don't identify with every aspect of Margie's, Sarah's, and Ann's approaches to dieting, chances are you can understand the principles at work—and learn to apply them to your unique circumstances.

Using Margie, Sarah, and Ann as examples, the upcoming chapters will help you to figure out:

• How to figure in (or discount) the effects of aging, pregnancy, menopause, and other hormonal factors on your weight and shape

• How to eat the proper number of calories for your body type and energy level

• How much dietary fat will make you feel full, and how much dietary fat will make you fat

• How to fit regular exercise into your schedule

Once you've assessed your situation, you can use the meal plans, cooking techniques, food tables, exercise programs, and self-coaching tips that follow to achieve your personal weight-loss and body-shaping goals—once and for all.

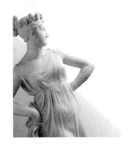

What You Can and Cannot Change

Margie believes that her two pregnancies have left her heavy forever. Sarah believes that menopause—combined with a lifetime of dieting—has ruined her chances of ever being thin again. And Ann believes that her thighs are a genetic inheritance over which she has no control. Are they right?

Well, yes and no. The women's beliefs are, for the most part, half-truths. The whole truth encompasses two realities: Biology plays a role in our size and shape, but we determine how much of a toll it will ultimately take. While pregnancy, dieting, and genetics do play a significant role in what we weigh and how we look, our lifestyles and eating habits weigh in even more.

"At 20, you usually have the body you were born with, but at 40 or 60, you have a body that reflects the way you lived your life," says Edith Hogan, R.D., a registered dietitian in Washington, D.C., and spokesperson for the American Dietetic Association. "One key to successful weight loss is learning to work with, not against, who you are and what you've been given. Some things you can change, and some you can't."

The Hormone Connection

Before we explore the details of Margie's, Sarah's, and Ann's diets, we have to explain a little bit about the science of body shape. While calories, fat, and energy expenditure determine to a great extent how much weight you'll gain throughout your life, one other factor figures into the equation—hormones.

Hormones are naturally occurring chemicals that circulate throughout our bodies. Their job is to carry a message from one organ of the body to another, influencing how the second organ will behave. In women, for example, the ovaries secrete estrogen and progesterone, reproductive hormones that play a big role in pregnancy, breast development, and 400 other bodily functions—including fat storage. They also produce testosterone and dehydroepiandrosterone (DHEA), albeit in much smaller amounts than men generate.

To a degree, hormones influence our weight and shape. Margie, Sarah, Ann, and most women, for that matter, already know that menstruation, pregnancy, and menopause are hormone-related and often result in weight changes. Until recent years, many doctors (and women) thought that changes caused by hormones were a *fait accompli*. Everyone assumed that we had very little power over our body types, our fat storage, and our life cycles.

That thinking has changed. Research shows that the way we eat, our activity levels, and our ability to handle stress will all affect our hormones—and, in turn, our hormones will affect our weight and body shape, says Elizabeth Lee Vliet, M.D., founder and medical director of HER Place women's health centers in Tucson and Dallas, and author of *Screaming to Be Heard: Hormonal Connections Women Suspect and Doctors Ignore*. Margie, Sarah, and Ann—and women like them—can learn how to help their bodies handle hormonal changes over the years.

Margie: Pregnancy, Cellulite— and Winter

Three things about her weight bug Margie. First, after each of her two pregnancies, she retained 10 extra pounds. Second, she always gains about 7 pounds during the winter, bringing her total close to 30 extra pounds for six months of the year. Third, the fat she has accumulated on her hips and thighs isn't attractive; Margie has cellulite, and it keeps her from wearing shorts in the summer, even though she's not quite as heavy then.

Margie assumes that these weight changes are inevitable. After all, she figures, most women are heavier after they've had a couple of kids—and everyone seems to gain weight during the winter. A lot of her friends have cellulite, too, and she seriously doubts that those creams that are sold in department stores will help. Margie wants to eat well and exercise, but she thinks her particular problems have no solutions.

Here's what she needs to know.

Pregnancy. If a woman is at her correct weight when she becomes pregnant, doctors recommend that she gain between 25 and 35 pounds during her pregnancy, to support and nurture her developing child. Underweight women should gain between 28 and 40 pounds, while overweight women are advised to gain between 15 and 25 pounds. No matter how heavy she is, a woman should never diet while she's pregnant unless she is doing so under the guidance of a doctor or dietitian.

Of 30 pounds gained during pregnancy, for example, only 7 of those pounds are comprised of fat. Amniotic fluid, other tissues, and the baby itself make up the rest and are lost during the birth. So a new mother should only have a few pounds to lose after her baby is born. Women will also notice changes in the shape of their breasts (especially if they breastfeed) and belly, which has stretched to accommodate a full-term child. Likewise, their hips may also widen a bit just before birth. These changes aren't due to fat accumulation, but to changes in the tissues and bones during pregnancy and lactation.

What Margie—and you—can change: If you retain any more than four extra pounds for more than a year or two after giving birth, it's due to your diet and lifestyle, not the pregnancy, says Hogan. Most women should be able to get back to, or just a couple of pounds above, their pre-pregnancy weights.

While you can't change the actual shape of your breast tissue, weight training can give your breasts a little more lift by increasing the strength of your pectoral, or chest, muscles. Extra folds of skin can't be exercised off, but losing unwanted fat through diet and exercise can get rid of tummy rolls. Hips that widened to accommodate pregnancy cannot be changed, unless the extra width is from a layer of fat. (If you can pinch it, it's fat.)

Cellulite. Although cellulite looks different from other fat, it really isn't. It looks dimpled because of the way the fat is connected to the muscle underneath—strands of connective tissues pull tight where the fat is thickest (usually on the hips, buttocks, and thighs). Not everyone who has a lot of body fat has cellulite, and conversely, some otherwise slender women have cellulite. The tendency to develop cellulite seems to have a lot to do with genetics and age, says Dr. Vliet. Women are more prone to cellulite than men, presumably because of a gender-linked predisposition to gain weight in the hips, buttocks, and thighs.

What Margie—and you—can change: You can certainly change the amount of fat on your body. This book shows you how. And when you reduce the amount of fat, then you'll reduce the appearance of cellulite. If, however, you lose excess body fat but what remains is still in the form of cellulite, over-the-counter products and exercise may temporarily help to improve its appearance, says Dr. Vliet. But no over-the-counter cream or beauty salon treatment will actually get rid of cellulite. She adds that cutting down on processed foods, which tend to be higher in fat and salt, and sodas as well as increasing your water intake and exercise may diminish your risk of developing cellulite in the first place.

Winter weight gain. If it's cold where you live during the winter, almost everyone you know probably does gain at least some weight. For one

Three Women, Three Body Types

If you're like a lot of women, you can probably identify with either Margie, Sarah, or Ann. We may vary in age, weight, and height, but we tend to carry extra weight in three different areas, which are shown here.

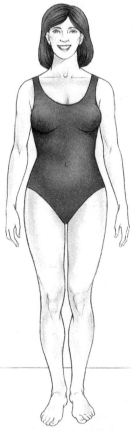 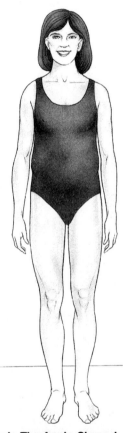 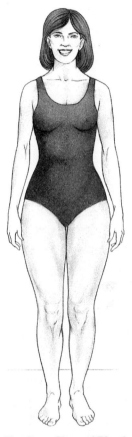

Margie: The Baby-Making Physique

Having children changes the shape of your hips and belly (especially if you deliver by cesarean section) and usually adds a couple of pounds to your weight. Of the three body types, this is the easiest to change, since controlling your weight before pregnancy and after can help prevent pregnancy-induced weight accumulation after having one or more children.

Sarah: The Apple-Shaped Physique

Post-menopausal women like Sarah are likely to become "apple"-shaped, since hormonal changes prompt their bodies to store fat around their abdominal organs. Because intra-abdominal fat carries greater health risks than lower-body fat, it's smart to minimize weight gain here even if appearance isn't an issue for you.

Ann: The Pear-Shaped Physique

For most women who are years away from menopause, like Ann, most body weight settles below the abdomen on the thighs, buttocks, and hips. Of the three body types, this is the most challenging to trim—but it can be done.

thing, we tend to be less active then, says Dr. Vliet. But hormones also play a part. Less sunlight means that our bodies produce more melatonin, a hormone that regulates our sleep-wake cycles. "Like bears, we 'hibernate' to some degree," Dr. Vliet explains. "But remember, part of the bear's ability to hibernate depends on its ability to store fat, which is helped by melatonin."

Other hormonal influences, such as a decrease in the levels of both estradiol (a naturally occurring female hormone) and a mood-regulating chemical in the brain called serotonin, also play a role, Dr. Vliet says. For some women, carbohydrate cravings seem to increase in the winter, and they also contribute to the accumulation of extra winter pounds.

What Margie—and you—can change: To prevent winter weight gain, fight the urge to stay indoors, says Dr. Vliet. Instead, get out in the sun and exercise. "Eating high-fiber foods and numerous smaller meals within a healthy winter diet will also keep your weight closer to that which you enjoy during spring and summer," she adds. High-fiber foods tend to be lower in fat and calories, and eating smaller portions more often increases your metabolic rate.

Sarah: Age, Menopause, and Yo-Yo Dieting

Sarah has spent her lifetime struggling with her weight. Now that she has hit (and passed) the age of 50, the latest changes in her figure are all the more discouraging. With menopause, her body has morphed from a generous hourglass shape to a round apple, and she feels flabbier than ever.

Meanwhile, just the idea of another diet is enough to send her running for the hills. And rightly so. "Sarah's metabolism has most likely slowed down in response to her years of dieting and being inactive," says Blenda Eckert, R.D., a registered dietitian in Clarksville, Maryland. "Another episode of simply cutting down on calories won't help Sarah lose weight anymore. Her age and her history of inappropriate dieting will work against her."

Does that mean Sarah has to give up? Absolutely not. She just has to do things differently this time. Here's what Sarah and women like her need to consider.

Aging and menopause. At one time, doctors thought there was nothing women (or men) could do to fight the aging process—bellies got bigger, muscles went flabby, and everyone ate less but gained more weight.

Now, the effects of aging are no longer considered inevitable, says Diana Dell, M.D., assistant professor of obstetrics and gynecology at the Duke University Medical Center in Durham, North Carolina. "The things that really change as you grow older are your muscle mass and activity level, which, in turn, affect your body shape and weight. If you build and maintain muscle and stay active, then your weight won't change very much."

The hormonal changes that accompany menopause do, however, affect a woman's metabolism and, as a result, her weight. "Ovarian hormones, such as estrogen and progesterone, are not just reproductive hormones," says Dr. Vliet. "They also have a metabolic role in the body and help you to build muscle and bone. So when these hormones decline, so do muscle and bone mass, and the body stores more fat."

With the drop in female hormones, the small amounts of adrenal hormones that both men and women produce come into play, changing a more feminine, hourglass figure into a more "male," or apple-shaped, physique.

Estrogen-replacement medications such as Alora that supply estradiol can help to prevent muscle and bone loss as well as the weight gain associated with menopause, says Dr. Vliet. Progesterone, on the other hand, promotes weight gain and is often combined with estrogen, for various reasons. Estrogen-like compounds found in some plants, such as soy, may contribute to weight distribution and the maintenance of a healthy female body shape.

What Sarah—and you—can change: Regardless of whether or not you take some form of hormone-replacement therapy, if you overeat and don't exercise, you won't slim down or shape up. It's a simple rule—energy begets energy. If you ask your muscles and bones to move, then they'll stimulate the process of using fat for fuel.

The solution is to do activities that are aerobic (such as walking) and weight-bearing (also walking and strength training), says Dr. Vliet. Both of these activities will mimic the gifts a youthful body contributes to metabolism. In other words, for women Sarah's age, moving regularly and building muscle are imperative.

Yo-yo dieting. Repeated weight losses and gains change the structure and number of your fat cells, which can ultimately make it much easier for you to regain weight you've worked hard to lose. Fat cells first increase in size during a weight-gain period, but when they reach their maximum size, they divide, creating two fat cells where once there was one. Once created, fat cells never disappear; they can only shrink.

What Sarah—and you—can change: As Sarah and other yo-yo dieters have discovered, repeated weight losses and gains make it increasingly difficult to lose weight, because they end up with more fat cells than when they started. Still, fat cells will always be able to change size—to grow or shrink—so losing weight is not impossible.

"This time around, Sarah needs to focus on her lifetime plan to keep weight off, not just her short-term diet to lose weight quickly," says Michael Steelman, M.D., a weight-loss specialist in Oklahoma City, Oklahoma.

Experts agree that exercise keeps weight from returning—and exercise is exactly what was missing from Sarah's past efforts.

Ann: PMS, Body Shape, and Heredity

Despite usually staying within 10 pounds of her goal weight, Ann is plagued by a week of PMS every month that adds another few pounds to her frame before menstruation. She feels so bloated and fat that she has accumulated a second wardrobe of "period pants and skirts." A size larger than her regular wardrobe, these clothes help Ann feel more comfortable at a time when she's already prone to crying.

But two other things bother Ann even more than her premenstrual weight gain. She harbors a secret that both embarrasses and frightens her: Her mother is overweight—very overweight, more than 100 pounds. So even though she only has 10 pounds to lose now, to Ann, they're a sign of what's to come. At this point, she has cellulite on her thighs and her body is quite pear-shaped. She obsesses about her weight and "heavy thighs" and feels doomed that one day she will follow in her mother's footsteps.

Ann's worries are valid, but her situation isn't hopeless. Here's where she stands.

Premenstrual bloating. Seven to 10 days before their periods begin, most women gain a few pounds because of water retention. Progesterone levels instigate these temporary weight gains that disappear once their periods start. It's a natural part of the reproductive cycle, although not all women experience bloating and other premenstrual symptoms.

What Ann—and you—can change: A few simple changes can minimize premenstrual bloating, says Dr. Vliet. Her suggestions are aimed at reducing the tendency to retain water. She recommends cutting some salt from your diet, increasing your activity level, eating more fiber, and consuming more magnesium, a mineral that plays a role in fluid balance. "Our lifestyles play a large role in whether or not the changes that come along with our menstrual cycles will be positive or negative," she says. If problems persist, Dr. Vliet recommends having your hormone levels checked.

If you've consistently gained an extra pound or two *after* your period, then you've been eating too much before and during your period, not retaining water.

Pears and apples. Although women come in all shapes and sizes, they tend to accumulate fat in two ways—in the shape of pears or apples.

"A pear gains weight in her lower body—the hips, thighs, and backside—while an apple gains weight around her abdomen," says Dr. Vliet. "The balance of female versus male hormones determines who becomes a pear and who becomes an apple."

Like Ann, most women are pears until middle age. "Your body shape changes as you grow older because of the hormonal changes that occur as the years go by," Dr. Vliet explains. "After menopause, we produce less estrogen and progesterone, and that causes us to begin to gain weight the way men do, over the tummy." This is due to the relative excess of testosterone and DHEA as estradiol declines, she says.

Ann believes that all the extra calories from her late-night food fests accumulate on her thighs. The truth is that the first few pounds might head to her lower body, but the rest distribute themselves all over. "Everyone has a particular pattern of weight gain," says Dr. Steelman. "You can't control or change those genes, but no one gains weight in just one place."

What Ann—and you—can change: Whether you're trying to prevent flabby thighs when you're young or head off a bountiful belly when you're older, the best strategy is to not gain weight in the first place. If, like Ann, you've already accumulated a few extra pounds, you can still affect the shape of your lower body with resistance training and abdominal exercises—if you also keep the fat off through diet and exercise, says Rick Kahley, an exercise physiologist and certified personal trainer in Macon, Georgia.

Genetics. Ann is obviously aware that genetics plays a significant role in body weight. If you have two obese parents (meaning that they weigh 20 percent or more than they should), the chance that you will be obese is about 80 percent. If, like Ann, one of your parents is obese, your chance is 23 percent. If neither of your parents is obese, you have less than a 10 percent chance of being obese. Likewise, some families or ethnic groups have a genetic tendency to gain weight or, conversely, have a high basal metabolic rate.

Two factors seem to be a part of heredity and weight gain. First, scientists have identified a gene (called the obese gene) that is responsible for leptin, a hormone that lets you know that you're full and can stop eating. Researchers believe that in some people, this gene doesn't work properly, and their cell receptors don't receive, or can't recognize, signals that help them stop eating.

Among relatively few women, the second possible factor is adaptation. Until this century, food wasn't plentiful for most human beings. So historically, our bodies have learned to store what they get to make sure they still have energy available during times when food is scarce. Over the course of several generations, some ethnic groups—Pima Indians, in particular—have become more adept than others at storing food as fat, in order to protect against times of famine, says Dr. Vliet.

"In a certain sense, it's almost unreasonable to consider which ethnic groups are more prone to obesity than others," says Dr. Vliet. "Our obesity rates are so high that they encompass all people who are inactive and eat too many calories."

What Ann—and you—can change: It takes work to fight your genes, but it can be done. "If Ann commits herself to staying in good physical shape, then she won't gain the fat that she's afraid of," says Grace Mello, R.D., a registered dietitian in Westerly, Rhode Island. "Ann and her sisters and parents may share the same basic shape. But if one works out regularly and eats well and the others don't, you will see a difference in their figures."

Biology Is Not Destiny

Margie's, Sarah's, and Ann's concerns are all legitimate. And, yes, hormones and our genetic backgrounds do influence our size and shape. We can't change our height, our sex, or the basic physics of our bodies, but we have a lot of control over our weight.

"The best thing anyone can do is commit to habits that research has shown lead to weight loss and weight maintenance," says Eckert. "People who have been successful at weight loss tend to have a positive outlook about their food intake and exercise habits, weigh themselves about three times a week, exercise consistently, and keep a record of what they eat and their activity."

Why do these things work? Because many overweight people don't accurately judge how much they eat against how little they exercise. "Behavior and habits are really the deciding factors for most people regarding weight," says Hogan. "The eating, exercise, and attitude habits you practice throughout your life have much more of an impact on your weight than genetics."

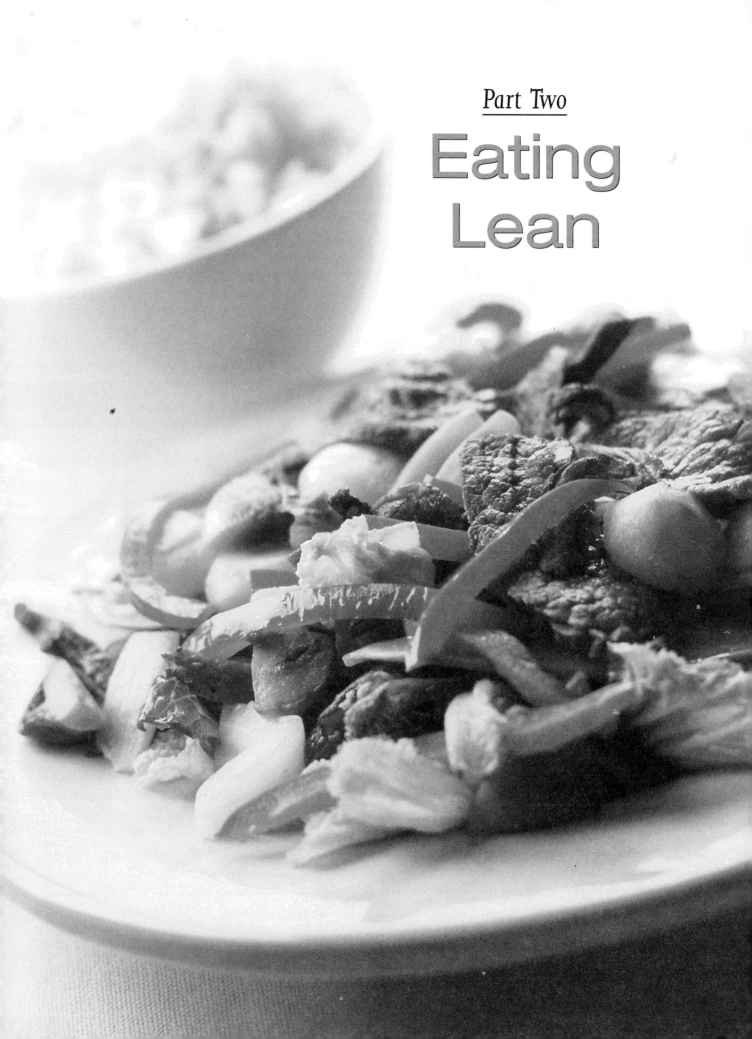

Part Two
Eating
Lean

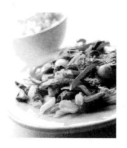

10 Winning Principles of Eating Lean

Stop treating food as the enemy! You can't live without it, so you might as well make peace with it. And the sooner you accept that no foods are inherently bad and that you can enjoy a rich and rewarding relationship with food, the sooner your battle against excess weight will be won.

Of course, barring sudden illness, weight loss doesn't just happen. As with everything else, you need a plan—and a set of guiding principles. Below are 10 that weight-loss experts swear by.

Keep in mind that for results to be permanent, you have to lose weight *your* way. What put your sister, mother, or best friend in size 10 jeans won't necessarily do the trick for you. So mold the following principles into a program that you can actually enjoy—and stick with.

1. Take stock of what you're eating now. You say that you don't understand why those extra pounds cling to your body like ivy to a brick wall? You're eating low-fat, getting lots of fruits and vegetables, avoiding empty calories, and choosing foods high in nutrients like iron and calcium. Or are you?

The only way you'll really know is to write down what you eat for several days. Don't grouse! A food diary is an effective weight-loss tool, says Suellyn Crossley, R.D., a registered dietitian and director of Healthy Weight Management at Florida Hospital Celebration Health in Orlando. She has all of her clients keep one for at least three days.

2. Shop smart. "You have to eat to lose weight!" says Megrette Hammond, R.D., a registered dietitian in Nottingham, New Hampshire,

who specializes in eating disorders and motivation issues. The trick is to eat differently than you do now. The easiest way to do that is to become a smart shopper, preferably one with an M.S. degree—a Masters in Substitution. Simple substitutions let you cut calories and grams of fat without missing them.

3. Balance your fat intake. Obsessing about each and every gram of fat isn't the goal. The goal is awareness of fat in foods so you can learn to balance high-fat items with low-fat ones. This is summed up best by Toni Bloom, R.D., a registered dietitian in San Jose, California, who counsels people all day long. "There's definitely room in every diet for high-fat foods. But you have to know which foods actually do have more fat so that you can plan to eat less of those," she says.

4. Learn the difference between hunger and thirst. "People often think they're hungry when they're actually thirsty," says Christine Palumbo, R.D., a registered dietitian in Naperville, Illinois. She recommends that you drink a glass of cold water when the urge to nibble hits. Then wait to see if your hunger disappears after a few minutes.

"Water gives you a sense of fullness," explains Ann S. Litt, R.D., a registered dietitian in Bethesda, Maryland, who tells all of her weight-loss clients to learn to love water.

5. Fill up on fiber. Fiber's not sexy, but it can help you fit into that slinky little red dress you've been hankering for. That's because, logically enough, high-fiber foods are filling. They prevent you from overeating. "Fiber-rich foods take up more space in your stomach, so you feel satisfied

Why You Crave Fat

Think of it as Mother Nature's cruel joke. Your brain is actually programmed to crave fat. In fact, there are several appetite-control chemicals in the brain that turn on your desire for fat, says registered dietitian Elizabeth Somer, R.D., author of *Food and Mood* and *Age-Proof Your Body*.

"The first of these chemicals is galanin, which is released from the hypothalamus about midday and stays on through the evening hours," Somer says. It entices you to choose fatty foods like hamburgers or pasta with cream sauce for lunch instead of chicken breast or spaghetti marinara.

Ironically, if you eat too much fat at lunch, galanin escalates and makes you likely to overeat fat later in the day as well. "So if you have a salad with lots of high-fat dressing, you're more likely to crave a big bowl of ice cream at 9:00 P.M.," Somer explains. Fat cravings are also stimulated by endorphins, proteins in the brain. They make eating fat pleasurable, so you're likely to want more of that food later on.

Carbohydrates also play a role, increasing the release of serotonin in the brain, which provides a calming effect and elevates mood. Many high-fat foods, such as ice cream, candy, cakes, and cookies, are high in carbohydrates.

Don't blame your brain entirely, though. "We are basically cave dwellers in Calvin Kleins," says Somer. "Our body chemistry is geared to a time when calories could be in short supply at any turn." But with supermarket shelves stuffed to the gills, famine isn't likely. We just eat like it is.

Two more causes of fat cravings: Hormonal fluctuations in the 10 days before our menstrual periods often cause women to experience an increased desire for fatty, sugary foods. So can skipping meals. According to Somer, people who skip breakfast and eat erratically are more prone to cravings, mood swings, and fatigue later in the day.

So what's the solution? "Work with your cravings, not against them," advises Somer. If you know that you're prone to cravings in the midafternoon, plan a nutritious snack that will satisfy the craving.

What if it's chocolate you lust after? Just have it! You already know what happens if you don't—you eat something else but don't feel satisfied. Then you eat something else. A bunch of calories later, you reach for the chocolate. You're far worse off than if you'd eaten the chocolate in the first place. Try to limit yourself to a few pieces of chocolate, though, or try something lighter—perhaps chunks of fresh fruit dunked in chocolate syrup.

longer," says Debra Indorato, R.D., a registered dietitian and the owner and consulting dietitian for Approach Nutrition and Fitness in Allentown, Pennsylvania.

How much fiber do you need? For general health as well as cancer prevention, the National Cancer Institute recommends 20 to 35 grams a day. Most people are lucky if they get half that, but it's not difficult to work fiber into your diet. Fruits, vegetables, dried beans, cereals, and whole-grain breads have plenty.

6. Eat all day long. That's music to a weight-watcher's ears! And it's the exact opposite of the old "starve yourself thin" line of (faulty) reasoning. Indeed, most weight-loss experts agree that eating small meals more frequently throughout the day really keeps you satisfied—and prevents a detour to binge city later in the evening. "When people front-load their calories (by eating earlier in the day) and then eat every three to four hours, they appease their appetites," says Bloom. "If you don't honor your day appetite, you'll have a wicked evening appetite to contend with."

7. Stop eating when you're satisfied. Losing extra pounds and keeping them off will be easier once you learn to distinguish between fullness and satiety. Fullness is the weight of food in your stomach. "You can feel full from 10 heads of lettuce, but will you be satisfied?" asks Hammond. Probably not, so you just keep on eating.

Satiety is the level of satisfaction you get from eating. And the best way to be satisfied is to eat foods with a variety of flavors, colors, and textures. Forget a cheeseburger and fries, with their similar color and texture. Think instead of chicken parmigiana, baby carrots, fettuccine, and a tossed salad with mixed lettuce and chopped yellow bell peppers.

8. Don't skip meals. Meal skipping is a classic form of deprivation among career dieters. When you eliminate entire meals, you deprive your body of adequate calories for energy, not to mention valuable disease-fighting nutrients and phytochemicals. Dietitians Crossley and Indorato both see skipping breakfast as a major deterrent to successful weight loss.

9. If you want it, eat it—sometimes. Deprivation doesn't work. Never has. Never will.

"You don't need to deprive yourself while trying to lose weight," Indorato says emphatically. "You can still eat your favorite foods." She actually has her weight-loss clients list all their favorite foods, especially those they absolutely cannot live without. Then she teaches them how to eat smaller portions of these foods and relish each bite.

10. Enjoy what you eat. "Slow down! Enjoy everything you eat," says Indorato. Many people eat so fast that they don't actually taste the food crossing their lips. And because of that, they aren't really satisfied—which sets them up for overeating later on. It's a vicious circle.

This concept is seconded by dietitian Litt. "I tell my clients to eat something they really like every day because it tastes good, not necessarily because it's good for them."

For more inside tips on how to eat lean, visit our Web site at www.banishbbt.com.

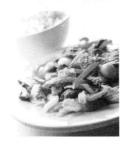

The Best and Worst Body-Shaping Foods

On any given day, you face dozens of food and beverage choices. Eggs or a muffin? Coffee or tea? Club sandwich or soup and salad? Chicken or fish? Pizza or tacos? Beer or wine?

Each decision, big or small, can be part of your strategy to lose weight—and that doesn't mean living on carrot sticks and diet soda. On the contrary, any food is fare game, say experts. Foods you've been shunning aren't forbidden at all. And some foods you thought were low-cal may be delivering hidden fat and calories.

"There really are no best or worst foods, only overall ways of eating that can be best or worst for you," says Roberta Duyff, R.D., a registered dietitian and food and nutrition consultant in St. Louis, Missouri, and author of *The American Dietetic Association's Complete Food and Nutrition Guide*, among other books. "You need to enjoy a variety of foods, and not too much or too little of any one food. Certainly go easy on high-calorie, high-fat foods. What counts is the fat and calories in your overall diet."

Other dietitians agree.

"All kinds of negative feelings and behaviors come into play when you eat so-called bad foods," says Kim Galeaz, R.D., a registered dietitian and food and nutrition consultant in Indianapolis. "Many people start to feel guilt, anxiety, and remorse. I'd like everyone to get over this 'good/bad' notion and start eating for enjoyment."

Not only are you "allowed" to eat your favorite foods, you *should* eat them, say experts.

"It's easier to stick to a healthful eating plan when you include some favorites," says Elizabeth Ward, R.D., a registered dietitian and nutrition consultant in Stoneham, Massachusetts, spokesperson for the American Dietetic Association, and author of *Pregnancy Nutrition: Good Health for You and Your Baby*, among other publications. "Lose your all-or-nothing dieting mentality, and gain some peace. Just because you ate more than you should at one meal doesn't spell dietary disaster. And keep in mind that you can eat more food when you include daily physical activity."

"You don't have to limit your choices to the best in any category, or even completely avoid those in the worst," says Kristine Napier, R.D., a registered dietitian and nutrition consultant in Mayfield Village, Ohio; consultant director of the Nutrition Enhancement Project at the Cleveland Clinic Heart Center, Preventive Cardiology Program; and author of *Power Nutrition for Chronic Illness*. The following lists should be used as they were intended—to guide you toward the better choices most of the time.

"'Best' selections are exceptionally helpful when you're trying to eat just a little leaner to counteract something with more calories you ate the previous day," adds Napier.

You can also use these examples to make trade-offs during the course of the day—a light dinner to compensate for selecting a special treat at lunch or celebrating with food at midday, for example.

For the fat and calorie content of foods not listed in this section, visit our Web site at www.banishbbt.com.

Bagels, Breads, Rolls, and Muffins

Remember when dieters axed the bun and ate the burger? Back then, carbohydrates were the bad guys, and protein was all the rage. (Sometimes, fat was the rage, too. Does the low-carbohydrate diet ring a bell? No bread but all the bacon you wanted.)

Those fads didn't make sense then, and they still don't. True, high-protein diets help you shed a few pounds quickly—simply because they dehydrate your cells. That fast weight loss of a couple of pounds is nothing more than life-sustaining water being wrung out of your cells. Worse, high-protein diets may place stress on your kidneys and

can spell big trouble when it comes to heart disease and cancer, especially if most of the protein comes from meat and other animal foods.

While convincing people that high-protein diets were the answer to dieting woes, media hype unfairly bad-mouthed carbohydrates, especially those in bread and related foods. It still comes as a surprise to many people that not all bread is fattening. In fact, if chosen properly, bread is one of the essentials in a lifelong weight-control routine.

The carbs in whole-grain foods, including whole-grain breads, are so rich in nutrients that

Best and Worst Bagels, Breads, Rolls, and Muffins

To qualify as a healthful selection, bread items should have fewer than four grams of fat per ounce. Also, look for breads with at least two grams of fiber per serving.

Best Choices			
Bread Item	**Portion**	**Calories**	**Grams of Fat**
Whole-grain bread	1 slice (1 oz.)	70	1.1
Whole-wheat pita	1 small pita (1 oz.)	74	0.7
Scandinavian flat bread	1 flat bread (1 oz.)	104	0.4
Tomato and basil tortilla	1 tortilla (1½ oz.)	110	1.0
Low-fat blueberry muffin	1 muffin (2 oz.)	162	6.2
Pumpernickel bagel	1 bagel (4 oz.)	250	1.0

Worst Choices			
Bread Item	**Portion**	**Calories**	**Grams of Fat**
Chocolate chip muffin	1 muffin (4 oz.)	370	15.0
Garlic bread	1 slice (3½ oz.)	360	17.0
Flaky biscuit	1 biscuit (3½ oz.)	357	16.5
Croissant	1 medium croissant (2 oz.)	231	12.0
Seasoned croutons	1 oz.	132	5.2

dietitians advise 7 to 10 servings daily. Whole grains are also high in fiber, which is a dieter's friend. High-fiber foods fill you up with fewer calories, alleviate hunger because they are metabolized slowly, and keep you from absorbing some of the calories in the other foods you eat.

Don't confuse simple carbohydrates with complex ones, however. Complex carbs are whole grains, fruits, and vegetables as they come from Mother Nature. Think of them as complex packages, the wrapping being the fiber and the insides a wealth of vitamins, minerals, protective substances called phytochemicals, protein, and even more fiber. Simple carbohydrates are stripped-down versions. Examples include white bread, white flour, pretzels, and white bagels. They're not loaded with fat, but they run shy in nutrients.

Shopping Smarts

For the bread you eat to qualify as the staff of life, you have to make the right choices when shopping. Here's what to look for.

Bread. Think color. Rich, variegated shades of tan, brown, and dark brown are often a clue that you're getting the whole-grain instead of the watered-down version. But they're not a foolproof indication. Molasses, caramel, and other coloring agents can help white bread masquerade as its healthier cousin. Make sure that the label confirms your choice. Look for words like "100 percent whole-wheat." ("Wheat bread" doesn't guarantee whole grain.) And check that some type of whole-grain flour is listed as the first ingredient.

Providing your tastebuds with a wide variety of flavors satisfies you with fewer calories. So shop where you can buy partial loaves of different whole-grain breads. That way, they won't go stale before you finish them. (Barring that, buy whole loaves and freeze part of each.)

Remember to have your bread sliced at the store. The employee can do it thinner than you can at home, which helps you control portion sizes. When you do cut your own bread, aim for one-ounce slices. (If you know that it's a 20-ounce loaf, for instance, try to get 20 slices.) One ounce of bread counts as one serving of whole grains.

If there's a bread machine collecting dust on your shelves, put it to use. Make your own whole-grain loaves with packaged mixes. Choose ones that have no more than one gram of fat but at least two grams of fiber per 100-calorie serving.

Bagels. Again, buy a variety. Rather than grabbing a whole bag of one type, pick up one rye, one pumpernickel, one whole-grain, one oat bran, and so forth. Even more important, pay attention to bagel size. Many bakery versions are the equivalent of five slices of bread and, at about five ounces, weigh in at around 390 calories. Depending on how you want to apportion your grain servings, cut these large bagels into halves or thirds. Bagels you buy frozen tend to be two ounces, the equivalent of two slices of bread. Watch out for some "bagel chips"—they tend to be heavily coated with oil or butter and not at all lean.

Muffins. Maybe muffins should be called masters of deception. They have such a healthy, homey image, yet too often they're high in fat. Some bakery muffins tip the scales at 15 grams of fat and 370 calories. Many fat-free ones are no calorie bargain either—the larger ones can weigh in with 350 to as many as 600 calories, but very few nutrients.

Regard some of those specialty muffins with a wary eye. Chocolate chip muffins are so tempting—and they're "breakfast food," so they must be good for you, right? Wrong! They're little more than chocolate cupcakes in disguise.

If you like to bake, try some of the lower-fat muffin mixes. By baking your own, you can control portion sizes. (You can even make mini-muffins.) When a box mix calls for oil, use half oil and half applesauce. To increase the nutritional value of the muffins, stir in grated carrots and some raisins. Both baking tricks increase flavor and moistness.

Dinner rolls and biscuits. The fancier they get, the fattier they are. Some of the worst offenders are the ready-to-bake rolls and biscuits in the dairy case. The "bigger is better" rule seems to apply, with many coming in he-man sizes. Frozen bake-and-serve products can also be problematic. Check the labels for fat and calories. As for frozen garlic bread—do you really want to squander 360 calories and 17 grams of fat (for a 3½-ounce slice) on an accompaniment? And *oui*, croissants can be even worse (even before you slather on the butter). Steer clear or at least reserve them for special splurges.

Make It *Better*

Good-for-Your-Waistline Muffins

MAKES 10 MUFFINS

Per muffin

119 calories

3.2 grams of fat

(23 percent of

calories from fat)

These muffins are great as an on-the-go breakfast. They have 251 fewer calories than the cupcakelike confections that masquerade as breakfast food. To cut the fat from your own muffin recipes, use two egg whites or one-quarter cup of fat-free egg substitute in place of each whole egg. Replace whole milk with fat-free milk, and reduce the oil to one tablespoon per cup of flour.

¾ **cup unbleached flour**	½ **teaspoon grated orange peel**
¾ **cup whole-wheat flour**	¾ **cup orange juice**
¼ **cup oat bran**	1 **egg white, lightly beaten**
1½ **teaspoons baking powder**	2 **tablespoons canola oil**
½ **teaspoon ground cinnamon**	2 **tablespoons honey**
⅛ **teaspoon ground allspice**	1 **medium carrot, shredded**

Preheat the oven to 400°F. Spray 10 muffin cups with nonstick spray (or line the cups with paper baking cups). Set aside.

In a medium bowl, stir together the unbleached flour, whole-wheat flour, oat bran, baking powder, cinnamon, and allspice.

In a small bowl, combine the orange peel, orange juice, egg white, oil, and honey. Add to the flour mixture and stir just until combined. Stir in the carrot.

Spoon the batter into the muffin cups, filling each about three-quarters full. Bake for 20 minutes, or until a toothpick inserted near the centers comes out clean. Remove the muffins from the muffin cups. Cool completely on a wire rack.

To store: Individually wrap each muffin in freezer paper or resealable freezer bags and freeze until ready to serve.

To serve: Thaw overnight at room temperature. Or thaw and reheat each muffin in a microwave oven on high power (100 percent) for 15 to 20 seconds.

English muffins, French bread, and pita bread. These items tend to be very low in fat with a reasonable number of calories. Try to find whole-wheat versions—even pitas now come in a variety of whole-grain and vegetable mixes. (But please avoid the temptation to fill those "nooks and crannies" in the English muffins with puddles of butter!)

Apple butter and fruit purees. These have not a lick of fat, but they do contain some vitamins and fiber. Buy them or make your own. To create one even the kids will enjoy: Scoop baked acorn squash from its shell and place in a food processor with a splash of milk and a sprinkle of ground cinnamon and brown sugar. Blend until smooth. Store in the refrigerator for up to a week. Use the same basic concept for cooked apples, pears, pumpkin, peaches, and more.

Weight-Friendly Substitutions

Traditional Scandinavian flat breads are easier to find than ever. Resembling thin crackers, these delightfully crispy breads are made with a combination of wheat, barley, potato, and rye flours. Serve them as the Scandinavians do—with soups, salads, and low-fat cheeses. They're fat-free, fiber-rich, and naturally low in calories—just 104 per one-ounce cracker, compared to 132 for croutons and 360 for garlic bread.

New Foods to Try

If you can't imagine spaghetti, lasagna, or other Italian foods without garlic bread, try checking a bakery for ciabatta. This low-fat "Swiss cheese of breads" has large holes peppered throughout its cloud-soft interior and is so flavorful it doesn't need butter, margarine, or olive oil. Warm the loaf briefly in a hot oven to make the outside even crisper.

Tortillas now come in a variety of whole-grain and vegetable versions that give a new dimension to wrap-style sandwiches. For a quick lunch, roll warm fat-free canned refried beans and chopped veggies in spinach, tomato and basil, jalapeño and cilantro, honey wheat, garden herb, or other flavor tortillas.

Some new products worth avoiding: pizza breads (such as cheese and pepperoni) and focaccia. Although focaccia is extremely popular, it's also high in fat.

Dining Out

In some restaurants, bread baskets rival the dessert cart. What used to be a basket of plain white bread has now become a bakery full of choices: little pecan rolls, mini-muffins, flaky biscuits, sesame seed rolls—accompanied by a crock of whipped butter. Worse, the basket arrives when you're hungriest and least able to resist. Before you know it, you've eaten a meal-size amount of bread and butter.

The best way to manage this terrible temptation is to head it off. Ask the server to remove the butter. You might even want him to take away the basket, leaving just one piece of bread or one roll per person. (Let him know that you'll ask for extra portions as needed—which means you really have to think about having another piece.) If you're with friends and they want the bread to stay, select something plain, like French bread or a breadstick. Then make sure they park the basket on their side of the table, out of your reach.

Beverages

When it comes to liquid calories, a lot of women who watch their weight fall into three camps.

Some can recite the fat and calorie count for hundreds of foods, but don't keep track of beverages they drink, which can squelch their weight-control efforts like a tidal wave.

Others are well aware that a can of soda is the equivalent of liquid candy, containing 150 calories and nearly as much sugar as two candy bars.

The fact is that whether the source of your calories is foods or beverages, if you take in more calories than your body needs, you will gain weight.

Water is the one beverage that helps, not hinders, your weight-loss efforts. Studies show that people who drink water before meals eat fewer calories and have an easier time taking off excess pounds. That's because water fills your stomach. And when your stomach is full, you don't eat as much.

When used appropriately, wet calories can help, not hinder, your body-shaping efforts. Here's how.

Best and Worst Beverages

From a strictly caloric standpoint, plain water is the best thing you can drink. Beverages that contain fat and sugar are the worst. If your tastebuds need excitement but your hips don't need the fat and calories, look for unsweetened beverages. Drinks that offer some nutrition in return for their caloric cost, such as an eight-ounce glass of skim milk, are also a wise choice. Serving sizes given here are typical for each drink.

Best Choices

Beverage	Serving Size	Calories	Grams of Fat
Still or sparkling water	8 oz.	0	0.0
Unsweetened, flavored water	8 oz.	0	0.0
Unsweetened, flavored iced tea	8 oz.	5	0.0
Vegetable juice	8 oz.	46	0.2
Calcium-fortified orange juice	8 oz.	120	0.7
Grape juice	8 oz.	127	0.2

Worst Choices

Beverage	Serving Size	Calories	Grams of Fat
Piña colada	8 oz.	466	4.8
Chocolate milkshake	12 oz.	430	13.0
Eggnog	8 oz.	342	19.0
Cappuccino with whole milk	12 oz.	288	10.0
Regular soda	12 oz.	150	0.0
Beer	12 oz.	146	0.0

Make It *Better*

Strawberry-Banana Smoothie

MAKES 4 SERVINGS

Per serving

85 calories

0.5 gram fat

(5 percent calories from fat)

Made properly, fruit smoothies make an excellent breakfast drink or midday pick-me-up. In contrast, the bottled versions are sticky sweet with fruit syrup, and you'll get stuck with lots of extra calories—often in excess of 300 calories per 8 ounces, and with very little nutrition to show for the calorie burst.

2   **cups frozen sliced strawberries**

1   **large banana, sliced**

½   **cup orange juice**

½   **cup nonfat vanilla yogurt or nonfat milk**

6   **ice cubes**

In a blender, combine the strawberries, banana, orange juice, yogurt or milk, and ice cubes. Blend until thick and smooth.

Shopping Smarts

For tips on buying milk and soy milk, see Milk and Dairy on page 78. Otherwise, follow these purchasing tips.

Water. Given that water has zero fat and calories and can keep you from overeating, bottled water should appear on every grocery list. Buy enough for a week. (If you drink tap water, fill four or five 20-ounce reusable sipper bottles and chill them in the refrigerator. Then carry water with you during the day.)

Still water is fine. If a little fizz helps you chug down more wet stuff, buy calorie-free flavored seltzer or club sodas. Just avoid the ones that are heavy in sugar and calories. They hide nearly as many calories as regular soda.

Coffee and coffee drinks. True, coffee contributes only 5 calories—if you drink it black. The real damage, however, comes from specialty coffees—the lattes, mochas, cappuccinos, and other tall treats sold in coffee bars and shops (and even some

gas stations). Choose poorly, and you've just blown your dessert calories for the next month. An eight-ounce regular café mocha splashes in at 493 calories and 49 grams of fat. Order it with nonfat milk and sans whipped cream (substitute the foam from steaming the nonfat milk), add artificial sweetener, and sneak by with just 120 calories. You're out the door with a chocolate fix—and loads of slimming, virtuous self-esteem.

Iced tea. If you're going to drink iced tea, drink plain old-fashioned iced tea—made from tea bags and flavored with lemon. It has just two calories, plus you get plenty of water in the bargain. Grab a 16-ounce bottle of flavored, sweetened iced tea, and you're grabbing the equivalent of a soda.

Juices. With few exceptions, juice doesn't really count toward the three to five daily servings of fruits and vegetables that experts recommend as rich sources of vitamins, minerals, fiber, and other protective nutrients. It's mainly sugar.

Two exceptions are calcium-fortified orange

juice and vegetable juice. Calcium-fortified orange juice helps satisfy the essential bone-building calcium requirement for women who don't drink milk. And vegetable juice offers a wide variety of nutrients for few calories (46 calories in eight ounces).

Alcohol. Experts agree that people who drink red wine in moderation seem to enjoy some protection against heart disease. Still, if you're watching your weight, that benefit comes at a caloric price—7 calories per gram of alcohol, or about 103 calories per 5-ounce glass. If you drink wine out of goblets, used in many homes and restaurants, you'll consume even more. And if you drink hard liquor, like gin or vodka, you'll quaff 97 calories or more in a shot, depending on the proof, plus whatever mixer you choose. Liqueur (like coffee liqueur) is even higher, at 160 calories per 1½-ounce shot. As for those fruity tropical drinks like piña coladas—well, you might as well be drinking a chocolate milkshake.

The other trouble with alcohol? It can erase your willpower—resulting in even more excess calories than the alcohol alone.

If you don't drink and you're watching your weight, don't start to imbibe. Both black and green tea, which have zero calories, may provide heart-protecting benefits similar to red wine. And if you do drink, keep the calories from alcohol to a minimum.

Weight-Friendly Substitutions

If you just have to have a higher-calorie beverage, try the following substitutes.

- Instead of regular lemonade (99 calories per 8 ounces), substitute artificially sweetened lemonade drink (5 calories).

- Instead of wine (103 calories per 5 ounces), have a wine spritzer (62 calories per 5 ounces).

- Instead of a chocolate milkshake (430 calories for 12 ounces), order a café mocha skim, no whipped cream (120 calories per 12 ounces).

New Foods to Try

Sugar-free powdered beverages are blossoming in many flavors—from pedestrian lemonade to peach, raspberry, and strawberry flavor explosions. Mix up a pitcher and keep it in the fridge year-round to satisfy a sweet tooth. Remember, though—these are substitutes for sweetened beverages, not a license to drink whatever you want freely.

Dining Out

A couple of beers, a glass of wine, an iced tea, after-dinner coffee or liqueur—extra calories can accumulate so easily when you're dining out. Managing liquid calories begins before you leave home. Enjoy a tall glass of water before you leave your home or office for a meal out. You'll eat less food and drink, starting with the bread basket.

When you do order something to drink, order fancy sparkling water with lime instead of an alcoholic drink, which can quickly erase your willpower just as you have so many scrumptious foods to choose from. If you've eaten lightly all day to save calories for a special dinner out (which is a great idea), beware: Alcohol is absorbed more quickly on an empty stomach; just a little alcohol can quickly become too much.

If a fancy dinner just wouldn't be special without wine, order something expensive by the glass: You'll be less likely to have two or three.

Burgers and Hot Dogs

What's more American than a doggie at the ball game or a burger on the grill for the Fourth of July? If these foods appeared only on such special occasions, they wouldn't pose too much of a weight problem. Unfortunately, they've turned into everyday guests in many homes—and they don't bring much with them to the table.

Hot dogs offer protein and little else (except fat, to the tune of 16 grams for a regular frank). Burgers can be better nutrition-wise, pairing iron, vitamin B_{12}, and zinc with their protein. But with 21 grams of fat in a McDonald's Quarter Pounder, they're no dietary bargain either. Face it, it's hard to find comfort in your comfort food when you're biting into a third of your day's total fat allowance—and that doesn't even include the fries.

Shopping Smarts

Luckily, you don't have to give up these quick mealtime staples. You just need to be more discerning when choosing them. Here are things to keep in mind at the store.

Burgers. Take a good look at that package of "lean" ground beef. What you really want to know is *how* lean. Regular ground beef is about 73 percent lean (which means 27 percent fat)—a three-ounce cooked patty has 18 grams of fat. Ground round (85 percent lean) is a little better. But ground sirloin (90 percent) and ground top round (97 percent) are wiser choices. A cooked ground sirloin patty has 6 grams of fat—one-third of what that regular ground beef gives you.

If you can't find really lean ground meat, ask the butcher to grind some sirloin or top round for you. (Make sure he trims off excess fat first.) An alternative is to use ground turkey breast or chicken breast—or to mix them with some ground beef to lower the fat content. Be aware that meat marked simply ground turkey or ground chicken contains dark meat and skin in addition to breast meat, so it's not nearly as low in fat as plain ground breast.

Grill or broil your burgers so any fat in them can drip off. (Or use a ridged grill pan made for the stove top.) If you must use a regular skillet, blot the cooked burgers with paper towels to remove surface fat.

Hot dogs. Your best choices in hot dogs are those with three grams or less of fat. Look for the words "reduced-fat," "low-fat," or "fat-free" on the label. Don't think that because it says turkey or chicken on the package, it's automatically low in fat. Regular turkey and chicken dogs can still pack six to nine grams of fat each.

Lean Menu-Makers

The more company that hot dog or hamburger has on your plate, the better. But make sure they're worthwhile accompaniments, like the ones below.

Tomatoes and onions. They're loaded with phytochemicals and vitamins that may cut the risk of cancer and heart disease. So don't skimp when adding sliced or chopped tomatoes and onions. Plus, you'll reach the five-a-day vegetable goal easier!

Lettuce. Go green! Load up on romaine, green- or red-leaf lettuce, and even fresh spinach leaves. They're a better vitamin value than iceberg lettuce.

Coleslaw. Make your own healthy slaw. Combine a bag of broccoli coleslaw or shredded cabbage mix with light or fat-free coleslaw dressing.

Fries. Regular french fries, the ubiquitous side for hamburgers and hot dogs, can sabotage your fat-banishing efforts. (A medium order of fast-food fries can cost you 21 grams of fat.) Scan the freezer section for fries with no more than 8 grams of fat per serving. Typically, straight and crinkle fries have less fat than shapes like cross-cut and spiral fries. Oven-bake rather than fry them, and cook them longer than the package says if you want to get them crispy.

Cheese. Craving a cheeseburger? Opt for a

slice of reduced-fat or fat-free American cheese on top instead of full-fat Colby or Cheddar.

Buns. Look to whole-grain hot dog and hamburger buns for a fiber boost.

Beans. Use vegetarian chili and baked beans for less fat and no cholesterol.

Weight-Friendly Substitutions

Try meatless vegetable patties. Although not necessarily fat-free—they range from zero to eight grams of fat—they're very low in saturated fat and have no cholesterol. With so many different flavors and brands available, you're sure to find at least

Best and Worst Burgers and Hot Dogs

Ground beef burgers supply ample amounts of iron, zinc, and vitamin B_{12}, which are crucial to women's health. But you don't want all this good nutrition at the expense of too much fat. Your best bets are burgers made from ground top round or sirloin, or ground chicken or turkey, with 10 grams of fat or fewer and 260 calories or fewer for a three-ounce cooked patty. Hot dogs don't make the grade for a nutrient-dense meat—eat them only occasionally and aim for the lower-fat versions (beef, pork, poultry, or veggie) with no more than 7 grams of fat.

Best Choices			
Burger or Hot Dog	**Portion**	**Calories**	**Grams of Fat**
Fat-free hot dog	1 hot dog	40	0.0
Turkey hot dog	1 hot dog	85	6.0
Light hot dog	1 hot dog	110	8.4
Veggie dog	1 hot dog	118	7.0
Lean smoked sausage (broiled)	3 oz.	120	3.6
Soy/veggie burger	1 patty (about 3 oz.)	137	4.1
Burger made from ground top round (broiled, no bun)	3 oz.	153	4.2
Burger made from ground sirloin (broiled, no bun)	3 oz.	166	6.1
Small hamburger (fast-food)	1 burger	260	9.0

Worst Choices			
Burger or Hot Dog	**Portion**	**Calories**	**Grams of Fat**
Large hamburger (fast-food)	1 burger	420	21.0
Burger made from ground chuck (broiled, no bun)	3 oz.	290	22.0
Small frozen burgers	2 burgers	270	14.0
Polish sausage (kielbasa)	1 sausage (about 3 oz.)	264	23.1
Bratwurst	1 sausage (about 3 oz.)	256	22.0
Burger made from regular ground beef (broiled, no bun)	3 oz.	246	17.6
Regular hot dog	1 hot dog	180	16.2

Make It *Better*

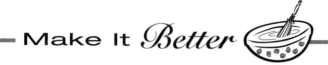

California-Style Turkey Burgers

MAKES 12 SERVINGS

Per burger

289 calories

2.6 grams of fat

(8 percent of calories

from fat)

One of these tasty burgers has 13.4 fewer grams of fat than a same-size burger made of ground round. To make the leanest patties possible, purchase boneless, skinless turkey breast. Cut it into chunks and grind it in a food processor using on/off turns. If you're serving fewer than 12, you can freeze the extra turkey mixture for future quick patties. Just form the patties, stack them (separated with pieces of wax paper), wrap well, and freeze.

3 pounds ground turkey breast

1 cup minced onions

1 cup celery

1 cup minced red bell peppers

¼ cup tomato paste

2 cloves garlic, minced

1 teaspoon ground black pepper

12 crusty rolls

Shredded lettuce

Tomato slices

In a large bowl, thoroughly mix the turkey, onions, celery, red peppers, tomato paste, garlic, and black pepper.

Form into 12 patties. Grill (or broil or sauté in a nonstick frying pan). Serve in the rolls with the lettuce and tomatoes.

one you like! Look for plain burger flavor, spicy black bean, mushroom, sautéed onion, garden vegetable, and more. Some are even made with soy protein, which has been said to lower the risk of developing cancer, osteoporosis, and heart disease.

Besides ready-made patties, various all-vegetable meat substitutes come in one-pound logs so you can shape your own burgers or hot-dog lookalikes.

New Foods to Try

Look for veggie hot dogs, many of which have seven grams of fat or less. Their main benefit is soy protein. Also try low-fat sausages, which have lots of seasonings to compensate for the fat that has

been removed. Serve any type of burger or hot dog with mayo-Dijon spread.

Dining Out

Forget "double animals," like cheese on a burger or meat chili on a hot dog. By doubling up on animal products, you add unnecessary fat and calories. Ask for more onions, lettuce, and tomatoes instead.

And whoa! Be careful with burger size! While most are four to six ounces, some are upward of nine ounces. Order the smallest size possible and eat only half if it's giant-size. Take the rest home for tomorrow's lunch. Better yet, ask if they have a veggie burger. Many restaurants carry them to cater to vegetarians.

Cereals

Cold or hot, cereal is a great way to start your day. Studies show that women who skip or skimp on breakfast tend to nibble more during the mid- and late morning, perhaps eating even more calories than if they'd eaten breakfast in the first place. So eating breakfast may help you lose weight.

Of course, a breakfast of bacon and eggs won't help your weight-loss goals. Served with buttered toast, fried eggs and two strips of bacon will gird you with 28 grams of fat and 395 calories. In contrast, a bowl of bran flakes, a half-cup of fat-free milk, and a half-cup of sliced strawberries will supply 1 gram of fat and 200 calories.

Breakfast cereals are made from grains—wheat, oats, corn, barley, rice, quinoa, or a multigrain mixture. Except for some granolas, which may contain saturated vegetable fat like coconut oil, most ready-to-eat cereals are low in calories from fat. For the most part, cereal serves as one of your best sources of complex carbohydrates (which, say nutrition experts, should account for 55 to 60 percent of your daily calories).

Best and Worst Cereals

Most cereals are low in fat and can also be a source of many vitamins, minerals, and fiber. A good cereal supplies at least 5 grams of fiber per serving, which is usually 30 grams or about one ounce.

Focus on whole-grain cereals and those with bran or fortified with fiber. If you like granola, choose low-fat versions, and compare the number of calories per serving, which reflects added sugars. Read labels and select cereals that contain the lowest amounts of sugar per serving.

Best Choices

Cereal	Portion	Calories	Grams of Fat	Grams of Fiber
Bran cereal with extra fiber	½ cup	50	0.5	13.3
100 percent bran	⅓ cup	80	0.5	8.0
Instant oatmeal with bran and raisins	1 packet (1.4 oz.), prepared	158	1.9	5.5
Unsweetened shredded wheat	2 biscuits	160	0.5	5.0
Raisin bran	1 cup	190	1.0	8.0
Nugget-type wheat cereal	½ cup	200	1.0	5.0
Wheat bran flakes with dried fruit and nuts	1 cup	210	3.0	5.0

Worst Choices

Cereal	Portion	Calories	Grams of Fat	Grams of Fiber
Cheese grits	½ cup	197	12.0	0.0
Granola (with oil)	¼ cup	131	6.9	2.9
Sugar-coated cereal	1 cup	120	1.0	0.0

Some cereals provide as much as 8 to 12 grams of fiber—about a third of the 25 to 35 grams a day experts recommend. Bran cereals—made from the outer layers of wheat, oats, or other cereal grains—have the highest amounts of fiber. Overall, a daily diet high in fiber (from cereal bran, whole grains, vegetables, fruits, and legumes) can help control your weight in several ways. For one thing, fiber itself has no calories. And since fiber is found only in foods from plant sources, high-fiber foods are often rich in nutrients and low in fat. Third, fiber-rich foods often

Make It *Better*

Three-Grain Granola

MAKES 4 SERVINGS

250 calories

1.5 grams of fat

(5 percent of calories

from fat)

3.5 grams of fiber

Despite its reputation for being healthy, granola—especially the commercial variety—is often alarmingly high in fat and calories. It can contain as much as 8.6 grams of fat and 225 calories per half-cup serving. Toasting the grains and adding honey help to make up for not using any added fat.

2 **cups puffed rice**

1⅓ **cups bran flakes**

½ **cup old-fashioned rolled oats**

¼ **cup raisins**

2 **tablespoons toasted wheat germ**

½ **cup unsweetened apple juice**

2 **tablespoons honey**

Preheat the oven to 300°F. In a medium bowl, combine the puffed rice, bran flakes, oats, raisins, and wheat germ.

In a small bowl, stir together the apple juice and honey. Pour over the puffed rice mixture and toss until moistened.

Spray a 15" × 10" baking pan with nonstick spray. Spread the puffed rice mixture in the pan. Bake for 30 minutes or until golden brown, stirring twice during baking.

Transfer the granola to a large piece of aluminum foil. Let the mixture cool, then break it into pieces.

To store: Transfer the granola to a container. Cover loosely and store at room temperature until ready to serve. (Do not cover tightly because the cereal will not stay crisp.)

To serve: For each serving, place three-quarters cup granola in a cereal bowl and add one-half cup fat-free milk.

Note: If you want to splurge a little, stir one-quarter cup flaked coconut into the cereal mixture before baking. You'll get an extra 35 calories and 2.4 grams of fat in each serving.

take the place of higher-fat foods. And high-fiber foods are bulky, making meals more filling.

As a bonus, different types of fiber offer different health benefits. While the insoluble fiber in bran may help protect you from colon cancer, the soluble fiber in oatmeal may help lower your cholesterol. To reap all the benefits of fiber, vary your choices of whole-grain cereal from day to day.

But wait, there's more: If they're fortified, breakfast cereals may supply a significant percent of your Daily Value (DV) of some vitamins and minerals, including B vitamins (like folate) and iron. Some are calcium-fortified, helping you maintain strong bones underneath your nicely toned figure. Topping your cereal with milk or yogurt multiplies that benefit.

Here's how to make cereal part of a weight-smart breakfast.

Shopping Smarts

Finding packaged cereals with the least fat and calories—and the most fiber—is easy: Read the ingredient list and Nutrition Facts information on the box. Pay attention to serving sizes: They vary from one-half to one cup or more.

Ready-to-eat cereal. Ready-to-eat cold cereal is a calorie bargain—provided you watch out for added sugars in presweetened cereals. To keep the number of calories down, don't get into the habit of adding a spoonful or two of sugar on your own.

Cooked cereal. Start with the best known—oatmeal, cream of wheat, and grits. Then look for other varieties, such as buckwheat, barley, oat bran, or a mixture of whole grains. Quick-cooking and instant varieties save time—just add milk, heat, and eat. Make them with low-fat or fat-free milk for less calories.

Lean Menu-Makers

Cereal boxes list nutritional data for cereal with milk—for good reason. That's how most women eat cereal. To make the most of cereal, stock your "breakfast center" with other nutrient-rich ingredients that can be added with the milk.

- Fresh apples, peaches, pears, apricots, kiwifruit, bananas, berries—whatever fruit you like (to slice or spoon on top)
- Canned fruit in natural juices (mandarin oranges, peaches, pears, figs, and applesauce)
- Dried fruit (cranberries, cherries, apricots, apple slices, and currants)
- Chopped nuts (almonds, walnuts, pecans)—use in small amounts
- Bran (to fortify your cereal with extra fiber)

Dining Out

Open any restaurant menu for breakfast, and the first thing you'll see is the usual fare—fried eggs, bacon or sausage, hash browns, cinnamon buns, and pancakes or waffles loaded with butter and syrup. As an occasional treat, they won't pack on the pounds. But if you travel a lot, a steady diet of high-fat, high-calorie breakfasts can quickly add inches to your hips and waistline.

Cold cereal with milk and fruit is almost always on breakfast menus, even at fast-food places. If not, ask for it. Look for hot cereals, such as oatmeal or cream of wheat, too. When you're traveling, plan to eat a smart breakfast and a lunch, rather than a late all-you-can-eat brunch. Chances are, you'll eat fewer calories overall because you won't be starved when you finally sit down for brunch.

Cheese and Cheese Dishes

More than a party food, cheese is apt to show up anywhere on the menu: in omelettes, sandwiches, soups, salads, casseroles, egg dishes, even desserts. Cheese varies in flavor and texture depending on many factors: the milk used (from cows, goats, or sheep), how the curds (or milk solids) are handled, whether it's aged (and if so, how), and whether any ingredients were added for flavoring. The results vary from plain old American cheese to rich, tangy feta cheese made from goat's milk.

A compact form of milk, cheese has a similar nutritional makeup—plenty of protein and calcium, and a good supply of riboflavin. But a serving of cheese also has more fat and cholesterol than a one-cup serving of milk does. For aged or most firm cheeses such as Cheddar or Swiss, a serving is 1½ ounces, or about the size of six dice. That amount provides 300 to 400 milligrams of calcium (30 to 40 percent of the Daily Value), 10 to 12 grams of protein (about 20 percent of the Daily Value), and 12 to 14 grams of fat. A serving of processed cheese such as American cheese is 2 ounces. This supplies about 350 milligrams of calcium (35 percent of the Daily Value), 12 grams of protein (25 percent of the Daily Value), and 18 grams of fat. Cottage cheese delivers calcium, too—about 75 milligrams in a half-cup serving; the fat content varies.

It's all too easy to nibble away at cheese, consuming more than we think. As a result, the calories and fat can add up. Cheese makers offer fat-free or reduced-fat versions of many popular types of cheese, including cream cheese and Brie. If you prefer the flavor and cooking qualities of full-fat cheeses, eat small portions so that you can keep your fat and calorie intake within "budget." Grate or shred cheese, rather than use slices or chunks, to make a smaller amount go farther. And make sure that most of your other food choices, including dairy foods, are lean, low in fat, or fat-free.

Here are other ways to go easy with cheese—and still enjoy its flavor and nutritional benefits.

Shopping Smarts

Low-fat cheeses are good sources of calcium, so you get this bone-building mineral even while you save fat and calories. Whether you buy regular or reduced-fat cheese, in chunks or shredded, check the Nutrition Facts label, especially if you're salt-sensitive. The sodium content will vary. Also, cheese is perishable, so check expiration dates.

If you buy sliced cheese or wedges at the deli counter, feel free to request nutrition information. By law, it must be available.

Here's how to select the low-fat cheeses that best meet your needs.

Cheddar, Swiss, and other aged cheeses. You'll find fat-free or reduced-fat versions of some, but not all, types of aged cheese. The melting qualities, texture, and flavor differ from brand to brand. Some brands work better than others as substitutes for full-fat cheese. In general, low-fat cheeses have better cooking qualities than their fat-free counterparts.

For pizza, lasagna, and other Italian dishes, look for low-fat or fat-free mozzarella. For a fun snack, try fat-free string cheese, which is a variation of mozzarella.

Processed cheese. American cheese, cheese spreads, and other pasteurized blends aren't ripened or aged. As a result, they don't have the same distinct flavor and texture as aged cheese. But they're versatile and keep longer than aged cheese.

Cottage cheese, ricotta, and cream cheese. Often viewed as a diet food, cottage cheese may not be quite as low-calorie as many people think—it depends on the fat content. For the lowest fat and calorie counts, look for fat-free or 1 percent milk-fat cottage cheese. For salad dressings and dips, whip fat-free cottage cheese as a thickener or as a substitute for sour cream. Reduced-fat and fat-free

Best and Worst Cheeses

USDA experts consider a serving of cheese to be 1½ ounces of natural cheese (like Cheddar) or 2 ounces of processed cheese (like American). But Nutrition Facts labels list a serving of cheese as somewhat less—only 1 ounce. So to keep things simple, that's the benchmark used here. By law, low-fat varieties have three grams of fat or fewer per serving, fat-free have fewer than 0.5 gram of fat per serving, and reduced-fat cheese has at least 25 percent less fat per serving than traditional cheese. If you are trying to watch your fat intake, low-fat cheeses make excellent choices. Generally, cheeses that are lower in fat are also lower in calories. Here's how some popular choices stack up.

Best Choices

Cheese	Portion	Calories	Grams of Fat
Fat-free Parmesan cheese	2 tsp.	20	0.0
Parmesan cheese	2 tsp.	20	1.5
Fat-free cream cheese	1 oz.	30	0.0
Fat-free mozzarella	1 oz.	35	0.0
Low-fat American processed cheese	1 slice	40	1.0
Fat-free Cheddar cheese	1 oz.	45	0.0
Low-fat Cheddar cheese	1 oz.	50	1.5
Low-fat mozzarella	1 oz.	50	1.5
Reduced-fat feta	1 oz.	50	3.0
Reduced-fat cheese spread	1 oz.	60	3.0
Low-fat ricotta	¼ cup	70	3.0
Fat-free cottage cheese	½ cup	90	0.0
Low-fat (1 to 2 percent) cottage cheese	½ cup	90	1.5

Worst Choices

Cheese	Portion	Calories	Grams of Fat
Mascarpone	1 oz.	124	13.0
Blue cheese	1 oz.	120	12.0
Cheddar cheese	1 oz.	120	10.0
Cottage cheese (4 percent)	½ cup	120	5.0
Ricotta	¼ cup	110	8.0
Cream cheese	1 oz.	100	10.0
Brie	1 oz.	100	9.0
Cheese ball or log with nuts	1 oz.	100	4.0
Cheese spread	1 oz.	90	6.0
Feta	1 oz.	80	6.0
American processed cheese	1 slice	70	5.0

ricotta work well in baked dishes, such as lasagna and pastitsio (a Greek version of lasagna).

Also a soft, unripened cheese, cream cheese—the popular ingredient in cheesecake—is very high in fat. Some varieties are herb, fruit, or salmon flavored. These are nice for dips as well as spreads, provided that you choose reduced-fat versions. Don't count on cream cheese for calcium, though—it supplies very little.

Soy cheese. Made from soy protein, soy cheese (sometimes called tofu cheese) is a lower-fat, cholesterol-free alternative to dairy cheese. It doesn't taste much like cheese, however. Experiment to see if it appeals to you.

Lean Menu-Makers

If you find yourself turning to cheese entrées as a way to put meatless meals on the table, be careful. Cheese is no lower in fat than meat—and may be higher. But with some careful planning, cheese dishes can serve as protein-rich centerpieces of your brunch, lunch, or dinner menu. Start with lower-fat versions of these traditional cheese dishes, and pair them with a variety of the foods suggested here.

Macaroni and cheese

- Waldorf salad (made with fat-free dressing) and hearty seven-grain bread
- A salad of sliced tomato, fresh basil, and low-fat mozzarella with a slice of crusty baguette bread
- Crisp garden salad with lemon-pepper vinaigrette and Boston brown bread

Toasted cheese sandwich on whole-grain bread

- Add sliced tomatoes to the sandwich and serve it with coleslaw tossed with fat-free dressing. For an interesting variation, try broccoli slaw, which is shredded broccoli that is sold in packages like coleslaw.
- A cup of tomato soup, with banana peppers, a nectarine, and tabbouleh salad (a Middle Eastern grain salad available as a mix) prepared with less oil
- Cucumber and jicama (a root vegetable) cut into sticks, and a pear

Cheese quiche

- Sautéed leeks or wilted spinach stirred into the quiche mixture before baking and broiled peach halves
- Sliced melon and an herb breadstick
- Steamed asparagus and a toasted slice of sourdough bread
- Sautéed zucchini and a baked cinnamon apple

Weight-Friendly Substitutions

These low-fat kitchen tips can help you enjoy the flavor and texture of cheese without overdosing on fat and calories.

- In cheese spreads, extend a small amount of stronger-flavored cheese, such as Asiago, blue cheese, feta, sharp Cheddar, or Romano cheese, with fat-free yogurt or cottage cheese.
- Substitute reduced-fat or fat-free cheese for full-fat cheese in your favorite recipes. Reduced-fat and fat-free cheeses will melt better if you layer them between other foods or cover the dish while it's baking. Use top-quality, full-flavored cheese for half the amount of cheese in the recipe, and a fat-free counterpart for the other half. Try it with Cheddar cheese first.
- Use sliced soy cheese in sandwiches and lasagna and other baked dishes. Or shred it for casseroles and salad or soup toppers.
- Substitute soft tofu (a block of milky white soybean curd) for cream cheese in dips, medium-soft tofu in cheesecakes, and sliced, firm tofu in sandwiches.
- Try Neufchâtel cheese, light cream cheese, and fat-free cream cheese in cheesecakes.

Dining Out

When you order pizza, skip the double-cheese option. Instead, ask for less cheese and more veggies. If you do treat yourself to pizza with pepperoni or sausage, limit yourself to just one or two slices: Combined with cheese, high-fat toppings really add up.

Cheese sauces on nachos, baked spuds, and other foods can add quite a lot of fat, too, especially if you're heavy with the ladle. Ask for fat-free salsa instead.

Many delis offer low-fat cheese for made-to-order deli sandwiches—just ask. For fast-food sandwiches, skip the cheese; order milk to get the calcium your body needs.

Make It *Better*

Baked Macaroni and Cheese

MAKES 4 SERVINGS

Per serving

415 calories

10.8 grams of fat

(24 percent calories

from fat)

This stripped-down version of the American classic has 153 fewer calories and 24 fewer grams of fat than a standard version. For even more flavor, sprinkle a little grated fat-free Parmesan cheese on top, along with herbs such as minced parsley. To make over your family's favorite cheese dish, use a reduced-fat Cheddar (or blend a strong-flavored, full-fat sharp Cheddar cheese 50-50 with a reduced-fat variety) and replace butter and whole milk with more reduced-fat cheese and skim milk.

8 ounces elbow macaroni	½ cup light ricotta cheese
1 tablespoon olive oil	2 tablespoons chopped green onions
1 tablespoon all-purpose flour	Salt
½ teaspoon dry mustard	Ground black pepper
1¼ cups skim milk	¼ cup toasted bread crumbs
1¼ cups shredded low-fat extra-sharp Cheddar cheese	

Preheat the oven to 375°F. Coat an 8" × 8" baking pan with nonstick cooking spray. Set aside.

Cook the macaroni according to the package directions. Drain well.

Meanwhile, heat the oil in a 3-quart nonstick saucepan over low heat; stir in the flour and mustard. Cook and stir for 1 minute. Gradually stir in the milk. Bring to a boil; cook and stir for 1 minute. Add the Cheddar. Remove the pan from the heat.

In a blender or food processor, puree the ricotta. Add to the sauce. Stir in the green onions and pasta; add salt and pepper to taste. Spoon into the baking pan. Top with the bread crumbs. Bake for 20 minutes, or until the top is golden brown.

Chicken and Turkey

Sliced, diced, roasted, or barbecued, poultry takes the prize for versatility. By choosing the right cuts, using healthy cooking methods, and being creative with herbs and spices, you can tempt your tastebuds, dodge fat, and reap healthy dividends from chicken and turkey.

Poultry is loaded with protein, an essential nutrient that repairs tissue, bolsters immunity, and helps keep your heart beating and your brain cells firing. While many other protein foods, such as beef and pork, can be high in fat, chicken and turkey shine because they're easily slimmed down by removing the skin, either before or after cooking. Three ounces of grilled or roasted skinless chicken breast (a serving about the size of a deck of cards) gives you 53 percent of the Daily Value (DV) for protein and just three grams of fat, which is a low 3.5 fat and 19.2 percent calories from fat. It also supplies generous amounts of niacin, vitamin B_6, and iron.

Best and Worst Chicken and Turkey Selections

Unadorned, chicken and turkey are low in fat and calories. But how we order or prepare the two—fried, barbecued, roasted, or souped up in dozens of ways—can drastically alter them (for better or worse). Here's a look at how some popular entrées measure up in calorie and fat content. (A healthy poultry entrée should contain no more than 500 calories and 15 grams of fat or less.) The portions listed are typical servings for each dish.

Best Choices

Entrée	Portion	Calories	Grams of Fat
Sliced, skinless roasted turkey	3 oz.	133	2.7
Barbecued, skinless chicken breast	3 oz., with 2 Tbsp. barbecue sauce	167	3.7
Grilled chicken kabobs	2 skewers	170	4.0
Lemon turkey cutlet	1 cutlet, sautéed with lemon and herbs	186	5.3
Oven-fried, skinless chicken	1 leg and thigh, with buttermilk and bread crumb coating	229	8.8
Grilled, skinless chicken breast	½ breast (3 oz.), with rosemary and black olives	245	8.0
Chicken fajitas	2 fajitas with grilled chicken and peppers	318	5.0

Worst Choices

Entrée	Portion	Calories	Grams of Fat
General Tso's chicken, breaded and deep-fried	2 cups (with 1 cup steamed rice)	730	24.0
Fried chicken (fast-food)	3 pieces (2 drumsticks and 1 thigh)	624	36.9
Buffalo wings (fast-food)	10 wings	583	40.0
Chicken nuggets (fast-food)	12 pieces	573	34.6

Make It *Better*

Oven-Fried Chicken

MAKES 4 SERVINGS

Per serving

229 calories

8.8 grams of fat

(36 percent of

calories from fat)

The simple step of switching to "oven frying" makes this all-American favorite healthier. This version has 5.4 fewer grams of fat than the equivalent serving of a fried chicken thigh. To trim calories and fat from your other favorite chicken recipes, remove the skin and use egg whites instead of melted butter to make coatings stick.

½	cup buttermilk	½	teaspoon dried thyme
1	cup fresh bread crumbs	½	teaspoon onion powder
1	teaspoon paprika	4	pieces skinless chicken legs and thighs
1	teaspoon ground black pepper		

Preheat the oven to 425°F. Coat a wire rack with nonstick spray. Place the rack on a foil-lined baking sheet.

Pour the buttermilk in a shallow pan. Put the bread crumbs in another shallow pan. Combine the paprika, pepper, thyme, and onion powder in a bowl. Season the bread crumbs with 1 teaspoon of the spice mixture. Add the remaining spices to the buttermilk.

Coat the chicken with the buttermilk. Roll the chicken pieces in the seasoned bread crumbs.

Place the chicken on the prepared rack. Coat the chicken with nonstick spray.

Bake for 15 minutes. Turn the chicken, coat it again with nonstick spray, and bake for 15 minutes more, or until golden brown.

Shopping Smarts

Years ago, buying and cooking poultry was simple: You bought a whole bird, then either roasted it or cut it up for other dishes. Today, you can buy chicken part by part, with or without skin, with or without bones, raw or precooked. Here's a look at how to make the best of what's available.

Boneless, skinless chicken breasts and thighs. Cut boneless breast meat into strips, then keep a package or two in your freezer. It will come in handy for stir-fries, fajitas, and chow mein. Both breasts and thighs are good in most sauté recipes because they add very little (if any) fat to whatever sauce you have in the pan.

Chicken breasts, legs, or thighs on the bone, with skin. These pieces are great for marinating and grilling because they hold in flavor and moisture. If you're going to baste the meat with a sauce such as barbecue sauce, remove the skin first to allow the sauce to cook in and flavor the meat more fully. Otherwise, remove it before eating.

Skinless chicken breasts or thighs on the bone. This type of chicken is best for oven frying or skillet dishes.

Whole chicken. Roasting chickens are meant for roasting, not frying or grilling. The whole bird generally has more fat than individual pieces without skin, so roast it on a rack to allow the fat to run off, and remove the skin before serving.

Chicken lunchmeat. All chicken lunchmeat isn't created equal, with some brands packing in as much fatty filler as bologna. Select lunchmeat with two grams of fat or less per ounce. And if you're cutting back on sodium for any reason, bear in mind that most lunchmeats—even the healthiest choices—are high in sodium.

Turkey breast. Choose the real thing, not the processed version. (Processed turkey is a combination of pressed white and dark meat, and it's loaded with salt.) Roast it covered to lock in the moisture, and enjoy the leftovers on salads and in sandwiches.

Turkey cutlets. Great lean sources of protein, these are perfect for grilling, sautéing, and baking. Cutlets cook quickly and need some moisture, so marinate them, then baste with your favorite nonfat sauce—such as barbecue, teriyaki, or sweet-and-sour—throughout cooking.

Ground turkey. Beware: Regular ground turkey is no leaner than most ground beef, so reach for the extra-lean version. Three ounces of regular ground turkey has more than 11 grams of fat, while the same amount of extra-lean light meat ground turkey has just 2.6 grams.

Turkey sausage, lunchmeat, and hot dogs. Choose carefully. Consumers assume that these items are low in fat, but many are not. Read the label to be certain that you're getting a lower-fat version, with less than two grams of fat per ounce.

Lean Menu-Makers

Nearly every cuisine, from Italian to Chinese, uses poultry in some form. It's the most versatile meat around, simple to prepare in dozens of tasty ways. But don't let added ingredients and side dishes wipe out the healthful, low-fat benefits that chicken and turkey have to offer. Here are some of the best accompaniments for common cuts of poultry.

Boneless, skinless chicken breasts or turkey cutlets

- Pasta (rotini, ziti, linguini, penne, gemelli)
- Grilled or steamed Italian vegetables (green peppers, mushrooms, eggplant, zucchini, scallions, Italian green beans)
- Rice pilaf (brown, basmati)
- Oriental vegetables (snow peas, red peppers, water chestnuts, bean sprouts, bok choy)

Chicken or turkey breasts, legs, and thighs on the bone, with skin

- Grilled onions and portobello mushrooms
- Steamed broccoli and cauliflower
- Steamed asparagus tips with lemon juice
- Glazed baby carrots or carrot coins
- Baked sweet potatoes
- Grilled pineapple slices

Whole bird

For roasted chicken:
- Boiled new potatoes
- Carrots and parsnips
- Peas and pearl onions

For roasted turkey:
- Steamed broccoli and carrots
- Baked acorn, Hubbard, or butternut squash
- Corn on the cob

Weight-Friendly Substitutions

Chicken and turkey are interchangeable in many recipes, and either one can stand in for other meats. Here are some suggestions.

- Enjoy extra-lean ground turkey as patties, in chili, and in any recipe as a substitute for ground beef.
- Grill chicken burgers instead of hamburgers.
- Cook ground turkey or chicken with taco seasoning for a low-fat taco filling.

New Foods to Try

If chicken and turkey dominate your menus, add variety by trying Rock Cornish game hens, pheasant, and quail. Game hens are available at many supermarkets, and you can ask a butcher to order pheasant or quail. Although they cost more, these low-fat, high-nutrition birds are a unique taste sensation. Three skinless ounces of each (about the size of your palm) has a skimpy 3.3 grams of fat and about 20 grams of protein. And there's no need to seek out exotic recipes for these birds: Game hens, pheasant, and quail can be roasted just as you would a chicken or turkey. Or, for a low-fat, high-flavor treat, try pheasant cacciatore, prepared with mushrooms, onions, and tomatoes and seasoned with Italian herbs such as garlic, basil, and oregano.

Two other members of the poultry family—duck and goose—are high in fat. Save them for special occasions.

Dining Out

When you're eating out, it often seems that the chef does everything possible to add fat to a dish. If you want chicken, ignore the menu and ask what's available in a boneless, skinless breast. If the item comes with a sauce, ask to have it served on the side.

If you order a grilled chicken breast sandwich, remember to ask for an unbuttered bun. (Did you ever wonder why the restaurant version is so moist?)

Salads with grilled chicken breast are a popular choice at many restaurants, but keep in mind that most salad dressings (especially Caesar) are loaded with fat. Substitute a reduced-fat dressing or order the dressing on the side. You can enjoy small amounts of regular dressing by dipping your fork in the dressing and then gathering a bite of salad.

Condiments and Spreads

A stroll through the aisle of any supermarket shows that we're a nation of condiment-lovers. Plain old ketchup, mustard, and mayonnaise are just a start. The condiment aisle is a kaleidoscope of flavors and textures: marinades, sauces, spreads, relishes, sauces, dips, salsas, mustards, and more. Travel around, and you might even stumble across separate stores devoted entirely to hot pepper sauces!

By definition, a condiment is "a savory, piquant, spicy, or salty accompaniment to food." Condiments and spreads concentrate flavor—and sometimes considerable fat and calories, if you're not careful.

If you're like a lot of women, you probably rely on condiments for breakfast, lunch, dinner, and parties. You might use them to perk up scrambled eggs. Moisten your morning toast or bagel. Give a turkey sandwich oomph and character. Embellish a baked potato. Top off nachos. By day's end, you can accumulate a fair amount of fat and calories from condiments and spreads alone. Chosen wisely, however, condiments can add excitement and flavor for very little fat and few calories. Here's how.

Shopping Smarts

If you've been trying to lose weight, you probably switched to fat-free or reduced-fat mayonnaise and "diet" margarine years ago. And you probably already read food labels closely for fat and calorie counts. Here are a few category-specific tips to help make the most of the zillion choices in the condiments and spreads aisle.

Fat-free or reduced-fat mayonnaises. Good start: Per tablespoon, low-fat (or light) brands contain 50 fewer calories and 6 fewer grams of fat than regular mayonnaise, and fat-free varieties run about 90 fewer calories and 11 fewer grams of fat than regular. For a flavor boost, stir in some minced garlic or onion from the spice rack.

Butters, margarines, and margarine-like spreads. Butter and full-fat margarines are about as concentrated in fat and calories as a product can get. Just one tablespoon of either contains about 12 fat grams and 108 calories. As a table spread, "calorie-reduced" or "light" tub margarine-like spread is your best bet, saving you 8.5 grams of fat and 73 calories per tablespoon over butter and full-fat margarine. Try different brands to find the flavor and texture that appeals most to you. Don't use reduced-fat spreads and margarines for cooking, though—they're high in water, so they won't brown foods, and they can ruin baked goods.

Look for margarine or margarine-like spreads made with olive or canola oils. These products are higher in monounsaturated fats and are less likely to clog coronary arteries than other vegetable oils, which are higher in saturated fat, a factor associated with heart disease. Also, look for varieties that are free of trans fatty acids (by-products of the manufacturing process that make margarine solid at room temperature and affect your heart like saturated fats do).

Mustards. Go ahead—eat most mustards with wild abandon. Brown, yellow, smooth, coarse—most contain a scant 4 to 10 calories per teaspoon and virtually no fat. Be adventurous—try Dijon, Parisian, stone-ground varieties, and those with added herbs. For a sweet touch, try honey mustard, but be aware that one tablespoon has 30 calories, not 4 or 5. So spread thinly.

Tartar sauces, horseradishes, and relishes. Once you've switched to fish without butter, lean roast beef, and fat-free hot dogs, you don't want to cancel out your calorie-saving efforts by smothering them in high-fat condiments. You won't go wrong here—provided you look for low-fat tartar sauce and prepared horseradish, not the cream sauce variety. No luck? Just mix some pickle relish or prepared horseradish with a tablespoon or two of fat-free mayo.

Jams, jellies, and marmalades. Standard fare in most households, fruit spreads are pure sugar—but not off-limits. Substituting one teaspoon of jam or marmalade for one teaspoon of butter or margarine on breads, bagels, and English muffins cuts calories from your spread by more than half—from 36 to 16. The key is to buy the best strawberry preserves, orange marmalade, raspberry jam—whatever is your favorite—and then enjoy just a little. Or try fruit butter for a lower-calorie, less sugary alternative.

Best and Worst Condiments and Spreads

As a general rule, try to limit the calories from condiments at any one meal to 50 calories or fewer. Be especially careful with jams and jellies (which weigh in at 40 to 50 calories or more per tablespoon) and peanut butter (at about 90 calories per tablespoon). If you use just a smidgen—no more than a couple of teaspoons of these spreads—you can enjoy toast, bagels, and crackers without going overboard on fat and calories.

Best Choices			
Condiment	Portion	Calories	Grams of Fat
Tabasco (hot pepper) sauce	1 tsp.	1	0.0
Fresh lemon juice	1 Tbsp.	4	0.0
Thick and chunky salsa	1 Tbsp.	5	0.0
Prepared horseradish	1 Tbsp.	6	0.0
Fat-free mayonnaise	1 Tbsp.	10	0.0
Sugar-free jam	1 Tbsp.	10	0.0
Yellow mustard	1 Tbsp.	12	0.0
Apple butter	1 Tbsp.	15	0.0
Bean spread	1 Tbsp.	15	0.0
Cocktail sauce	1 Tbsp.	15	0.0
Ketchup	1 Tbsp.	16	0.0
Sweet pickle relish	1 Tbsp.	20	0.0
"Light" tub margarine-like spread	1 Tbsp.	35	3.5

Worst Choices			
Condiment	Portion	Calories	Grams of Fat
Butter	1 Tbsp.	108	12.2
Margarine	1 Tbsp.	101	11.4
Full-fat mayonnaise	1 Tbsp.	100	11.0
Honey mustard dressing	1 Tbsp.	80	7.5
Horseradish sauce	1 Tbsp.	60	4.5
Sandwich spread	1 Tbsp.	55	5.2
Tartar sauce	1 Tbsp.	50	5.0

Bottled sauces. From good old Texas-style barbecue sauce to Oriental duck sauce, you'll find a virtual United Nations of flavor enhancers available for meat, chicken, and fish: steak sauce, teriyaki, miso (a soy product), hoisin, Szechuan—plus the standard soy sauce and ketchup. Calorically speaking, they're all pretty low—four to eight calories per teaspoon—and they ring up a scant portion of a fat gram (compare that to Mornay sauce, at triple the calories and at least two grams of fat per teaspoon). Slathered on lean beef, pork, or poultry, these sauces will serve your weight-loss effort well, since they tenderize meat as they break down animal protein.

Salsas. The Mexican word for "sauce," salsas are cooked or fresh mixtures of tomatoes, sweet peppers, hot peppers, and onions. Traditionally, there were just two salsa staples: "salsa cruda," which was uncooked tomato-based salsa, and "salsa verde," or green salsa made from raw tomatillos, green chili peppers, and cilantro. Today, the selection is wider, with varieties that are chunky or spicy, or that use all kinds of vegetables or even fruit.

When you think of salsa, think beyond a topping for chips: Spoon salsa on baked potatoes instead of sour cream, spread it on steamed broccoli and cauliflower, drop it by the spoonful on grilled chicken, fish, and veggie burgers.

Most salsas are fat-free, but double-check the label, and bypass any laced with cheese or oil.

Lean Menu-Makers

If you're like most women, meals at your house probably center around chicken, pasta, potatoes, cooked vegetables, and other basics. And you're probably short on time to prepare elaborate meals. The right condiments, sauces, and embellishments can serve as quick, low-maintenance ways to garnish mealtime standards without the fat and calories that come with elaborate sauces.

Mix up these flavor-boosting condiments and spreads, then serve them on chicken, fish, and veggies, and be bored no longer.

- Pasta sauce with peppers, mushrooms, and garlic
- Salsa with frozen chopped broccoli (proportions to taste)
- Two tablespoons of mustard mixed with one tablespoon of balsamic vinegar
- Two tablespoons of orange or apricot marmalade mixed with one tablespoon of soy sauce
- One teaspoon peanut butter, one tablespoon soy sauce, and one teaspoon each minced garlic and fresh ginger
- Fat-free mayonnaise and freshly chopped rosemary (one tablespoon each), and one clove garlic, minced
- Guiltless guacamole (two tablespoons mashed avocado; two tablespoons mashed frozen peas, defrosted; one tablespoon lemon juice; and minced garlic, salt, and pepper to taste)
- Roasted red peppers (half of a 7.5 milliliter jar, packed in water) pureed with two tablespoons fat-free cream cheese and two tablespoons freshly chopped basil
- Two tablespoons nonfat sour cream, one tablespoon lime juice, one tablespoon chopped fresh cilantro, and cayenne pepper to taste
- One fresh papaya, chopped; ¼ cup finely minced red bell pepper; ¼ cup finely minced green bell pepper; one teaspoon extra virgin olive oil; and black pepper to taste
- ¼ cup each of vanilla, lemon, and peach nonfat yogurt, combined (excellent on fish, chicken, and turkey burgers)

New Foods to Try

Consumers try ethnic dishes when they travel. Food companies experiment with new varieties of condiments to suit your taste. Growers respond by cultivating foods that are new to the American diet but are widespread and healthful options in other lands. As a result, you have more ways than ever to eat lean without ever getting bored or feeling that you're on a restricted diet. Consider these condiment concepts in your shape-up efforts.

Margarine-like sprays. For most of these sprays, the main ingredient is soybean oil. These brilliant inventions tally no calories or fat for the spritz necessary to coat toast, an English muffin, air-popped popcorn, or steamed veggies.

Creamy mustard blends. There's something about mayo's creamy/tangy/pungent consistency that merits it a high rating among comfort foods. A cross between mustard and mayonnaise, mustard-mayo blends give mayonnaise-lovers lots of the creamy taste, with just five calories and zero grams of fat per teaspoon (enough for a sandwich).

Soy butters. Made from roasted soybeans, reduced-fat soy butter has about one-third the fat of peanut butter. When it's paired with their favorite jam, jelly, or fruit butter, even your kids will eat it.

Ethnic sauces. To lend an ethnic flair to your family's standard meat-and-rice dishes, try a Thai or Jamaican sauce. These are usually found on the grocery shelf next to the soy sauce. You might be pleasantly surprised.

Fruit salsas. These salsas make gentler, uncommon, and delightful accompaniments for chicken, fish, and all sorts of ordinary and not so ordinary vegetables. Start with mango salsa and grilled chicken—there will be no going back.

Bean spreads and hummus. Shop around for bean-salsa dips or hummus (a savory combination of chickpeas and sesame butter). When spread on fat-free chips, low-fat crackers, or toasted pita bread, these savory spreads are a valuable alternative to cheese spreads—a big plus if you're entertaining vegetarian friends (or avoiding dairy yourself). For the best bet, read labels.

Flavored cream cheeses. For an alternative to ordinary cream cheese for bagels or crackers, try fat-free or light cream cheeses flavored with herbs or fruits. Fat-free strawberry cream cheese, for example, adds a new dimension to your Sunday morning bagel over the nonflavored varieties. Or try garden vegetable or roasted garlic to liven up a lunch bagel. You can also create your own version with veggies and your favorite herbs, or with finely diced fruit. Another bonus to adding fruits or veggies to make your own version: Less cream cheese goes farther, so you can use the real thing if you so desire.

Dining Out

More and more family restaurants are offering fat-free or reduced-fat condiments, giving hope to anyone who wants to avoid full-fat garnishments. Patrons might also ask for a squeeze of lemon instead of butter- or cream-based condiments. This is a standard tactic—use it, with no apologies.

If you can't avoid full-fat condiments from the menu, you can minimize the damage while maximizing flavor: When a menu item comes with any kind of spread or other condiment, always ask for it on the side. This gives you more control over a potentially high source of unwanted calories. Instead of spooning or pouring a condiment or sauce over your food, dip your fork tines in the condiment and then gather a bite. This tactic works well for creamy horseradish, Mornay, Hollandaise, tartar, and other butter- or cream-based sauces.

Oriental sauces, on the other hand, are usually scant on calories, so they can be used fairly liberally—most have less than five calories per teaspoon.

Deli Food

Whether it's on a neighborhood corner or in a supermarket, the deli is a convenient place to get meals in a flash. In fact, supermarket delis are in heavy competition with fast-food restaurants for your dinner dollars. Be aware, though, that you can end up with a plateful of calories with that garlic dill pickle: The typical deli sandwich has four to five ounces of meat and stands six inches tall. Add a hefty scoop of coleslaw or potato salad, and you might as well have a giant hamburger.

It doesn't have to be that way. If the choices are vast—with lots of pasta and vegetable salads and reduced-fat meats—making wise selections is easy. Most of the time, however, you'll need smart-substitution skills to figure out the best choices.

Shopping Smarts

Keep your wits about you and don't be afraid to ask questions. Here are some important things to keep in mind.

Meats. Despite their reputation, lunchmeats today are leaner than ever. So a deli sandwich isn't necessarily a bad choice. The lowest-fat lunchmeats are turkey breast, chicken breast, roast beef, turkey pastrami, and—yes!—ham, whether plain or honey-glazed.

You can't go wrong if you choose deli meats with no more than 2 grams of fat in an ounce. Ask for nutrition information if it's not out on the counter; delis must have it available. If nothing else, they can let you read the label on the big piece of meat. (Keep in mind that one ounce is the equivalent of about 30 grams. If the serving size is 57 grams and the total fat is 4 grams, you're right on the money.)

Remember healthy portion sizes. That pound of lean turkey breast you buy should make at least four sandwiches (four ounces of meat apiece). Even then, you've eaten more than half of the recommended six ounces of meat, poultry, and fish per day.

When buying rotisserie chicken or turkey breast, remove the skin. Almost all of the fat is located there.

Sandwiches. Deli sandwiches offer mountains of meat. To save calories, consider setting half the meat aside for tomorrow's sandwich. Or order half a sandwich.

Be skeptical when choosing an all-vegetable sandwich. Make sure those vegetables aren't bathed in oil and smothered with high-fat cheese, mayonnaise, avocado slices, guacamole, or a bunch of olives. Veggie sandwiches should be overflowing with fresh tomatoes, green bell peppers, sprouts, and onions.

Finally, be savvy about the bread. Croissants make delectable sandwiches, but those flaky rolls are ridiculously high in fat and calories. Choose hoagie rolls, sub buns, kaiser rolls, bagels, pita pockets, and bakery breads—preferably fiber-rich ones like whole-wheat or other whole-grain varieties.

Salads. Picking salads in the deli department is a real challenge. Chicken salad, egg salad, tuna salad, shrimp salad—their common bond is a ton of mayonnaise. You're better off with lean lunchmeat as sandwich filler. As for side salads, look for ones without a creamy dressing (for instance, choose pickled cabbage instead of creamy coleslaw and three-bean salad rather than macaroni salad).

Lean Menu-Makers

Since the produce department is usually just steps away from the deli in supermarkets, you can easily buy vegetables and fruit to round out your deli choices.

- Bagged salads are convenient complements to sandwiches and rotisserie chicken. Select those without dressing and grab a bottle of low-fat or fat-free dressing while you're in the store.

- Bagged baby carrots and broccoli and cauliflower florets are good raw or steamed. They're

Best and Worst Deli Food

The first rule for that dash to the deli: Aim for plain. Choose unadorned meats, sandwiches, and salads as opposed to foods drowning in fat, like chicken salad, creamy side salads, and sandwiches slathered with sauces and mayonnaise. The best lunchmeats are those with no more than two grams of fat per one-ounce slice. So, a three-ounce serving of lunchmeat on a sandwich should have about six grams of fat. Choose reduced-fat cheeses—those with no more than seven grams of fat in a one-ounce slice. Salads with minimal oil, like three-bean salad and German potato salad, are better choices.

Best Choices

Deli Item	Portion	Calories	Grams of Fat
Three-bean salad	½ cup	78	2.4
Reduced-fat cheese	1 oz.	90	7.0
Sliced turkey	3 oz.	92	1.3
Sliced ham	3 oz.	93	3.0
Sliced roast beef	3 oz.	94	2.5
Sliced turkey pastrami	3 oz.	120	5.3
Rotisserie chicken breast (without skin)	½ breast	142	3.1
German potato salad	1 cup	167	2.2

Worst Choices

Deli Item	Portion	Calories	Grams of Fat
Fried chicken	¼ chicken	673	40.4
Reuben sandwich	1 sandwich	497	30.0
Crabmeat salad	1 cup	450	22.0
Ham on rye sandwich with extra meat (more than 6 oz.)	1 sandwich	346	7.0
Chicken salad	1 cup	333	25.0
Potato salad	1 cup	325	17.2
Pastrami	3 oz.	297	24.9
Ham salad	1 cup	286	22.0
Macaroni salad	1 cup	225	10.0
Salami	3 oz.	223	18.0
Corned beef	3 oz.	213	16.1
Egg salad	½ cup	209	16.0
Creamy coleslaw	1 cup	195	14.6

an easy way to add nutrient-rich vegetables to a deli meal.

- Broccoli coleslaw is a nice change from regular coleslaw. Buy bags of broccoli slaw and add low-fat coleslaw dressing.
- Buy an apple, orange, or banana to round out your meal with no fat.

Weight-Friendly Substitutions

Always ask for lower-fat mayonnaise on sandwiches. You'll save at least half the calories. If it's not available, request naturally fat-free condiments like ketchup and mustard. (Flavored mustards such as honey and peppercorn are especially good.)

Look for baked potato chips instead of regular. They're much lower in fat. So are baked tortilla chips. And pretzels are generally fat-free.

A pickle may be all you need to satisfy that urge for a crunchy, salty snack to go with your deli sandwich. Delis usually have the best kosher dill pickles. Pickles are nothing but seasoned cucumbers, so they're completely fat-free and very low in calories.

Got a yen for pastrami? If it's well-trimmed, go for it. Otherwise, opt for pastrami made from turkey breast; it averages 3.5 grams of fat in two ounces.

Choose cheese wisely. If you're adding cheese to three ounces of meat on a sandwich, that's a protein overload—and probably a fat excess, too. Either skip the cheese altogether or reduce the meat to two ounces and go with one ounce of cheese. Naturally, low-fat cheese is preferable to regular. As for cream cheese spreads, see if a light version is available.

When it comes to potato salad, German is often lower in fat than American and mustard types. See if nutrition information is available or if someone can tell you how the salad was prepared.

New Foods to Try

New lunchmeats like lean roast pork are packed with protein and B vitamins and are a nice alternative to turkey breast.

Hummus spreads are moderate to low in fat. They pack protein and various helpful nutrients from the chickpeas. There are lots of flavors to pick from, too. Spread them on bread, crackers, or a pita for a change of pace from a deli sandwich.

Other meal solutions in the supermarket deli area can include stir-fry dishes and cold and hot pasta salads. Some supermarkets even have carry-out cafés that feature grilled sandwiches with unique vegetables like specialty mushrooms and roasted red peppers.

Dining Out

Remember to speak up if you'd like to make substitutions. Ask questions if you want to know how a sandwich or salad is prepared. (For instance, do they make their signature tuna salad with low-fat mayonnaise? Maybe if enough people ask, they will!)

If the meat is piled on Dagwood-style, save half the sandwich for tomorrow.

Reubens—a combination of grilled rye bread, Swiss cheese, sauerkraut, and tons of corned beef, often slathered with Thousand Island dressing—are loaded with fat. Nutritionally speaking, the best part of a Reuben is the sauerkraut. Made from cabbage, it's rich in health-building nutrients. Ask the deli server to go easy on the dressing, meat, and cheese, and to pile on extra kraut.

Desserts

Experts say that for long-term weight control, you don't need to even try to swear off dessert. You'll only feel deprived and go whole-hog when you do give in.

Chosen wisely, dessert can contribute nutrients that you need. Pudding made from a mix with low-fat or fat-free milk contributes calcium, for example.

The keys: Make dessert calories count. Keep an eye on fat and sugar. And rein in the portions.

Be aware that "low-fat" and "fat-free" aren't a license for second helpings. Eating twice as much can easily negate the benefit of choosing a low-fat version. Also, many reduced-fat treats more than make up for the calories from fat with added sugar. The fat-free versions may have more calories than the regular versions.

Shopping Smarts

To prepare low-calorie, low-fat desserts from scratch, stock the following staples. If time is short, buy convenience products. For products that promise to be low-fat or fat-free, check the Nutrition Facts on the back of the package, and compare the calorie and fat content to regular products. They may not necessarily have fewer calories.

Pantry staples. If you like to bake (or your family expects it), keep the following items on hand.

- Whole-wheat flour, oatmeal, and other whole grains, such as barley flour (to boost the fiber content in baked goods).
- Low-fat or fat-free dairy products for baked dishes. (You can substitute fat-free evaporated milk and buttermilk for cream.)
- Naturally sweetened fruit spreads, applesauce, and prune butter (to replace part of the fat in baked goods).
- Sugar substitutes. (Read the tips for use on the package. Those with aspartame aren't appropriate for cooked or baked desserts.)
- Vegetable oil spray (to coat baking pans).

Mixes. For quick homemade desserts, look for mixes with less fat or sugar (or, ideally, less of both): low-fat and sugar-free pudding mix, low-fat cake mix, low-fat brownie mix, low-fat cheesecake mix, angel food cake mix, and sugar-free gelatin, to name just a few.

Frozen desserts. Try lower-fat and fat-free varieties of ice cream as well as frozen yogurt, ices, and sorbets, all of which are available in a variety of tempting flavors.

Packaged treats. Tuck the following products into your shopping cart.

- Vanilla wafers, gingersnaps, or graham crackers. Enjoy as is or use for crumb crusts.
- Low-fat crumb crusts. Fill with low-fat pudding.
- Angel food cake from the bakery department. Just slice and spread fruit or frozen yogurt in between the layers.
- Low-fat, sugar-free cookies. Read the label to see if they're really low-calorie.

Lean Menu-Makers

The following are simple versions of traditional, more elaborate desserts. They capture the essence of the dessert with less fat and sugar than the original.

Apple pie

- Baked apple (a cored apple stuffed with an oatmeal and brown sugar mixture)
- Apple flan (sliced apples topped with orange juice concentrate and slivered almonds and baked just until tender)
- Crisp apple and cheese slices (freshly sliced apples and reduced-fat Cheddar cheese)

Hot fudge sundae

- Chocolate yogurt sundae (frozen chocolate yogurt topped with crushed gingersnaps)
- Chocolate smoothie (low-fat chocolate milk, chocolate or vanilla frozen low-fat yogurt, and a banana processed until thick and smooth)

Weight-Friendly Substitutions

To make your desserts more weight-friendly, try cutting back on high-fat and sugary ingredients. Be aware, though: In many desserts, espe- cially baked desserts, substitutions affect the tex- ture, volume, and flavor of the end result. Experi- ment a bit to get results that satisfy you. You may like your new version even better!

Best and Worst Desserts

Technically, no dessert is off limits. You can have any dessert you like—provided you don't eat the whole thing, eat it every day, or have it several times a day. Also consider your food choices for the rest of the day. That said, if dessert is a fre- quent guest on your menu, these guidelines will help steer you toward choices that have less fat and fewer calories, es- pecially when eaten in moderation. Select prepared desserts or choose recipes that have 25 percent fewer calories per serving than the traditional versions. If you can find desserts that are also low-fat, that's even better.

Best Choices

Dessert	Portion	Calories	Grams of Fat
Poached fruit topped with toasted oatmeal	1 peach and 2 Tbsp. oatmeal	55	0.0
Fat-free pudding (prepared from a dry mix with fat-free milk)	½ cup	70	0.0
Meringue cookies	4 cookies (about ¾ oz. total)	73	0.0
Sorbet	½ cup	80	0.0
Angel food cake with fresh fruit	1 slice (¹⁄₁₂ of cake)	85	0.0
Biscotti	1 cookie (about ¾ oz.)	100	3.0
Low-fat frozen yogurt	½ cup	110	2.5
Gingersnaps	4 cookies (about 1 oz. total)	120	2.5
Strawberries with low-fat frozen yogurt	¼ cup sliced berries with ½ cup frozen yogurt	122	2.5

Worst Choices

Dessert	Portion	Calories	Grams of Fat
Cheesecake	1 slice (¹⁄₁₂ of 9-inch cake)	457	33.3
Pie	1 slice (⅛ of 9-inch pie)	411	19.0
Hot fudge sundae	2 scoops	406	24.6
Tiramisu	4 oz.	390	23.0
Crème brûlée	4 oz.	362	27.2
Cobbler	4 oz.	360	18.4
Chocolate chip cookies	4 cookies	312	18.0
Premium ice cream	½ cup	270	18.0
Frosted cake	1 slice (⅛ of 18-oz. cake)	243	11.1
Fudge brownie	1 brownie (2-inch square)	112	6.9

For baked desserts

- Replace up to half of the fat with an equal amount of fruit puree, such as mashed banana, applesauce, or prune butter. It imparts a naturally sweet taste, too, and adds to the moist texture. You can expect especially good results in bar and drop cookies.

- Experiment with vanilla yogurt in place of butter or margarine in muffins and quick breads. Use reduced-fat cream cheese in cheesecake.

- Instead of buttery cakes, prepare angel food cake, which is made with egg whites and no fat.

- Use fresh fruit or fruit canned in juices, rather than syrup, in fruit crisps and cobblers.

For toppings

- Instead of frosting, top cakes with fresh sliced fruit, a spoonful of lemon yogurt, or your favorite flavor of frozen yogurt.

- For a thick sauce, puree fruit with a little juice to the consistency you want. Try different types of fruits (mango, kiwifruit, blackberry, or apricots) or a mixture. If you wish, thin the sauce with a splash of white wine.

- Dust cakes with confectioners' sugar mixed with instant coffee, spices, or cocoa.

For crusts

- Prepare desserts with a single, not a double, crust. Or use a low-fat, prepared crumb crust.

- For a crumb crust instead of a pastry crust, coat the pan with vegetable oil spray, then dust it with graham cracker crumbs.

- Top fruit crisp or pie with uncooked oatmeal instead of a pastry crust.

For custard or pudding desserts

- Prepare effortless puddings with a fat-free or low-fat mix. Layer them with fruit for creamy parfaits, or pour them into a low-calorie crust.

- Prepare custard or rice pudding with low-fat milk, and egg whites or egg substitutes. Flavor with cinnamon and cranberries. Serve topped with freshly sliced fruit.

For any desserts

- Enhance the flavor with fresh ginger, grated citrus rind, mint, and spices, and cut back on sugar, honey, and other sweeteners.

- Substitute low-fat and nonfat plain yogurt—cup for cup—in recipes that call for sour cream. (In fact, using the low-fat version of any dairy product helps cut calories.)

- For cakes and other baked chocolate desserts, replace melted chocolate with cocoa powder. Shave a little chocolate on top for flavor but few calories.

New Foods to Try

Dessert-lovers are notorious for trying new recipes. As you browse through your favorite cooking magazines, try recipes for:

- Meringue shells flavored with cocoa powder. Fill with vanilla low-fat yogurt and fresh fruit.

- Soufflés made with egg whites and fat-free milk.

- Poached fruits flavored with interesting spice blends.

As a ready-to-eat frozen dessert option, look for fruit juice bars, including sugar-free varieties, frozen yogurt bars, and fruit sorbet, a frozen fruit ice. Sorbet, similar to granita, is easy to make, too.

Dining Out

If you love to dine out and you love dessert, you may fare better at fine restaurants than fast-food places or diners and family-style restaurants, where choices typically come with heavy whipped toppings, syrupy fruit fillings, and thick frostings.

Try these strategies for a sweet ending to your meal out.

- Ask for fresh fruit. If it's not on the dessert menu, check the appetizer menu or ask the server.

- Check the dessert menu for other lower-fat fruit desserts, perhaps a poached pear topped with a fruit sauce and a crumble of strong-flavored cheese. A few plump berries dipped in chocolate

Make It *Better*

New York Cheesecake

MAKES 12 SERVINGS

Per serving

121 calories

5.2 grams of fat

(37 percent of

calories from fat)

A cheesecake that's low in fat? You bet! Light cream cheese, low-fat ricotta cheese, and a fat-sparse cookie crust reduce the fat without reducing a forkful of flavor. (If you don't have amaretti crumbs, substitute graham crackers.) To make over your favorite cheesecake recipe, substitute light, reduced-fat, or fat-free cream cheese for full-fat cream cheese, fold in stiffly beaten egg whites to add volume, use a dusting of crumbs on the bottom of the pan as a crust, and top with fruit instead of a syrup fruit topping.

8 ounces light cream cheese	¼ cup golden raisins
1 cup low-fat ricotta cheese	3 tablespoons cornstarch
2 eggs, separated	1 tablespoon grated orange rind
¼ cup honey	⅓ cup amaretti cookie crumbs

Preheat the oven to 400°F. In a large bowl, combine the cream cheese and ricotta until smooth. Stir in the egg yolks, honey, raisins, cornstarch, and orange rind, mixing until thoroughly combined.

In a medium bowl, whip the egg whites with clean beaters for about 2 minutes, or until they form stiff peaks. Fold the whites into the cheese mixture.

Coat a 9" pie plate with nonstick spray and cover with the amaretti crumbs. Pour the cheese mixture into the pie plate. Bake for 30 minutes, or until golden and set.

---

may be just enough to satisfy a chocolate craving.

- Ask for sorbet (which has less fat, but is not necessarily low in calories) as a light, refreshing dessert—or a small, plain scoop of your favorite ice cream.

- Avoid temptation. A sneak peek at the dessert tray makes it hard to resist. If you don't look, you're less likely to order.

- If you can't resist crème brûlée or tiramisu, order one dessert—with spoons for everyone at the table.

- For a little sweetness without too many calories, order coffee with either a splash of liquor or a crunchy biscotti.

Eggs and Egg Dishes

Sitting unadorned in your refrigerator door, a large egg contains about 5 grams of fat and 75 calories, including just 1½ grams of saturated fats. Further, it offers a decent amount of protein—about 6 grams—plus riboflavin and other B vitamins, vitamin A, iron, and other minerals. So it's a high-quality source of protein for vegetarians. In addition, eggs are quick to fix when time is short, economical when you're on a tight budget, and flexible enough to combine with what you have in the fridge.

So far, so good. The problem, as many women know, is not fat or calories, but cholesterol—a fatlike substance produced by the liver. All animals—including chickens—manufacture cholesterol. Your body does, too. Although cholesterol has no calories, a high intake of dietary cholesterol is linked to high levels of blood, or serum, cholesterol. Experts have found that too much cholesterol in your bloodstream is associated with heart disease. They advise limiting in-

Best and Worst Egg Selections

Eggs are a good source of protein and average about 75 calories and 5 grams of fat apiece—without added or accompanying fat. If you're watching your cholesterol intake as well as your figure, consider that a whole egg supplies 213 milligrams of cholesterol. Experts advise consuming no more than four eggs or egg yolks a week. Keep in mind that many egg dishes can be made with low-fat or cholesterol-free ingredients.

Best Choices

Egg	Portion	Calories	Grams of Fat
Scrambled egg substitute	equivalent to 1 egg	35	0.0
Poached egg (yolk well-cooked)	1 egg	75	5.0
Hard-cooked egg	1 egg	78	5.3
Egg salad made with fat-free mayonnaise	½ cup	98	5.3
Vegetable omelette made with egg substitute	substitute equivalent to 2 eggs	125	4.0

Worst Choices

Egg	Portion	Calories	Grams of Fat
Eggs Benedict	1 serving (2 eggs)	452	31.0
Cheese omelette made with full-fat cheese	1 serving (2 eggs)	356	32.6
Egg salad made with regular mayonnaise	½ cup	190	16.3
Deviled egg	2 halves	145	12.0
Fried egg	1 egg	92	6.9
Hollandaise sauce	¼ cup	86	8.0

Make It *Better*

Basil and Mushroom Omelette

MAKES 1 SERVING

158 calories

6 grams of fat

(34 percent of

calories from fat)

Parmesan cheese and basil add a lot of flavor to this slimmed-down omelette. You could also make an omelette substituting egg whites for whole eggs and using other vegetables and herbs of your choice (such as broccoli and thyme).

1 **cup sliced mushrooms**	¼ **teaspoon ground black pepper**
¾ **cup fat-free egg substitute**	
	1 **teaspoon margarine**
1 **tablespoon water**	1 **tablespoon grated Parmesan cheese**
½ **teaspoon dried basil**	

Place the mushrooms in a 2-cup glass measure and cover with vented plastic wrap. Microwave on high for 2 minutes, or until the mushrooms are wilted. Drain off any liquid.

In a medium bowl, whisk together the egg substitute, water, basil, and pepper.

In a medium nonstick frying pan over medium heat, melt the margarine. Swirl the pan to coat the bottom. Add the egg mixture. As the eggs begin to set, pull the outer edges toward the center with a fork or spatula; allow uncooked portions to run underneath. Continue until the eggs are just barely set.

Sprinkle with the mushrooms and Parmesan. Fold the omelette in half. Transfer to a serving plate.

Note: If you don't have a microwave, cook the mushrooms in a little bit of fat-free broth until they soften and give up their natural juices. Then cook a few minutes longer to evaporate the liquid.

take of dietary cholesterol to 300 milligrams a day.

Eggs have more cholesterol than just about any food—213 milligrams in one large egg, all of it in the yolk. Experts recommend limiting your intake to four whole eggs or egg yolks a week from all kinds of food—omelettes, quiche, and so forth. Be aware that eggs are also used in baked goods and mayonnaise. (On the other hand, you can eat all of the egg whites you want—they have zero cholesterol.)

As you're rationing your egg yolks, you also want to keep a lid on high-fat, high-calorie ingredients added during the preparation of egg dishes. Butter or margarine, mayonnaise, cream, and cheese—all often found in egg dishes—can add significant amounts of fat and calories. And as it turns out, consuming a lot of saturated fat—the kind found primarily in butter and other foods of animal origin—not only contributes to your waistline but also may help to raise blood cholesterol levels. With careful planning, you can prepare eggs-traordinary meals while watching fat and calories.

Shopping Smarts

Basically, you have two choices when buying eggs—whole eggs or egg substitutes. Here's what to use and when.

Whole eggs. Whether the shells are white or brown makes no difference in nutrient or calorie content. Four jumbo eggs equal five large eggs or six small eggs. Obviously, jumbo eggs have more of everything—calories and nutrients—than smaller varieties. Most recipes are written using large eggs.

Egg substitutes. These are blends of egg whites, nonfat milk, cornstarch, and vegetable oil, plus some vitamins and minerals. They look like raw scrambled eggs, and they have no cholesterol and as little as 35 calories per quarter-cup. Check the Nutrition Facts panel for calorie and nutrient content since some have fat, but others don't.

You'll find egg substitutes in the frozen foods and refrigerated cases in your supermarket. You can use them to replace some or all of the whole eggs or egg yolks in your breakfast or in baked goods. Try several brands to find the ones you like, since the flavor and texture vary. Once the package is opened, keep it refrigerated, and use the substitute within three days.

Egg replacers. For totally vegetarian meals, health food stores often sell egg replacers, a mixture of potato starch, flour, and leavening, which can substitute for whole eggs or egg whites. Just be aware that, without egg whites for consistency, dishes made with egg-free products may lack the texture and flavor you expect from eggs.

Convenience foods prepared with eggs. Supermarket shelves are full of partly and fully prepared products made with eggs: frozen quiche and quiche mixes, pudding mixes, pudding cups, and custard pies, to name a few. These contribute protein and other nutrients you need. Check the Nutrition Facts label, and take cholesterol, fat, and calories into account when comparing these products.

Lean Menu-Makers

Whether you use whole eggs, a combo of whole eggs and egg whites, or egg substitutes, don't let high-calorie accompaniments overshadow their benefits. Here are some serving suggestions for popular egg dishes.

Omelettes or crepes

- Fill with stir-fried vegetables, such as spinach, asparagus, peppers, onions, mushrooms, and tomatoes, and serve with an oat bran muffin
- Stuff with cooked, shredded chicken and serve with a broiled tomato and raisin bread
- Prepare with flaked crabmeat and serve with fresh berries and a whole-wheat baguette

Scrambled eggs

- Top with tomato salsa and wrap in a wheat tortilla
- Serve with a sliced tomato and sprouts and layer on a whole-wheat English muffin for a breakfast sandwich
- Stuff in a pita pocket with shredded carrots and sprouts, and serve with grapes

French toast

- Make with toasted whole-grain bread, and top with sliced kiwifruit and berries and a dollop of thick yogurt

Weight-Friendly Substitutions

The easiest way to work eggs into your menu without going overboard on calories or cholesterol is to prepare them without added fat.

For breakfast eggs

- Extend scrambled eggs by adding chopped, steamed vegetables just before the eggs are done cooking, and use one egg per person.

- To lighten up scrambled eggs without adding fat, blend in a stiffly beaten egg white or pureed nonfat cottage cheese.
- Cook scrambled eggs and omelettes in a non-stick pan that has been lightly coated with vegetable oil spray. That way, you won't need to add butter or margarine.
- Prepare a hard-cooked egg instead of a fried egg for breakfast. To save time in the morning, prepare hard-cooked eggs the night before while dinner is cooking, then refrigerate.

For egg salad

- Blend the eggs with thick low-fat yogurt, pureed cottage cheese, or fat-free mayonnaise instead of full-fat mayonnaise. Add a touch of dry mustard, horseradish, paprika, or chives for flavor. Prepare the yolks of deviled eggs the same way.
- To extend egg salad, mix in chopped celery or red or green bell pepper to boost the volume, and serve it nestled in a sliced whole tomato.
- Substitute chopped firm tofu for hard-cooked eggs for a mock egg salad.

In other dishes

- Replace whole eggs with egg whites or egg substitutes to cut cholesterol and save on fat. As a rule of thumb, two egg whites or one-quarter cup of egg substitute can replace one whole egg. This tip is as good for omelettes as it is for baked goods.
- For the color and flavor of egg yolks, but less cholesterol and fat, use one whole egg and substitute two egg whites for the other egg when a recipe calls for two eggs or more.
- For totally egg-free baked goods, substitute half of a small, ripe mashed banana or one-quarter cup pureed fruit for each egg called for in the recipe.

New Foods to Try

Using egg substitutes, try recipes for these dishes, all of which lend themselves to the use of substitutes.

- Huevos rancheros (Mexican scrambled eggs mixed with salsa and green onion, and topped with low-fat cheese)
- Egg drop soup (Chinese chicken broth, slightly thickened with eggs)
- Frittata (Italian omelette with the ingredients mixed into the eggs, not folded inside. It's finished in the broiler, making it firmer.)

Dining Out

If you regularly eat breakfast away from home, go easy on the full American breakfast. When ordering eggs, order one or two, rather than the three-egg omelette. To keep the total fat and calorie count down, enjoy fruit on the side, rather than bacon, sausage, or hash browns. And ask for unbuttered whole-grain toast.

Many restaurants can prepare egg dishes with egg substitutes—even if they're not listed on the menu. Ask. For made-to-order omelettes, ask for the lower-fat, nutrient-dense fillings: chopped tomatoes, broccoli, onion, salsa, lean ham, and perhaps lower-fat cheese if available. Request that very little or no butter be used.

Watch for other restaurant items made with significant amounts of whole eggs or egg yolks: baked custard (flan), custard pie, crème brûlée, crepes, pumpkin pie, quiche, souffle, and tapioca pudding. Enjoy them—but share with a friend.

Fast Food

Believe it or not, you can still eat smart at fast-food restaurants (especially if they're not the mainstay of your diet.) Among the standard greasy, salty fare are healthier options. Your mission is to seek them out—and recognize them when you see them. Here's how.

Shopping Smarts

Ask the person at the counter for nutrition information for the food served. Many places either have brochures on hand or post the information on the wall. Most of the major chains also have that type of information posted on their Web sites. If you have access to a computer at home or at a library, print out those pages and keep them in your car. That way, you can make your choice before you even walk in the door.

If you have to wing it, focus on bread, vegetables, fruit, and milk. Pass up pastries, sugar, and fries. For example, instead of fatty fries, order nutrient-dense vegetables, like a side salad. A carton of milk would meet your dairy needs. Juice is better than soda.

Burgers. "Mega," "super," and "jumbo" portions may give you a lot of food for your money. But you also get "mega" fat and calories. A Big Mac has 560 calories and 31 grams of fat; a Whopper has 660 calories and 40 grams of fat—nearly an entire day's allotment. Instead, think in terms of reasonable portions—kid-size, if necessary. The regular hamburgers at McDonald's and Burger King have half the calories and a third of the fat of their overstuffed big brothers. Finally, ask for burgers to be prepared without special sauces or to have the sauce served on the side.

Mexican. If you must eat at fast-food restaurants, vary your choices so you'll get a wide variety of nutrients. Mexican establishments like Taco Bell offer items featuring refried beans, a fiber-filled change from meat. You're better off choosing a bean burrito with 12 grams of fat than a Big Beef Burrito Supreme weighing in at 23 grams of fat.

Chicken and fish. These items aren't always a healthier choice than burgers. Pay attention to how they're cooked. Are they grilled without extra sauces and toppings? Or are they breaded and fried? There's a huge difference in the amount of fat and calories between the two. If chicken comes with the skin on, remove it and throw away lots of fat. (At Kentucky Fried Chicken, for instance, a roast chicken breast without skin has 4 grams of fat; one with skin has 11 grams.)

Baked potatoes. Wendy's has baked potatoes—get a plain spud and top it with healthy salad-bar choices like peas, onions, tomatoes, and green peppers. Or order a small bowl of chili to top your spud. At 7 grams of fat, it's a better choice than asking for the menu-item chili and cheese baked potato (22 grams).

Salads and sandwiches. Subway has a wide variety of salads with fat-free dressings. (Try the roasted chicken breast salad: It has 162 calories and four grams of fat.) Many bagel places feature bagel sandwiches as well as soups.

Accompaniments. Ask about low-fat versions of accompaniments like mayonnaise, salad dressing, and milk. They may be available, just not listed on the menu. You'll find low-fat chips and lots of vegetable choices for sandwiches at Subway, for instance.

Lean Menu-Makers

That burger looks mighty lonesome all by itself. Find it some worthwhile companions, like these items.

Milk. Round out any fast-food meal with a carton of milk. Even if it's 2 percent fat instead of 1 percent, you're getting more calcium than you would with a soda and way fewer calories than a shake offers. Or ask for orange juice for a vitamin C boost. Even though juice is a breakfast item, most fast-food places serve it any time of the day.

Best and Worst Fast Food

Even when your choices are limited, you'll save fat and calories by choosing small portions of simple items. Rule #1: Think small, not supersize. Rule #2: Keep it plain—not cheesy, saucy, or smothered. Rule #3: Look for lower-fat choices.

Best Choices

Fast Food	Portion	Calories	Grams of Fat
Soft taco	1 taco	220	10.0
Bagel (with 2 Tbsp. fat-free cream cheese)	1 bagel (2½ oz.)	225	1.1
Grilled steak soft taco	1 taco	230	10.0
Baked potato (with ½ cup broccoli and 2 pats of butter)	1 potato	244	8.5
Small hamburger with bun (without condiments)	1 hamburger	260	9.0
Sub sandwich with lean turkey, ham, and vegetables (no mayo)	1 sandwich (6 in.)	280	5.0
English muffin sandwich (with egg, Canadian bacon, American cheese, and buttered muffin)	1 sandwich	290	12.0
Grilled chicken sandwich (without mayonnaise)	1 sandwich	370	9.0
Bean burrito	1 burrito	380	12.0
Pancakes and syrup	1 serving (3 pancakes)	440	9.0

Worst Choices

Fast Food	Portion	Calories	Grams of Fat
Taco salad with shell	1 salad (19 oz.)	850	52.0
Nachos (with meat and cheese)	1 serving (11 oz.)	770	39.0
Giant cinnamon roll	1 roll	730	24.0
"Supersize," extra-large burger with bun (with mayo, lettuce, and tomato)	1 burger	660	40.0
Biscuit sandwich (with egg, sausage, and American cheese)	1 sandwich	620	43.0
Fried fish sandwich (with tartar sauce)	1 sandwich	560	28.0
"Supersize," extra-large French fries	1 serving	540	26.0
Fried chicken sandwich (with mayo)	1 sandwich	500	25.0
Cheese Danish pastry	1 pastry	410	22.0

Chips. They needn't be on the forbidden list. Choose low-fat, baked potato chips at sub shops and the like. If baked chips aren't available, see if another low-fat salty snack is. Pretzels, for instance, might satisfy you. (If it really is the taste of salt you're after, get extra pickles. They have zero fat and barely any calories.) When only chips will do, at least opt for a lower-fat variety like Sun Chips (6 grams of fat per ounce instead of 10).

Vegetables. Don't hold the lettuce. Or the tomatoes, onions, or green peppers. In fact, get extra—and get them in place of cheese.

Fruit. Is there cut fruit on the salad bar? A bowl of apples behind the counter? (No, apple pie isn't a good alternative.) If there's really nothing on the premises, scout out fruit elsewhere for a healthy snack later.

Weight-Friendly Substitutions

Think small. Small *anything* is better than super-size or jumbo. You still may be getting too many calories and grams of fat for your liking, but at least the amount's not ridiculous. Small fries at McDonald's, for example, tally 210 calories and 10 grams of fat—compared with super-size fries at 540 calories and 26 grams of fat.

A better idea: Go with a side salad and reduced-fat dressing instead of fries. And ask for plenty of tomatoes! They're virtually fat-free.

In general, keep your food choices simple. Choose plain and unadorned instead of "supreme" or another superlative that connotes a heavy helping of cheese, sour cream, guacamole, special sauce, or bacon bits.

New Fast-Food Restaurants to Try

There's more out there these days than burger joints. Here are some places to look for good food in a flash.

Bagel shops. Many bagel shops offer lunch items in addition to bagels. Lots of lower-fat options are available, like lean lunchmeat, smoked salmon, and hummus. Skip such high-fat choices as Gouda or Asiago cheese and spreads like olive and pine nut. Soups such as zesty lentil, chicken noodle, and chicken tortilla are filling yet easy on the calories. Black bean soup or red beans and rice is even healthier because it has more fiber.

Wrap places. Wrap sandwiches are popular, and sandwich shops everywhere offer them. They fill their wraps with grilled lean beef or chicken and lots of vegetables like tomatoes, peppers, onions, and even roasted potatoes. Don't forget beans (everything from black beans to pinto beans). They're a nutritional gold mine.

Supermarkets. What could be faster than running in and grabbing a lunch-size salad in a bag, some string cheese, a box of crackers, and a couple pieces of fresh fruit? Other good ideas: dried fruit, bite-size cereal, and small cartons of milk or juice. If you need a bowl or plate, or even a plastic spoon or fork, head to the deli department and ask for one. They normally provide these items free of charge.

Breakfast on the Road

What are the makings of a healthy fast-food breakfast? Choose higher-fiber bagels like eight-grain or whole-wheat. Then, since you need more than carbohydrates for a balanced breakfast, spread that bagel with light cream cheese or hummus, if available.

If you want an egg sandwich, have it on a bagel or an English muffin instead of a high-fat biscuit or croissant. Eggs are a filling protein choice and have just five grams of fat each. Keep fat and calories down by watching cheese and meats. One slice of cheese is okay. Canadian bacon and ham are lean meat choices. Sausage and bacon, however, put you in fat overload.

Finally, choose low-fat muffins instead of Danish pastries, doughnuts, and cinnamon rolls.

Fish and Seafood

If you're a career dieter, you probably sail right over to the fish entrées listed on the menu when you dine out. And well you should: Fish can be a helpful ally in your battle against fat on your belly, butt, and thighs. Fish is almost all protein, and because your body metabolizes protein much more slowly than carbohydrates, fish keeps you satisfied for hours. Protein also "feeds" your blood sugar over four to six hours rather than just an hour or so like carbs do. The result? Protein helps you eat less over the long haul. Also, it rebuilds muscle and powers the millions upon billions of chemical

Best and Worst Fish and Seafood

Fatty fish like salmon, tuna, and swordfish have slightly more fat and calories than white fish like haddock and cod. But those calories are worthwhile—they supply omega-3 fatty acids, which are beneficial to heart health.

Whether you're cooking fish at home or ordering it out, the key is to keep the added fat and calories from butter and cream sauces to a minimum, limiting the total number of calories from any fish entrée to 150 and the number of grams of fat to 5. The exception: casseroles containing fish, where you need to allow for calories from rice, noodles, milk, or other added components of the dish.

Best Choices			
Entrée	Portion	Calories	Grams of Fat
Steamed crabmeat	3 oz.	87	1.5
Haddock (broiled or baked)	3 oz.	95	0.8
Albacore tuna packed in water	3 oz.	105	1.5
Steamed shrimp with 2 Tbsp. cocktail sauce	3 oz.	114	0.9
Tuna (broiled or grilled)	3 oz.	118	1.0
Broiled lobster tail with lemon juice	6 oz.	166	1.0

Worst Choices			
Entrée	Portion	Calories	Grams of Fat
Fried clams with 2 Tbsp. tartar sauce	¾ cup	600	42.4
Popcorn shrimp (fried)	6–8 shrimp	454	24.9
Steamed lobster tail with 2 Tbsp. butter	6 oz.	370	24.0
Lobster salad	½ cup	286	16.6
Battered fried fish	3 oz.	197	10.4
Chunk-style tuna packed in oil	3 oz.	158	6.8

reactions that your body performs every millisecond, which is important in sustaining you during your body-shaping workouts.

Compared to other sources of protein, like meat or cheese, fish is relatively lean—from 2 to 8 percent fat, depending on the species. (In comparison, a well-marbled porterhouse steak weighs in at 48 percent fat.) The trouble arises when fish comes gift-wrapped in batter, butter, or other high-calorie coatings.

Shopping Smarts

You don't have to go to the best fish market in town every time you want to have fish. While fresh fish certainly remains the most delectable way to enjoy fish, there are now several convenient ways to make including fish in your diet easier. Fortunately, options are now available in frozen and "convenience" fish beyond breaded and fried fillets or oily canned selections that quickly negate the reason you've chosen fish.

Canned fish. If you're an old hand at the diet game, you already know that three ounces of water-packed tuna has 53 fewer calories and 5.3 fewer grams of fat than oil-packed tuna. And over the years, you've probably eaten enough tuna to stock a fleet of Peruvian fishing boats. So, no doubt, you'll welcome a little variety in your fish repertoire, such as tuna's cold-water cousins-in-a-can: salmon, clams, sardines, and anchovies. Look for water-packed versions of salmon and clams. If you like sardines and anchovies, save them for special occasions. They supply as many as 180 calories and 12 grams of fat for three ounces (even for sardines packed in mustard sauce).

As for tuna salad, if you make it at home with fat-free mayo, you're in the clear. Tuna salads from the supermarket deli case, though, are pretty heavy on the regular mayonnaise.

Frozen fish. At one time, the only way to get frozen fish without loads of breading was to go ice fishing. What came out of the water with a scant 74 calories and less than a solo gram of fat per three-ounce serving gained weight when it hit the deep fryer, turning a bantam-weight finback into a heavyweight with 197 calories and 10.4 grams of fat. Further, your choices were pretty much limited to "white bread" varieties like haddock, cod, flounder, and halibut.

Today, supermarkets compete with fish markets and offer a virtual smorgasbord of fish. In addition to the old standards, you can find just about any finfish that's fit to eat—swordfish, perch, orange roughy, monkfish, snapper, catfish. Throw a couple of fillets on the grill with some lemon and herbs, and you've added zero fat and calories but a whole lot of zip in just minutes. Or whip up a fish stew or chowder with fat-free milk. Serve with a salad and oyster crackers, and it's chow time.

If you can afford it, help yourself to shrimp, lobster, or crab. Although these crustaceans are higher in cholesterol than most other types of fish, studies have shown that eating shrimp, for example, lowers triglyceride levels and raises high-density lipoprotein (HDL) cholesterol levels (the good variety). Ten large steamed or broiled shrimp have just 54 calories and barely a half gram of fat. If it is consumed without butter, even lobster—the Cadillac of seafood—is totally figure-friendly.

Imitation fish. Check the frozen fish case for fully cooked, packaged fish labeled as imitation crab, imitation lobster, and imitation scallops. Commonly made from white fish, they are exceptionally low in fat; in fact, most varieties are fat-free. Just open a package and top your salad with a generous three ounces of imitation crabmeat chunks. You'll reel in just 87 calories, 10 grams of protein—and only 1 gram of fat. For a quick entrée, combine packaged fish with a bag of frozen vegetables in a stir-fry. If you're allergic to shellfish, always read the label, though, to make sure the brand you've chosen doesn't include any of the real stuff for flavor, as some do.

Lean Menu-Makers

From salsas to cocktail sauce, there are plenty of fat-free and low-fat ways to spice up your fish fillet. Both jarred tomato-based and fruit-based salsas are

Make It *Better*

Tuna Noodle Casserole

MAKES 4 SERVINGS

Per serving

583 calories

12.8 grams of fat

(20 percent of

calories from fat)

This time-honored favorite may not be glamorous, but it can save the day on weekday nights when you haven't had time to shop for groceries but don't want to give in to a fast-food meal out of desperation. Round out this one-dish supper with stewed tomatoes—a great source of heart-healthy lycopene—or a satisfying salad of dark, leafy greens, green peppers, beans, and other nutrient-dense veggies.

8   ounces no-yolk or whole-wheat noodles

1   16-ounce package frozen broccoli florets, thawed

1   12-ounce can water-packed white tuna, drained and flaked

1   10¾-ounce can fat-free, reduced-sodium condensed cream of mushroom soup

1   cup low-fat (1%) milk

1   cup shredded reduced-fat Monterey Jack cheese

8   ounces fat-free plain yogurt

½   teaspoon ground black pepper

¼   teaspoon celery seeds

¼   teaspoon crushed red-pepper flakes

½   cup crushed reduced-fat snack crackers

¼   cup grated Parmesan cheese

Preheat the oven to 350°F. Coat a 13" × 9" baking dish with nonstick spray.

Cook the noodles in a large pot of boiling water according to the package directions. Drain and return to the pot. Remove from the heat; toss with the broccoli and tuna.

In a large bowl, mix the soup, milk, Monterey Jack, yogurt, black pepper, celery seeds, and red-pepper flakes. Pour over the noodle mixture and stir carefully. Transfer to the baking dish.

Mix the crackers and Parmesan; sprinkle over the casserole. Bake for 30 minutes or until lightly browned.

excellent additions to a grilled fish fillet. If you're adventurous in the kitchen, try making your own chunky salsa, stirring together chopped mango, orange or tangerine chunks, kiwifruit bits, chopped green onions, and perhaps a dash of chili powder.

Marinara sauces work well with many types of fish, especially the very lean varieties such as cod.

- Starting with fresh or frozen fillets, spray a non-stick pan with vegetable oil spray, then add the fillets and cover with marinara sauce. Cover and simmer until fork-tender. For a complete meal, add your favorite frozen vegetable or vegetable blend and let it cook in the sauce.

- Fat-free salad dressings double extremely well as interesting fish marinades. Experiment with your favorite dressings—and try one of our favorites, fat-free poppyseed, as a salmon or char marinade. Give the fish at least an hour in the refrigerator to absorb the flavor, and then grill or broil.

- While most cocktail sauces are very low in fat, tartar sauces aren't—they're basically mayonnaise. If you're hankering for a good lower-fat tarter sauce, try making a simple version at home: Add pickle relish to fat-free mayonnaise (to taste) and spritz in some lemon juice.

- For low-fat crabmeat salad, layer romaine lettuce with crabmeat and sandwich between two deliciously golden-brown whole-wheat bread slices. Make the spread with low-fat mayonnaise, extending one tablespoon (an acceptable amount) with a little lemon or lime juice (and an artificial sweetener or dash of sugar as necessary). You might also want to try a shake of ground red pepper for interest. Fold in a grated carrot and chopped red onions.

Dining Out

If you're looking for something low-fat at your local fast-food restaurant or diner, think twice before ordering the tuna salad plate. You might use water-packed tuna and fat-free mayo at home, but restaurants do not. One 12-inch fast-food tuna salad sandwich on white bread, for example, has 30 grams of fat per sandwich and 752 calories—and most diners follow suit. You'd have to swim moderately hard for over an hour to work off that sandwich. Instead, swim past the tuna salad on over to the grilled chicken.

Ever wonder why the broiled fish fillet from your favorite seafood restaurant is so moist? It's no secret: Many restaurants add melted butter or herbed oils to broiled fish. To enjoy the lean benefits of fish, just ask the server to bring your fillet sans fat. The same is true for accompanying sauces. While there may be a fairly fat-innocent sauce out there at some restaurant, most hide behind a high-fat profile. If you'd like to try the sauce without going overboard on fat, order it on the side and try dipping your fork tines in the sauce and gathering a bite on your fork.

As for batter-fried fish, both the fast-food and the full-service restaurant versions are high in fat because the batter soaks up fat like a sponge. A batter-fried fish entrée from a full-service restaurant serves up 197 calories and 10.4 grams of fat. One order of fast-food fish and fries comes in even higher with 420 calories and 26 grams of fat. You can compensate for the calories with exercise, but bear in mind that one indulgence demands nearly an hour of bicycling at a fast pace. If you find yourself with no other options at dinnertime, flicking off the batter with your fork before you eat the fillet can control the damage.

Clam chowders and lobster bisques are made with cream, so if you must indulge, order by the cup, not the bowl—and split it with your dining partner. One cup of bisque, for example, comes in with nearly 200 calories and at least eight grams of fat—that's about 25 extra minutes on the stairclimber at a fast pace.

Fruit and Fruit Dishes

If you love sweets but can't afford to indulge in dessert frequently, fruit also can help satisfy your sweet tooth: If offers no fat and fewer calories than rich, sweet desserts. Keep a bowl of fruit on hand to snack on, rather than a box of candy. Or drink calcium-fortified orange juice instead of soda.

To maximize the benefits of eating fruit, follow these tips.

Shopping Smarts

A generation ago, certain fruits were available only in summer. While fruit usually is sweeter and more flavorful in season, you can now buy almost any fruit all year long. Choose fruit to match your "food-style."

Fresh fruit. Nothing beats a fresh, crisp apple or a juicy peach. When it comes to fresh fruit, quality is what counts. Look for firm fruit, without bruises or signs of decay.

For a quick salad, dessert, or snack, you can buy cut-up fruit in the produce department or salad bar of your local supermarket.

Canned or frozen fruit. To ensure that you always have some kind of fruit on hand, even when you don't have time to get to the store, stock up

Best and Worst Fruit Selections

Try to eat two to four servings of fruit a day. Half a cup of chopped fresh, frozen, or canned fruit counts as a serving. So does six ounces of fruit juice. For more nutrients, choose fruit juice, rather than fruit drink.

Best Choices

Fruit	Portion	Calories	Grams of Fat
Frozen unsweetened fruit	½ cup	26	0.0
Canned fruit packed in juice	½ cup	50	0.0
Unsweetened applesauce	½ cup	52	0.0
Mixed fruit	½ cup	58	0.0
Fresh fruit	1 medium	60	0.0
Poached fruit	1 serving (half a peach or pear)	65	0.0
Fruit juice	¾ cup	79	0.0

Worst Choices

Fruit	Portion	Calories	Grams of Fat
Double-crust apple pie	1 piece (⅛ of a 9" pie)	411	19.4
Fast-food fruit pies	1 pie	266	14.4
Flavored applesauce	½ cup	100	0.0
Frozen sweetened fruit	½ cup	100	0.0
Fruit-flavored drink	¾ cup	95	0.0
Canned fruit in heavy syrup	½ cup	90	0.0

on canned and frozen fruit, like applesauce, canned peaches, pears, and pineapple. Also, keep some canned tropical fruit salad on hand—it's great stirred into fat-free yogurt for an instant, nutritious dessert.

From a nutritional standpoint, canned and frozen fruit are as good as fresh fruit. In fact, if the fruit is processed at its peak, the amount of nutrients in processed fruit may be greater than those in fresh fruit that has been around a while. Look for canned "lite" fruit, which contains less added sugar. Fruit canned in natural juices has fewer calories than fruit in syrup. Check the Nutrition Facts on the label to compare. Some frozen fruit is packed in syrup, too. For ease of use, look for those that pour freely out of the package.

Dried fruit. Because moisture is removed, the natural sugars in dried fruit are concentrated. As a result, dried fruit has more calories than an equal amount of fresh fruit. Eaten out of hand, like nuts, you can quickly consume quite a few calories in dried fruit. Instead, toss smaller amounts of raisins, dried bananas, cranberries, apricots, and apples into salads, breakfast cereals, pancake batters, and mixed dishes. Dried fruits are nutrient-packed, so by all means, include some in your shopping cart.

Fruit juice and fruit drinks. Check out the Nutrition Facts labels and ingredient lists for 100 percent juice and juice blends. Be aware that fruit-flavored drinks are mainly water and sweeteners.

Fruit bars, pastries, and spreads. Fruit is an ingredient in all kinds of packaged and prepared foods—from frozen fruit bars and dried fruit snack bars, to fruit spreads, jams, and jellies, to pie fillings. Because many of these offer little in the way of fruit, and much in the way of calories from added sugar, they don't really count as fruit choices. Opt for the real thing instead.

Lean Menu-Makers

Fruit can be the highlight of your menus in ways that never occurred to you, whether as a sweet complement in mixed dishes or a nutritious and flavorful snack. Consider these imaginative ways to eat lean with fruit.

Fruit as the main event

- For breakfast, spread a seasonal array of sliced fruit or berries on a toasted waffle and serve with hot chocolate
- For lunch, serve mixed fruit in half of a cantaloupe with low-fat or fat-free yogurt and fruit-nut bread
- Serve a bowl of chilled fruit soup (berry, melon, peach, mango) with a bagel and herbed yogurt cheese
- For an elegant but light supper, fold mixed fruit into a warm crepe and top with fruit yogurt

Fruit as a mealtime supplement

- Add chopped fruit to main-dish salads—pears in chicken salad, apples in tuna salad, and peaches in seafood salad
- Add fruit to soup—grated, tart apples in lentil soup and orange juice concentrate in carrot soup
- Include dried fruit in grain dishes—dried cranberries in couscous, dried apricots in wild rice, and dried apples in poultry dressing
- Accompany entrées with fruit salsa—pineapple salsa with salmon, peach salsa with chicken, and papaya salsa with pork chops
- Add fruit to vegetable salads—raspberries in spinach salad, chopped apples in broccoli slaw, and tangerine segments in a mixed-greens salad

Weight-Friendly Substitutions

What could be easier than substituting a fresh, crisp apple for apple pie? There's no easier substitution than just plain fruit! It can be a menu item by itself—with no fat or sugar added. When you want something more, these quick tips can help you enjoy the nutritional benefits of fruit without adding extra sugar and fat.

As a sweet, refreshing beverage

- For no calories, replace sugary fruit drinks with ice-cold water slightly flavored with a lemon, lime, or orange slice.

Make It *Better*

Apple-Cranberry Crisp

MAKES 8 SERVINGS

Per serving

186 calories

5.2 grams of fat

(25 percent of

calories from fat)

Instead of viewing dessert as a sinful indulgence, consider it an opportunity to reach your daily quota for fruit. This appetizing meal finale focuses on fresh fruit, oats, whole-wheat flour, and apple juice concentrate, with a minimal amount of fat and sugar. If you can't get dried cranberries, substitute other dried fruit, such as chopped prunes or apricots.

- ¾ cup old-fashioned rolled oats
- ⅓ cup whole-wheat flour
- ¼ cup packed dark brown sugar
- ⅛ teaspoon salt
- ⅛ teaspoon ground allspice
- 3 tablespoons chilled unsalted butter or margarine, cut into small pieces

- 3 large Empire, Idared, or Granny Smith apples, cored and sliced into ¼"-thick wedges
- ½ cup dried cranberries
- 3 tablespoons frozen apple juice concentrate
- 1 tablespoon sugar

Preheat the oven to 425°F.

In a medium bowl, combine the oats, flour, brown sugar, salt, and allspice. Using your fingers or a pastry blender, lightly mix in the butter or margarine until the mixture is crumbly.

In an 8" or 9" square baking dish, toss together the apples, cranberries, apple juice concentrate, and sugar until well-mixed. Sprinkle the oat mixture evenly over the top.

Cover with foil and bake for 20 minutes, or until the mixture is bubbly and the apples are tender. Uncover and bake for 5 to 10 minutes longer, or until the topping is lightly browned.

- Enjoy "just plain" juice instead of soft drinks for the nutritional benefits. Mix two juices together for your own refreshing blend.
- For a thick, creamy drink, blend fresh fruit with fat-free milk, buttermilk, or fat-free yogurt in place of ice cream. Half of a banana is a good thickener, too.

In fruit salads and side dishes

- Sweeten fruit with a light splash of juice rather than spoonfuls of sugar. Combine mixed fruit compote with peach nectar or sliced pears with orange juice.
- Prepare fruit gelatin salads from sugar-free mixes.

As a topping or sauce

- Puree fruit with a little juice to make a "syrup" for French toast, pancakes, and waffles. Besides strawberries and peaches, try papaya, blackberries, and other less common fruits for your syrup.

- For a thick sauce, just puree fruit with herbs or spices. The sauce is great over broiled or baked chicken or seafood. For starters, blend mango with rosemary or peaches with cardamom.

To enhance flavor without adding calories

- Add grated orange, lemon, or lime rind to soups, stews, salads, and baked goods.

- Use spices that create the sensation of sweetness in fruit and fruit dishes, such as cinnamon, ginger, nutmeg, and cloves. For example: cinnamon on broiled peaches, ginger in applesauce, nutmeg in fruit soup, and ground cloves in poached pears.

- Sweeten fruit and fruit dishes with sugar substitutes. Be aware, though: Aspartame loses its sweetness with heating. Sugar substitutes may not give the result you expect in baked dishes.

New Foods to Try

Produce departments display a greater variety of fruit than ever before—you could go for a couple of weeks without eating the same fruit twice. Yet the average shopper sticks mostly with apples, bananas, and oranges, according to consumer studies. When you can, try new varieties of common fruits, like fuji apples, finger bananas (they're sweeter!), and blood oranges. Buy a Crenshaw melon, fresh figs, or Rainier cherries. And try uncommon fruits: perhaps an Asian pear, cherimoya (custard apple), persimmon, or prickly pear.

Check the supermarket shelves, too, for fruits you've never tried, perhaps loquats, mangosteen, lychees, or lingonberries.

To keep old standbys interesting, get creative: Blend applesauce with another fruit and canned raspberry-flavored peaches. New fruit blends of refrigerated and canned juices make beverage choices more fun and flavorful!

Dining Out

Working fruit into meals eaten away from home takes a little resourcefulness, but it can be done. For a light meal any time of day, order a fruit plate. Make it a more varied meal with a cup of vegetable soup, a whole-grain roll, and low-fat milk.

At restaurant buffets, select cut-up fruit rather than stewed fruit, which is often prepared with plenty of sugar.

When dining out means fast food, bring whole fruit— perhaps a tangerine, peach, or bag of cherries or grapes—with you. Skip fast-food fruit pies!

When you're mall-walking, take a break and rest your feet while sipping a fruit smoothie, thickened with low-fat or fat-free yogurt or a banana, or a frozen fruit juice drink. Avoid the temptation of the deluxe size—an 8- to 12-ounce serving is probably all you need.

At a sit-down dinner, look for fruit options instead of a high-fat, high-calorie dessert. Order a fruit cup from the appetizer menu or ask for fresh fruit, perhaps a bowl of berries.

Gravies and Sauces

Good gravy, girlfriend! What's that on your mashed potatoes? Isn't gravy one of the biggest dieting no-nos there is? Well . . . not necessarily. True, good old-fashioned homestyle gravy made with a mess of meat drippings isn't such a hot idea. The calories and fat in it add up mighty fast. But lighter versions are now available—and that goes for many of our other favorite fatty sauces as well.

Before you take that as license to smother everything you eat in silken sauces, remember that many foods taste fine without embellishment. By preparing meat, poultry, fish, and vegetables in ways that preserve their natural flavors, you do away with the need to gussy them up. But for those times when something extra is called for, follow this advice.

Shopping Smarts

In addition to looking for lighter versions of your sauce favorites, think of entirely new ways to jazz up the plain meat, vegetables, or even dessert on your plate. Then go to the market with these tips in mind.

Gravies. If you haven't perused the gravy section lately, you may be surprised at what's there. The major manufacturers offer all sorts of nonfat gravies. In addition to regular beef, pork, chicken, and turkey gravy, you'll find mushroom, zesty onion, au jus, slow-roasted types, rotisserie flavors, and more. Many are fat-free, and even the ones that aren't typically have only a gram or two of fat per quarter-cup serving.

The flavor is surprisingly good, although they may be a little on the salty side. If the texture is too thick for your taste, thin the gravy with water, broth, or wine when you heat it.

Creamy sauces. Let's face it: Béarnaise and hollandaise are diet-busters. A typical béarnaise sauce has 12 grams of fat in just two tablespoons. Hollandaise can run about that much, too. If it's

creaminess you're after, try reduced-fat condensed soups. Thinned-down cream of chicken, mushroom, celery, and broccoli make good toppings for simply prepared chicken, fish, and rice. Horseradish stirred into nonfat mayonnaise, yogurt, or sour cream makes a superb sauce for roast beef. Replace the horseradish with dill for fish, shrimp, and other seafood. An envelope of dry salad dressing, such as ranch or roasted garlic, combined with two cups of fat-free sour cream and a little milk is good on baked or mashed potatoes.

Salsas. Mexican for "sauce," salsa perks up everything from fish fillets and chicken breast to meat loaf and baked potatoes. There are literally dozens of varieties available, including green ones made from cactus or tomatillos. Most are nearly fat-free; check the label to be sure.

Other savory sauces. Make leftover vegetables work for you. Puree cooked red peppers, broccoli, or carrots with broth or wine. Start with one cup of vegetables and one tablespoon of broth or wine. Add more liquid if you want a thinner sauce or more vegetables if you want a thicker one. Add the seasonings of your choice. The sauce can be used as a topping for meat, poultry, or seafood. Or try defatted broth as a light, refreshing glaze for meat or poultry. Simply boil it in a saucepan until it's reduced to half or less of its original volume. (Use reduced-sodium broth to keep the glaze from becoming too salty.)

Tomato sauce is good for more than just pasta. Chicken breasts, fish fillets, and baked potatoes taste great with a tomato sauce topping. Look for ones with 2 grams or less of fat per half-cup serving. As for pesto sauce, be careful. Even the reduced-fat type isn't what you'd call low in fat. Just two tablespoons have 15 grams of fat. The good thing about pesto is its assertive flavor—a little goes a long way. Thin it with defatted broth or stir a spoonful into nonfat sour cream, yogurt, or pureed cottage cheese. Then serve it with poultry, seafood, steamed vegetables, and baked potatoes.

Dessert sauces. Forget about custard sauce when serving angel food cake, reduced-fat pound cake, poached pears, and other desserts. Instead, try nonfat chocolate, vanilla, or butterscotch pudding (make it thinner by using an extra half-cup of milk when you cook it). Or go with flavored yogurt (add a little grated orange rind to kick up the flavor a notch). You might also want to try sweetening nonfat sour cream or plain yogurt with brown sugar. Don't overlook cranberry sauce (try orange- or raspberry-flavored), chunky applesauce, crushed pineapple, and pureed raspberries or strawberries. Also consider fat-free butterscotch, caramel, and chocolate sauces for ice cream and frozen yogurt.

Best and Worst Gravies and Sauces

If you're sizing up a sauce or gravy, those with fewer than 110 calories and three grams of fat are decent choices. Even meat gravy can make the grade—provided you don't empty the whole gravy boat over your plate. Dress it, don't drown it.

Best Choices			
Gravy or Sauce	**Portion**	**Calories**	**Grams of Fat**
Tomato sauce	¼ cup	18	0.2
Fat-free gravy	¼ cup	20	0.0
Au jus gravy	¼ cup	24	0.3
Reduced-fat cream of mushroom soup	¼ cup	35	1.5
Regular meat gravy	2 Tbsp.	40	3.0
Horseradish sauce made with nonfat mayonnaise	2 Tbsp.	44	0.9
Raspberry sauce	¼ cup	50	0.3
Nonfat caramel sauce	2 Tbsp.	100	0.0
Cranberry sauce	¼ cup	100	0.1
Nonfat chocolate sauce	2 Tbsp.	110	0.0

Worst Choices			
Gravy or Sauce	**Portion**	**Calories**	**Grams of Fat**
Alfredo sauce, ready to serve	¼ cup	170	10.0
Pesto sauce	2 Tbsp.	155	15.0
Curry sauce with coconut milk	⅓ cup	140	15.0
Hollandaise sauce	2 Tbsp.	135	14.0
Béarnaise sauce	2 Tbsp.	120	12.0
Custard sauce	¼ cup	114	5.6
Creamy horseradish sauce	2 Tbsp.	110	10.0
Regular meat gravy	¼ cup	80	6.0
Cheese sauce	2 Tbsp.	60	4.4
Béchamel sauce	2 Tbsp.	51	5.0

Make It *Better*

Thigh-Friendly Mushroom Gravy

MAKES 8 SERVINGS

Per ½-cup serving

33.5 calories

0.1 gram of fat

(3 percent of calories

from fat)

If the guys in your household insist on gravy with their turkey and mashed potatoes, you can all ladle up without wrecking your weight-friendly eating plan. This velvety stand-in for giblet gravy will save you 46 calories and 6 grams of fat.

½ cup sliced celery	1 0.35-ounce package dried mushrooms (found in produce section)
½ cup chopped carrots	
½ cup chopped onions	
3 cloves garlic, minced	¼ cup all-purpose flour
Pinch of dried sage	¼ teaspoon hot-pepper sauce
Pinch of dried thyme	
2 cans (14 ounces each) fat-free, reduced-sodium chicken broth	½ cup fat-free, reduced-sodium chicken broth (optional)

Coat a large nonstick saucepan with cooking spray. Add the celery, carrots, onions, garlic, sage, and thyme. Coat with cooking spray. Cover; cook over medium heat, stirring occasionally, for 10 minutes.

Add the broth and mushrooms. Cover; simmer for 30 minutes. Using a slotted spoon, remove the mushrooms. Chop finely.

Pour the gravy mixture into a blender and add the flour. Puree. Return to the pan, and add the hot-pepper sauce and mushrooms. Reheat to a boil. Add extra broth, if desired, to thin.

Lean Menu-Makers

Flavorful foods require little in the way of extra gravies and sauces. It pays to use the freshest, best-tasting ingredients your money can buy and to prepare them in ways that preserve their flavors. For example, searing meat and fish over high heat at the beginning of cooking seals in juices and gives the surface an appealing brown color. Little is needed to embellish foods cooked this way.

Other flavor-enhancing techniques: Lightly steam or microwave vegetables until just crisp to conserve color and taste—you won't miss the cheese sauce. Stir-fry vegetables with a splash of reduced-sodium soy sauce and bypass butter or margarine. Pan-roast chopped veggies like potatoes, zucchini, and broccoli with a bit of high-quality olive oil and balsamic vinegar to bring out bold flavors often hidden by high-fat toppings. Before grilling, gently rub the surface of meat with a mixture of dried herbs or a spice blend like Cajun-style seasoning to impart big flavor.

Weight-Friendly Substitutions

Turn your back on unwanted calories with these saucy stand-ins.

- Knock off calories in creamy sauces by substituting evaporated skim milk for cream. Another idea: For every cup of cream sauce, slowly whisk one tablespoon of flour into one cup of cold fat-free milk until smooth, then stir over medium heat until the mixture comes to a boil. Continue to stir for a minute or two to get rid of the raw-flour taste. Season with salt and pepper plus your choice of herbs, mustard, Parmesan cheese, shredded low-fat cheese, or horseradish. You can use the same technique with defatted broth or a combination of broth and milk. For glossy, somewhat transparent sauces, substitute cornstarch for the flour, but use one-half tablespoon of cornstarch for every one tablespoon of flour in the original recipe.

- Prepare your favorite packaged sauce mixes with fat-free milk and half the butter or margarine.

- When making gravy, degrease the meat or poultry juices with a fat-separating pitcher before continuing with the recipe. Thicken the juices with either cornstarch first dissolved in a little cold water, or flour.

- Instead of adorning vegetables with cheese sauce, toss them with lemon juice, fat-free Italian dressing, or a dash of hot sauce.

New Foods to Try

Admittedly, old food habits die hard. You may think it impossible to cut back on gravy and savory sauces, especially if you cook for someone who grew up eating gravies and sauces with his meals. But other flavor enhancers can take their place. Flavored vinegars, such as tarragon and raspberry, add zest without fat. So do mustards, such as honey, peppercorn, and Dijon. They go great with meat. If they're not "saucelike" enough for you, mix them with nonfat sour cream. For more ideas, see Condiments and Spreads on page 44.

Dining Out

The gravy you get in a restaurant will not be low in calories or fat. Asking for it on the side translates into significant calorie savings—as long as you don't eat the whole serving. Try dipping the tines of your fork into the sauce and then spearing your food. You'll get the taste of the gravy without actually eating a lot of it.

Additionally, it helps to brush up on your sauce vocabulary, so you know what you're getting when you dine out. And by all means, get as much information as possible from your server about ingredients and preparation methods before ordering. Here's a selection of sauces commonly offered in restaurants.

- Alfredo. Butter, heavy cream, and Parmesan cheese dominate this sauce. You can have it—once in a blue moon.

- Au jus. A fancy way of saying meat juices, especially beef. A good choice.

- Béarnaise. Tarragon-flavored first cousin to hollandaise. This thick sauce gets its start with egg yolks, wine, and butter. Use sparingly.

- Béchamel. Flour, cream, and butter make up this one. Go easy.

- Bourguignonne. Mainly red wine with a bit of bacon. One of the lower-fat sauces.

- Curry. Contains coconut milk, which is high-fat. Proceed with caution.

- Hollandaise. Thick and creamy, with egg yolks and butter. Reserve for special dining occasions.

- Peanut. A staple of Thai cuisine, peanut sauce provides heart-healthy monounsaturated fat—just too much of it. Have only a smidgen.

- Velouté. This sauce is flavored by meat, poultry, fish, or vegetable broth, instead of cream or milk. But it still has fat as its base, so use only occasionally.

Meat

Got a beef with beef? Well, lighten up! Beef has. So have other meats like pork, lamb, and veal. If you've been eating poultry and fish every night in the name of slimming down, you can stop now. Leaner cuts abound in the meat case, and they add up to calorie savings. For example, seven cuts of beef and eight cuts of pork have a little more fat than skinless chicken breast, but less than skinless chicken thighs.

Giving up meat can, in fact, be a woman's

Best and Worst Meat Selections

When you're choosing meat, it's generally a good idea to zero in on cuts or entrées with fewer than 350 calories and nine grams of fat per serving. But of the two, fat content is a better benchmark. For example, bacon doesn't have a lot of calories, but most of those calories come from fat, not protein.

Best Choices

Meat	Portion	Calories	Grams of Fat
Lean roast beef from deli	3 slices (3 oz.)	120	4.5
Canadian bacon	3 slices (3 oz.)	129	5.8
Pork tenderloin	3 oz.	139	4.1
Roasted beef eye of round	3 oz.	141	4.0
Beef top round	3 oz.	169	4.3
Flank steak	3 oz.	176	8.6
Broiled pork sirloin chops	3 oz.	181	8.6
Lamb shish kebabs	3 oz.	190	7.5
Beef and broccoli stir-fry	4 oz.	346	3.9

Worst Choices

Meat	Portion	Calories	Grams of Fat
Barbecued ribs	6 oz.	674	51.6
Moo shu pork	1 serving (about 11 oz.)	501	13.0
Bacon double cheeseburger	1	460	28.0
Bean, cheese, and meat burrito	2 burritos (7 oz.)	331	13.3
Veal cutlet	4 oz.	322	19.0
Beef stroganoff	6½ oz.	300	13.5
Salami (made with beef and pork)	3 slices (3 oz.)	214	16.5
Frankfurter (made with beef and pork)	1	182	17.0
Bacon	3 slices (⅔ oz.)	109	9.4

downfall. Meat supplies the nutrients busy women need to keep going. Three ounces of cooked meat provides about 50 percent of the Daily Value for protein, approximately 25 percent of the zinc and niacin, and up to about 17 percent of the iron.

Balance, variety, and moderation are the cornerstones of a nutritious eating plan you can stick with in the long run. That includes modest portions of beef, pork, veal, lamb, ham, and even lunchmeat. Most women need only about six ounces of meat, chicken, or seafood a day. Three ounces of lean meat a few times a week will do you more good than harm.

Shopping Smarts

When shopping for meat, think, "Buy less, eat less." Start by keeping high-fat meats out of your shopping cart and concentrating on leaner versions. If you get a good buy on lean meat, use a small amount now and freeze the extra in three-ounce portions. That's about the size of a deck of cards. Here are the best buys at the meat counter.

Beef. Find out whether the beef your market sells is graded prime, choice, or select. Prime has the most fat marbled throughout; select, the least. Choose cuts with the word loin or round in the name for the fewest calories and least fat. Eye of round, top round, round tip, top sirloin, bottom round, top loin, and tenderloin are the lowest-fat choices. When selecting ground beef, go for the highest percentage of lean that you can find. Ground top round (97 percent lean) and ground sirloin (90 percent) are better choices than ground round (85 percent) and regular ground beef (73 percent).

Pork. The leanest cuts are tenderloin, sirloin chops, loin roast, top loin chops, loin chops, sirloin roast, rib chops, and rib roast. Check your market for Smithfield Lean Generation Pork, which is specially bred to be low in fat—it's 35 to 61 percent leaner than traditional pork. Despite its reputation, ham is also lean, as long as the exterior fat has been trimmed off. Bacon? Regular, no. Canadian bacon, yes—it's made from cured pork loin.

Veal. The cuts that are lowest in fat include arm, blade, steak, rib roast, loin chops, and cutlets. Cook veal in ways that keep it lean—that means not making a habit of veal cordon bleu (veal stuffed with ham and cheese) or veal Oscar (veal topped with crab and buttery béarnaise sauce).

Lamb. Look for arm chops, loin chops, shank, and leg roast. Grill the chops, braise the shank, and make vegetable-rich stew with the leg meat.

Lean Menu-Makers

You may have heard it before, but it bears repeating: Treat meat as a condiment, not as the centerpiece of your meals. Combine it with lots of grains and vegetables for satisfying, lower-calorie meals. Additionally, alter your meat preparation and cooking techniques to curb calories. Here's how.

- Grill, broil, or roast meat on a rack. Fat will drip off into the pan and won't be reabsorbed by the meat.

- Use nonstick cookware and nonstick spray to minimize the need for added fat when sautéing or browning meat.

- Another idea for sautéing or browning meat: Use a small amount of fruit juice, wine, or broth.

- Brown ground beef as usual, breaking up the meat as it cooks. Transfer to a colander to drain well, then remove even more fat by rinsing with warm water. Pat the beef dry with paper towels before continuing with your recipe.

- Always trim as much fat from meat as possible before cooking.

- Tenderize lower-fat cuts of meat by marinating them in acidic liquids such as juice (orange, lemon, grapefruit, white grape, pineapple, tomato, or vegetable), vinegar, wine, or vinegar-based reduced-fat salad dressing. Or combine juice with broth for a less fruity marinade.

- Combine three ounces of lean beef or pork per serving with a generous amount of vegetables for a stir-fry. Cook the meat with a minimum of oil in a nonstick pan. Add the vegetables and stir-fry until crisp-tender. Serve over cooked rice.

Make It *Better*

Banish-the-Fat Beef Stew

MAKES 4 SERVINGS

Per serving

335 calories

6.9 grams of fat

(18 percent of

calories from fat)

When it comes to beef, a little bit goes a long way toward helping you reach your shape-up goals, especially when it comes "packaged" with tons of soul-satisfying potatoes and vegetables. You probably have most of these ingredients on hand. This streamlined recipe is great for nights when your only other time-saving alternative might be a fast-food burger and a shake.

4   small red potatoes, each cut into 6 wedges

1   medium turnip, peeled and cut into chunks

1   medium parsnip, peeled and cut into chunks

1   cup frozen peeled pearl onions

3   medium carrots, peeled and cut into chunks

1   cup drained canned tomatoes

1¾   cups defatted reduced-sodium beef broth

1   tablespoon red wine vinegar

2   cloves garlic, crushed

1   bay leaf

½   teaspoon dried thyme

½   teaspoon freshly ground black pepper

12   ounces lean, trimmed beef top round or sirloin, cut into ½" cubes

1   tablespoon all-purpose flour

1   tablespoon olive oil

In a large, heavy saucepan, combine the potatoes, turnip, parsnip, onions, carrots, tomatoes, broth, vinegar, half the garlic, the bay leaf, ¼ teaspoon of the thyme, and ¼ teaspoon of the pepper. Break up the tomatoes with the edge of a spoon. Cover and bring to a boil over high heat. Reduce the heat to medium and simmer for 25 minutes, or until the vegetables are just tender.

Meanwhile, toss the beef cubes with the remaining garlic and the remaining ¼ teaspoon each of the thyme and black pepper. Dredge the seasoned beef cubes with the flour.

In a large, heavy skillet, warm the oil over high heat until it's very hot but not smoking. Add the beef and sauté for 5 minutes, or until the beef is browned on the outside and medium-rare on the inside.

Add the beef to the vegetables, reduce the heat to medium-low, and simmer for 5 minutes, or until the vegetables are fully tender and the flavors are blended. Remove the bay leaf before serving.

- Skewer meat to make it go farther. Shish kebab any combination of meat (three ounces per serving is plenty) and vegetables. Serve over couscous or rice.

- Prepare your favorite stew with half the required meat, substituting diced potatoes and carrots in its place.

- Concoct a steak Caesar salad by tossing together lean roast beef cut into strips, chopped romaine lettuce, a little grated Parmesan cheese, low-fat croutons, and fat-free Caesar salad dressing.

Weight-Friendly Substitutions

Even when you're using lean meat, don't get carried away. Make a habit of cutting the amount you use by trying protein-rich substitutes, like the following.

- Use marinated firm tofu in traditional meat and vegetable stir-fries. Serve over rice.

- Make tacos and burritos with only half the meat. Toss in rinsed canned beans to make up the difference. Likewise, prepare your favorite chili recipe with half meat and half beans.

- Substitute the following for one ounce of meat: one large egg, one-quarter cup egg substitute, one ounce chicken or turkey, one ounce seafood, one-half cup cooked dried beans (including lentils and split peas), one-quarter cup nonfat or low-fat cottage cheese (two ounces), eight ounces nonfat or low-fat yogurt, or one ounce of tofu, tempeh, or textured vegetable protein.

- Use your slow cooker to make meat and vegetable meals. The long, slow cooking time tenderizes lean cuts of meat.

- Substitute rice for half the meat in stuffed peppers.

- Replace some of the ground beef in pasta sauces and meat pies with ground turkey breast.

New Foods to Try

Feeling adventurous? Consider game meats. Venison, elk, bison, and rabbit are exceptionally lean. Venison, elk, and bison may be made as pot roasts or as chops, and rabbit is tasty braised. If you're timid about trying them "straight up," use them in mixed dishes such as stews and tacos.

Soybean products, such as tofu and tempeh, have gone mainstream and are good replacements for some of the meat in recipes. Try them in stir-fries, chili, and pasta sauces. The same goes for textured vegetable protein crumbles, which mimic ground meat in shape and protein content.

Dining Out

Whether it's fast food or fine dining, there's generally enough meat in one serving at a restaurant to satisfy your entire day's allowance—if not more. Few women need more than 6 ounces of meat, chicken, or seafood a day, but restaurants serve far more—up to 16 ounces at some steak houses. Rather than staying home, step out with these strategies in mind.

Before you take a bite of your steak, cut it in half. Ask for a doggie bag, and put half the meat in it before you start eating. You'll avoid the temptation of finishing off food solely because it's sitting on your plate.

Steer clear of offers to "supersize" any meal, especially one that contains meat. It will always be too much for one person.

At breakfast or brunch, shave calories by requesting lean ham or Canadian bacon instead of bacon or sausage.

Go Japanese and save. Select shabu-shabu, a simmered dish with meat; sukiyaki, which is stir-fried; and yakitori dishes, which are grilled. Add plenty of plain rice and clear soup to fill you up. At Mexican restaurants, fajitas are a good choice because they combine meat with vegetables and a grain (tortillas). Skip the sour cream and guacamole.

Milk and Dairy

Milk is more than a beverage. It's a snack (cheese or yogurt), a condiment (cream cheese or sour cream), and a dessert (ice cream). For women, milk and dairy foods supply hefty amounts of calcium, much needed for strong bones, plus decent amounts of muscle-building protein and essential vitamins B_{12} and riboflavin. As a bonus, milk is fortified with vitamin D, which offers added bone protection. After all, you may want to banish your belly, butt, or thighs, but not at the expense of the bones underneath. So in your quest for a beautiful body, you want to include milk and dairy foods in your diet.

If you're not careful, however, milk, like all animal foods, can serve up fair amounts of fat and calories with the valuable vitamins and minerals it supplies. And if you have trouble digesting lactose, the sugar naturally found in milk, you can end up

Best and Worst Milk and Dairy Selections

From the examples shown here, it's easy to see how choosing the right milk and dairy foods can make a big difference in the amount of fat and calories you consume. As a general rule, when you're shopping in the diary aisle, look for milk that contains no fat and 85 calories per eight ounces, coffee creamer that offers 1.5 grams of fat and 45 calories per tablespoon, sour cream and cream cheese that contains no fat and 14 calories per tablespoon, yogurt that contains no fat and 100 calories per eight ounces, and fat-free frozen yogurt and ice cream that contains no fat and 140 calories per half-cup serving.

Best Choices

Food Item	Portion	Calories	Grams of Fat
Nonfat milk	1 cup	85	0.4
Low-fat buttermilk	1 cup	99	2.2
Sherbet	½ cup	102	1.5
Low-fat milk	1 cup	102	2.6
Unsweetened nonfat yogurt	1 cup	137	0.4
Soy milk	1 cup	141	2.8
Low-fat chocolate milk	1 cup	158	2.5

Worst Choices

Food Item	Portion	Calories	Grams of Fat
Sweetened yogurt	8 oz.	230	3.0
Premium ice cream	½ cup	220	15.0
Nondairy coffee creamer	2 Tbsp.	88	5.6
Cream	2 Tbsp.	60	6.0
Full-fat sour cream	2 Tbsp.	60	5.0
Half-and-half	2 Tbsp.	40	7.0

with bloating, abdominal cramps, gas, or diarrhea. In this chapter, you'll find out how to sidestep both problems, so that you can make milk a part of your Eating Lean plan. (For information on cheese, see page 36.)

Shopping Smarts

If you're watching your weight, you're probably already buying fat-free or reduced-fat milk. With 8.1 grams of fat and 150 calories per cup, whole milk gives you almost as many calories and fat as a handful of potato chips. Whole milk has only a rare place in your Eating Lean plan—as a substitute for cream in the occasional special recipe, for example. Instead, look for:

Reduced-fat milk. At 4.7 grams of fat and 121 calories per cup, 2 percent milk (reduced-fat) is a great intermediate step in coming down from whole milk to nonfat. Switching to fat-free (zero gram of fat and 85 calories per cup) or nonfat milk (less than 0.5 gram of fat and 85 calories per cup) can help you shed the pounds that shave off inches effortlessly. If you drink three glasses of milk daily, switching from 2 percent to fat-free milk will help you shed a pound every month or so. Note that skim milk is now called fat-free milk or nonfat milk on labels.

If you've avoided nonfat (skim) milk in the past because it tasted watery to you, look for protein-fortified products—the extra protein gives them the rich body of whole or reduced-fat milk, with less fat and calories.

Fat-free evaporated milk. Does your pumpkin pie recipe (or the recipe for some other sweet treat) call for evaporated milk? Substitute the fat-free variety—the only thing you'll miss is the calories. Fat-free evaporated milk works well in cream sauces, too, saving loads of calories.

Coffee creamer. Don't let the nondairy tag fool you—coffee creamers do contain fat. If you drink coffee on a regular basis, you're better off using milk. Suppose, for example, that you normally use one tablespoon of nondairy powdered creamer in your coffee daily, and you drink two cups of coffee a day. If you switch to two tablespoons of reduced-fat milk instead, you'll drop a pound effortlessly in about seven weeks. (And that doesn't count all the other pounds you'll lose making other, more significant changes in your diet.)

Or look for fat-free flavored coffee creamers, such as café mocha, Irish cream, and amaretto.

Sour cream. At 2.5 grams of fat and 28 calories per tablespoon, sour cream isn't so bad provided that you limit how much you use. By substituting the lower-fat version, you can either use more or save calories. Making guacamole or sour cream dip? Use reduced-fat sour cream (1.8 grams of fat and 20 calories per tablespoon) or nonfat sour cream (zero gram of fat and 13 calories per tablespoon). Switching from regular sour cream to nonfat practically slashes calories in half and wipes out a whopping six grams of fat in two tablespoons—the amount most people use on a baked potato.

Need a few tricks for enjoying less sour cream—especially if you don't like the low-fat versions? Stretch it out by mixing one tablespoon of the low-fat or full-fat version with salsa. On baked potatoes, try sour cream with picante tomato salsa. On fish, try sour cream with fruit salsa. Or add finely chopped onions, bell peppers, and a small dollop of the real thing. Perhaps you'll soon find that just a teaspoon of the regular or low-fat version is all you need with the extra flavor boost of interesting additions.

Cream cheese. A tablespoon of regular cream cheese has 5 grams of fat and 51 calories. In comparison, fat-free cream cheese harbors a mere trace of fat and 14 calories. (Light, or low-fat, cream cheese supplies 2.5 grams of fat and 35 calories.) If you're like many people, you may have a hard time making the switch to fat-free, preferring instead the low-fat variety. So compromise: Buy the low-fat and fat-free versions and mix them, creating a version with 1.4 grams of fat and 25 calories. As your tastebuds adjust over time, you'll be able to make the switch all the way down to the fat-free version.

You might also want to try fruit- or herb-flavored low-fat versions, like raspberry or strawberry flavored cream cheese.

Yogurt. Shopping for yogurt is more complicated than buying milk, cream, sour cream, or cheese. The choices are mind-boggling: full-fat, reduced-fat, nonfat. With fruit or fruit syrup—or plain. With sugar or with artificial sweetener. Along with those choices come a range of fat and calorie totals, from three grams of fat and 230 calories for full-fat, naturally sweetened yogurt to as little as zero gram of fat and 100 calories for the nonfat, artificially sweetened variety. Still, scouting out yogurt you like is worth the effort: For busy women, a container of yogurt makes an instant power-packed mini-meal or snack—a much healthier substitute for pastries or vending machine snacks. Further, many women find yogurt easier to digest than milk thanks to the active cultures responsible for fermenting milk into yogurt.

To select yogurt, start by homing in on products that are fat-free. Then check out the calories. Choose a product with no more than 120 calories in eight ounces or 100 calories in six ounces. Or look for plain, vanilla, or lemon nonfat yogurt and slice your own fruit into the container.

Frozen yogurt and ice cream. Saving up calories for a daily dessert helps you stay on the lean eating track. It takes only about 150 calories to satisfy this desire for pleasurable food—just the amount in appropriately chosen frozen yogurt or ice cream. Choosing well means not only ferreting out the best calorie bargain but also the rich flavor that still satisfies in a controlled portion. Experiment with flavors that interest you, such as black raspberry swirl nonfat frozen yogurt or caramel-praline crunch nonfat frozen yogurt. Limit your serving to a half-cup, which uses up under 150 calories and no grams of fat. This is a substantial savings from the 178 calories and 12 grams of fat in a half-cup of regular ice cream—and sometimes even more in richer versions loaded with chocolate and other goodies.

As for real ice cream, save it for topping the occasional hot low-fat fruit compote or crisp. Use only a quarter-cup and enjoy every rich bite slowly.

Lean Menu-Makers

If you don't care to drink milk "straight," there are plenty of other ways to work it into your eating plan.

Breakfast smoothie. Blend one cup of nonfat milk, one cup of frozen fruit (strawberries or raspberries work well), and one banana. This drink also makes a refreshing between-meal power snack.

Hot chocolate. Stir a tablespoon of unsweetened cocoa powder (which supplies less than one gram of fat) and a packet of artificial sweetener into a cup of hot nonfat milk. Or use a packet of fat-free, reduced-calorie hot chocolate mix. As an alternative, you might add a teaspoon or two of vanilla extract and some artificial sweetener to a cup of warm nonfat milk.

Digestion-Friendly Substitutions

Milk sugar, or lactose, is made up of two other sugars, glucose and galactose. The intestinal tract releases an enzyme, called lactase, to break apart the milk sugar; it then sends the sugar subunits through the rest of the metabolic pathway. When this works well, you don't even know it's happening. When a person doesn't produce enough lactase, however, she is often miserable, suffering from abdominal gas and sometimes diarrhea. Fortunately, there are several options for lactose-intolerant people.

■ Buy lactase-treated milk, such as Lactaid and DairyEase 100 (available in many grocery stores). Like other milks, it comes in a range of varieties from full-fat to nonfat, so ferret out that nonfat or fat-free label.

■ Purchase untreated milk and add lactase enzyme drops (available at drug stores).

■ Take a lactase enzyme in pill form (also sold in drug stores) before eating or drinking anything containing milk. Follow the label directions.

■ Try soy milk, which is naturally lactose-free. Soy milk's taste has improved dramatically over the years. To get the most bone-building power from soy milk, choose a variety that has been fortified with calcium, vitamin D, and vitamin B$_{12}$. Look for low-fat versions. (Nonfat soy milk isn't widely available.)

- If you're having a little trouble with intestinal upset after taking antibiotics, the antibiotics may have upset the natural balance of bacteria in your intestinal tract. If so, try acidophilus milk, which is fortified with *Lactobacillus acidophilus* bacteria, thought to restore nature's balance in the intestinal tract. Choose the 1 percent fat version. Low-fat buttermilk also works well to restore healthy bacteria in the gut.

- Buy calcium-fortified orange juice. If you don't or can't drink milk, reach for calcium-fortified OJ, either in the dairy case or as a concentrate in the frozen foods section.

New Foods to Try

Your options go beyond drinking plain milk out of a glass. Consider:

Milk-in-a-box. Individual serving–size milk drinks are an easy way to carry nonfat milk to work or on camping trips. If you like your milk cold, refrigerate or pack it on ice before serving.

Yogurt cheese. Looking for something very low in fat and unique in flavor to spread on your toast or bagel? Spread a coffee filter into a metal strainer and pour in a pint container of nonfat plain, vanilla, or lemon yogurt. Place the strainer in a bowl, cover, and place in the refrigerator overnight. In the morning, you'll find a thick, rich "cheese" that you can spread on breakfast bread.

Stir in herbs, chopped veggies, diced fruit—or any combination of these—for a fat-free party spread.

Chocolate milk. Want something chocolate right now? Keep a quart of low-fat chocolate milk in the refrigerator, and next to it a chilled eight-ounce glass, so when a chocolate craving strikes, you can pour yourself half a glass (four ounces) of chocolate milk and no more, using up just 79 calories.

Dining Out

Don't feel self-conscious about ordering milk when you dine out—it will help you get your requisite quota of calcium for the day. After all, kids do it all the time. If you want fat-free or nonfat milk, not just low-fat milk, be specific. Some servers assume that low-fat is the same as nonfat. While the occasional glass of low-fat milk is fine, the calories add up if you frequently order milk while dining out.

As for sour cream, cream cheese, and yogurt, very few restaurants carry the lower-fat versions. It's better to order these things on the side and use them sparingly. Restaurants serve up about one-quarter cup of sour cream on a baked potato, and they often hide a little butter underneath. So always order on the side and know how to eyeball a tablespoon or two.

Finally, putting cream in your coffee can break your fat budget pretty quickly, especially if you linger over a pot of coffee with a friend. Ask the waitress for a pitcher of skim milk and enjoy even a second pot.

Pasta and Toppings

Capellini, Farfalle, and Orzo. An Italian law firm? No. They're types of pasta—just three of dozens (including the all-American standard, spaghetti). And they're a dieter's dream, despite unfair accusations of being fattening.

Pasta is filling, low in fat, packed with energy-producing complex carbohydrates, and generally cholesterol-free. It's also a good source of B vitamins. You can't go wrong with all that nutrition for about 200 calories per serving. Where you *can* go wrong is topping your tagliatelle with fatty Alfredo, carbonara, pesto, or sausage or other meat sauces.

Shopping Smarts

Happily, you don't have to give pasta the boot when cutting calories. Just keep these things in mind when shopping.

Best and Worst Pasta and Toppings

When you're planning a pasta meal, aim for about 300 calories per serving and four grams of fat or fewer (although you can afford a few more calories if the fat content is much lower).

Best Choices			
Pasta or Topping	Portion	Calories	Grams of Fat
Sapsago cheese	1 oz. (2 Tbsp.)	16	0.5
Parmesan cheese	1 Tbsp.	23	1.5
Pasta primavera (with garlic and oil, not a cream-based sauce)	About 3 Tbsp. sauce over 1 cup cooked pasta	107	4.0
Pasta with clam sauce (water, clams, oil, and spices)	¼ cup sauce over 1 cup cooked pasta	169	5.5
Pasta	1 cup cooked	197	1.0
Linguini with red clam sauce	½ cup sauce over 1 cup cooked pasta	257	2.0
Pasta with marinara sauce	½ cup sauce over 1 cup cooked pasta	268	2.6

Worst Choices			
Pasta or Topping	Portion	Calories	Grams of Fat
Fettuccine Alfredo	½ cup ready-to-serve sauce over 1 cup cooked pasta	437	21.0
Cheese manicotti	11.7-oz. frozen entrée	394	15.2
Spaghetti carbonara	½ cup sauce over 1 cup cooked pasta	378	11.5
Cheese tortellini	4.5-oz. frozen entrée	268	10.9
Pesto sauce	¼ cup	157	13.1
Meat sauce	½ cup	68	2.0

Pasta. With so many shapes and sizes available, you can have pasta every night for weeks without ever repeating a meal. Buy strands like spaghetti and fettuccine, tubes like penne and ziti, various colored spirals, and shells of all sizes. Don't forget lasagna noodles and elbow macaroni for casseroles, cannelloni and manicotti for stuffing, and small shapes like orzo, stars, and acini di peppe for soups.

Check labels carefully when buying fresh pasta, especially stuffed types like ravioli, cappelletti, and tortellini. Fresh pasta often contains eggs and is generally higher in fat than dried. In addition, the fillings in stuffed varieties are usually high in fat.

Sauce. Stick with low-fat meatless tomato sauces rather than creamy ones like Alfredo and pesto. Even reduced-fat pesto can have four grams of fat in just one tablespoon. Fat content can vary widely among tomato sauces, so check labels. Look for sauces with four grams or less of fat per half-cup serving. Be especially vigilant when reading labels for creamy sauces. Often the serving size has been reduced to a quarter-cup—less than you might actually use.

Pasta-ready tomatoes are also a good choice and are very low in fat. Look for flavors other than Italian for a change of pace. Taco-style Mexican sauce can give your pasta a whole new identity.

Cheese. What's pasta without cheese (besides much lower in fat)? If it's just not Italian without a dusting of cheese, make it a really flavorful type. Packaged grated Parmesan and Romano are okay in a pinch—there are even some reduced-fat varieties. But freshly grated or shredded cheese has far more flavor, so you can actually use less and still get great taste. Buy a thin wedge of really good cheese (like Parmigiano-Reggiano or Pecorino Romano) and grate it at the table. Tightly wrapped, it will keep in the refrigerator or freezer for weeks, so you can always have some on hand. Almost as flavorful is Parmesan or Romano that has already been shredded; buy it in small quantities.

An interesting alternative to Parmesan is sapsago, a very hard cone-shaped cheese from Switzerland that's low in fat. It has a light green color and a pungent herbal flavor that adds unexpected punch to pasta.

Lean Menu-Makers

To make a calorie-conscious meal, start with about one cup of cooked pasta per serving. Top with a half-cup of fat-free marinara sauce that you've mixed with two ounces of lean ground beef or diced cooked chicken (leftovers work great for this) and a half-cup of sautéed onions and mushrooms. Add a salad of flavorful greens like Romaine, escarole, arugula, and radicchio with fat-free dressing—and there's dinner. Other ways to feast on pasta without piling on the pounds:

- Use a can of drained minced clams as a pasta topping. (Warm them in a saucepan with minced garlic and fresh parsley.) Reserve a little of the liquid to moisten the pasta with instead of oil.

- Mix heated marinara sauce with pureed low-fat cottage cheese. You'll get creaminess and pleasing texture without a lot of calories. Or instead of cottage cheese, mix in some crumbled firm tofu.

- Stir pureed red peppers into tomato sauce for an extra helping of beta-carotene (an immunity-enhancing vitamin) with hardly any calories.

- Prepare a quick soup by mixing cooked orzo, diced cooked carrots and celery, leftover diced chicken, and reduced-sodium chicken broth. Serve with a large fruit salad for a balanced meal.

- Toss together one cup of cooked spaghetti, one teaspoon of olive oil, one-half cup of cooked chickpeas, and one tablespoon of grated Parmesan cheese for a fast and easy entrée.

- Puree cooked vegetables with enough broth to make a light sauce. Season with herbs and toss with cooked pasta. Top with a sprinkling of Parmesan.

- Serve up to one-half cup of cooked pasta as a side dish. Toss with fresh or dried herbs and one teaspoon of butter or grated Parmesan.

Make It *Better*

Beef and Spinach Lasagna

MAKES 4 SERVINGS

Per serving

595 calories

12.5 grams of fat

(19 percent of

calories from fat)

A typical slab of lasagna can easily run you as much as 24 grams of fat. With this slimmed-down version, you can serve the whole family while you stick to your Eating Lean plan.

2 cups reduced-fat ricotta cheese

1 10-ounce package frozen chopped spinach, thawed and squeezed dry

½ teaspoon ground black pepper

½ teaspoon ground nutmeg

1 pound lean ground beef top round

1 teaspoon crushed red-pepper flakes

⅛ teaspoon salt

1 26-ounce jar fat-free tomato-basil sauce

1 8-ounce box no-boil lasagna noodles

5 leaves fresh sage, coarsely chopped

1 cup shredded fat-free mozzarella cheese

1 plum tomato, thinly sliced

5 large leaves fresh basil

¼ cup grated Romano cheese

Preheat the oven to 375°F. Coat a 9" × 9" baking dish with nonstick spray.

In a medium bowl, combine the ricotta, spinach, black pepper, and nutmeg. Mix well.

Place a large nonstick skillet over medium heat until hot. Crumble the beef into the skillet. Cook, stirring to break up the meat, for 4 to 6 minutes, or until the meat is no longer pink. Drain off any accumulated fat. Add the red-pepper flakes and salt to the beef. Mix well.

Spread ½ cup of sauce in the prepared baking dish. Place 3 or 4 of the lasagna noodles on the sauce so their edges don't overlap. Top with half of the remaining tomato sauce and all of the beef. Sprinkle with half of the sage. Top with another layer of noodles. Spread the ricotta mixture over the noodles and sprinkle with ½ cup of the mozzarella.

Top with a third layer of noodles and the remaining tomato sauce. Top with the tomato, basil, and the remaining sage. Sprinkle evenly with the Romano and the remaining ½ cup of mozzarella.

Cover tightly with foil and bake for 20 to 25 minutes, or until bubbling and heated through.

Weight-Friendly Substitutions

Here's how to cut fat in some of your favorite pasta recipes.

- Replace ground beef in pasta sauces with ground turkey breast. You'll save about 65 calories per three-ounce portion of meat.

- Let steamed mushrooms, onions, and bell peppers stand in for some of the meat in pasta sauce.

- For an awesome Alfredo sauce, substitute low-fat cottage cheese or ricotta cheese blended with milk for the cream in a traditional recipe.

- Slim down pesto sauce by substituting chicken broth for some of the oil and using fewer nuts and less cheese. Or dilute purchased reduced-fat pesto sauce with chicken broth. Whatever method you choose, use pesto sauce sparingly since it will never be truly low-fat.

- Make homemade macaroni and cheese with fat-free milk and reduced-fat sharp Cheddar cheese. Add chopped cooked vegetables for extra fiber.

- Whip up pasta salads with fat-free Italian dressing instead of mayonnaise. Add canned, packed-in-water tuna and chopped vegetables for a meal in a dish.

New Foods to Try

Think beyond spaghetti, ravioli, and lasagna. Try whole-wheat and spinach pastas. They contain up to three times the fiber of regular pasta. Fiber is a dieter's friend, since it keeps you full longer. All sorts of other colors and flavors are available, from squid ink to beet to garlic herb. The more tasty the pasta itself, the less sauce you need. And don't forget the non-Italian types of noodles, like Japanese soba (made from buckwheat flour), udon (made from wheat or corn meal), somen and ramen (made from wheat), rice, mung bean, and others.

Dining Out

In this country, Italian food is synonymous with large portions, and few pasta menu items are low in fat. Your best bet is pasta topped with plain marinara or fresh tomato sauce. If that's not appealing, order an appetizer-size portion of another pasta dish and supplement it with a large green salad with fat-free dressing or a large bowl of minestrone soup. If you can't get a smaller portion, eat only part of your entrée and take the rest home for another day.

Avoid cheese-filled cannelloni, tortellini, ravioli, and manicotti. Steer clear of anything labeled Alfredo or carbonara. Be aware that some sauces that look light actually have a lot of oil in them—ask about preparation. Stick with entrées featuring lots of fresh vegetables (like pasta primavera in a light oil sauce) as well as low-fat protein sources like fish, shrimp, and clams.

Pizza and Toppings

Everyone likes pizza. But how does it fit into your plan to slim down—and stay that way? Quite nicely, thank you.

Pizza is a nutritional powerhouse. The crust contains B vitamins and complex carbohydrates for energy. The tomato sauce supplies carbohydrates, vitamin C, lycopene (a natural substance that appears to protect against cancer), and little fat. The cheese provides protein as well as much-needed calcium to strengthen your bones. Topped off with vegetables, pizza serves as a meal in itself, providing fiber and vitamin A. For added protein, you can add lean meat or seafood. What more could a busy woman want?

A lot less fat. Fat is pizza's pitfall. That doesn't rule it out of your eating plan, however. With a bit of nutrition know-how, you can curtail pizza's calories and still satisfy yourself.

Shopping Smarts

It pays to purchase healthy pizza ingredients. That way, you can concoct a nutritious and satisfying meal on a moment's notice—and for a lot less than a pizzeria pie costs (in dollars and calories). Here's what to buy.

Crust. Look in the refrigerated case for prepared pizza crust. There are ready-formed ones and those

Best and Worst Pizza and Toppings

Pizza can fit in nicely with your Eating Lean plan. Your best bets give you less than 300 calories and 12 grams of fat per slice, including the topping. On the other hand, if you're on a 1,600-calorie-a-day menu plan and you treat yourself to a deep-dish personal pan pizza, that amounts to more than one-third of your calories for the day, even without a beverage. So plan accordingly.

Best Choices			
Pizza	Portion	Calories	Grams of Fat
Thin crust cheese pizza with peppers, mushrooms, and onions (fast-food)	1 slice (⅛ of pie)	190	8.0
Homemade pizza (with low-fat prepared pizza shell, fat-free sauce, 8 oz. part-skim mozzarella cheese, and 1 cup steamed vegetables)	1 slice (⅙ of pie)	211	3.1
Thin crust cheese pizza (fast-food)	1 slice (⅛ of pie)	225	10.0
Thin crust cheese pizza with 1 oz. of Canadian bacon	1 slice (⅛ of pie)	268	12.0

Worst Choices			
Pizza	Portion	Calories	Grams of Fat
Deep-dish cheese pizza	one 7-in. individual pie	625	44.0
Deep-dish pepperoni pizza (frozen)	one 7-in. individual pie	525	19.5
Stuffed-crust pizza with any meat topping (fast-food)	1 slice (⅛ of pie)	440	17.0

in a tube. Either way, check labels to find the lowest in fat. Sometimes plain crusts are also available in the freezer section. Don't forget the box mixes; prepare them with less oil than is called for in the recipe.

Sauce. There are lots of low-fat pizza and pasta sauces from which to choose. Look for ones with four grams or less of fat per half-cup. Try different flavors to give your pizza extra sparkle.

Cheese. Pick up reduced-fat shredded cheeses. Mozzarella is standard, but it needn't be your only choice. There are good Italian and Mexican cheese blends, for instance, that make terrific pizza. Limit cheese to eight ounces per large pizza. If there's a really flavorful full-fat hard cheese you love, such as sharp Cheddar, go ahead and get it. Just use less—it's easy when the cheese is packed with flavor. (Other assertive, nontraditional cheeses to try include Asiago, feta, and blue.)

Other toppings. Favor veggies like onions, bell peppers, mushrooms, and pickled hot peppers—even a few olives, if you like. Buy super-lean ground beef or ground turkey breast. They're better meat choices than pepperoni, sausage, meatballs, and salami. Brown the ground meat in a nonstick skillet and drain it well before sprinkling it over the crust. Canadian bacon and lean ham are good replacements for regular bacon.

If you'll be making pizza soon after you shop, stop at the supermarket's salad bar for already sliced onions, peppers, mushrooms, and other vegetables.

Frozen pizza. Steer clear of frozen deep-dish pizza; the fat is out of sight. If you must purchase frozen pizza, pick the thin-crust varieties. Enhance their nutrition by adding steamed or sautéed vegetables, lean ground beef, or diced cooked chicken. (Leftovers work great as pizza toppings.)

Lean Menu-Makers

Having nothing but pizzeria pizza for dinner is a mistake—and a lost opportunity. Instead, limit yourself to two slices and round out the meal with a substantial tossed salad (throw in lots of crisp vegetables) with low-fat dressing. Or you could serve a side-dish vegetable like steamed broccoli or baby carrots, in addition to a veggie topping.

Leftover pizza is a portable feast. Add a piece of fruit to a slice of reduced-fat pizza, and you have a healthy, light meal to eat on the run.

For an instant no-fuss pizza, top a sliced English muffin or slice of pita bread with fat-free pizza sauce and one ounce of reduced-fat cheese. Heat under the broiler or in a toaster oven until the cheese melts. Add fruit and some raw chopped vegetables to round out the meal.

Weight-Friendly Substitutions

Unless you're careful, pizza tends to be top-heavy with calories and fat. Here are some slimming substitutions.

- Sun-dried tomatoes can stand in for pepperoni. They have a similar look, but the intensely flavored tomatoes are much lower in fat. (Be sure to drain them of as much oil as possible.)
- Instead of sausage, try eggplant, portobello mushrooms, broccoli, jalapeño peppers, spinach, tomato slices, artichoke hearts, or zucchini. Pair drained crushed pineapple or fresh pineapple pieces with lean ham, or have shrimp or clams instead of meat.
- Skip the cheese and pile on more vegetables to take up the slack. If it's calcium you're concerned about, have a glass of fat-free milk or a scoop of low-fat cottage cheese with your pizza.

New Foods to Try

Select whole-wheat crust whenever possible. It adds fiber and a nutty flavor to your pizza pie. Low-fat tortillas and pita rounds make great personal-size pizza crusts.

Dining Out

It's Friday night, and cooking is the last thing on your mind. Your gang is clamoring for pizza. How can you refuse? Don't—even when weight control is your goal. Banishing your favorite foods in the name of banishing your belly is a foolish strategy that is doomed to failure in the long run. You can indulge in pizza without dietary disaster. Here's how.

Make It *Better*

Very Veggie Pizza

MAKES 6 SERVINGS

Per serving

211 calories

3.1 grams of fat

(13 percent of

calories from fat)

When you want pizza in a hurry, use a premade pizza shell from your supermarket and load it up with a helping of veggies sautéed in minimal amounts of fat. The payoff for your efforts: Compared to pizzeria pizza with regular cheese and pepperoni, you'll save 190 calories and 17 grams of fat per slice.

¼ **cup low-fat spaghetti sauce**	¼ **cup thinly sliced shiitake or white mushrooms**
1 **Italian bread pizza shell**	¼ **cup broccoli florets**
¼ **cup thinly sliced zucchini**	¼ **cup thinly sliced red bell pepper**
¼ **cup thinly sliced yellow squash**	½ **cup shredded part-skim mozzarella cheese**
¼ **cup thinly sliced red onion**	2 **teaspoons Romano cheese**

Preheat the oven to 400°F. Spread the sauce on the pizza shell. Set aside.

Spray a nonstick skillet with nonstick olive oil spray. Add the zucchini, squash, onion, mushrooms, broccoli, and pepper and sauté over medium heat until tender-crisp. Arrange on the pizza shell; top with the mozzarella and Romano. Bake for 4 to 5 minutes or until hot and bubbling. Let stand 5 minutes before cutting.

Deep-six the deep-dish pie. Sack the stuffed-crust pizzas. Put off the personal pan varieties. Stick with thin-crust choices, even if it means ordering a pizza that suits your needs while others are eating higher-calorie choices. Limit yourself to two slices. You can always take the leftovers home for other days.

Order only half the cheese. To make the pizza more interesting and nutritious, request double the amount of tomato sauce and at least two vegetable toppings.

To keep from getting carried away and eating too much pizza, always order a large garden salad with low-fat dressing and unsweetened iced tea or other low-calorie beverage or water. Nibble on the salad before your pizza arrives. If you know that a low-fat salad won't be available, eat a piece of fruit before you leave home so you're not ravenous when the pizza arrives.

If you just cannot resist a high-fat pizza, don't despair. Eat only a slice or two, then make up for the indulgence by curbing your calorie consumption and exercising a bit more in the following days. Remember that no single meal or food makes or breaks weight-control efforts. It's what you eat in the long run that counts the most. Cutting out all high-fat favorites actually creates a destructive dietary backlash that leads to weight gain.

Potatoes and Toppings

Pity potatoes. Although one of America's favorite foods, spuds don't get the respect they deserve—from dieters or anyone else. (Why are lazy people called couch potatoes? No respect for the humble spud.) The truth is that these tubers are tasty, versatile, convenient, and nutritious. But much like pasta, potatoes are often maligned because of the fattening company they keep.

That's too bad, because potatoes are a nutritional bargain. For about 150 calories, a baked white potato contributes complex carbohydrates and fiber, supplies more potassium than a medium banana, and

Best and Worst Potatoes and Toppings

When figuring out how to serve potatoes, aim for 180 calories or fewer per serving and fewer than four grams of fat, including the topping.

Best Choices			
Potato	**Portion**	**Calories**	**Grams of Fat**
Boiled potatoes	1 cup	113	0.1
Oven-baked sweet potato wedges	4 oz.	117	0.1
Mashed potatoes with fat-free milk	1 cup	124	0.2
Candied sweet potato wedges	3.75 oz.	144	3.4
Medium plain baked potato	5.5 oz.	145	0.2
Boiled red potatoes, skin on, tossed with 1 tsp. margarine or butter	1 cup	149	4.1
Medium baked sweet potato topped with 1 tsp. brown sugar	5.5 oz.	156	0.2
Medium baked potato with 1 Tbsp. light sour cream	5.5 oz.	165	2.0

Worst Choices			
Potato	**Portion**	**Calories**	**Grams of Fat**
Large baked potato stuffed with chili and cheese	7 oz.	482	22.0
Potatoes au gratin	1 cup	323	18.6
Potato chips	2 oz.	304	19.6
Large french fries (fast-food)	6 oz.	259	12.6
Mashed potatoes with butter and whole milk	1 cup	223	8.9
Scalloped potatoes	1 cup	211	9.0

Make It *Better*

Buttermilk Mashed Potatoes

MAKES 4 SERVINGS

Per serving

96 calories

0.5 gram of fat

(5 percent of calories

from fat)

This slimmed-down version of mashed potatoes will satisfy the staunchest meat-and-potatoes fan at your house. Compared to mashed potatoes made with butter and whole milk, you save 127 calories and 8.4 grams of fat per serving.

1 **pound (about 3 medium) baking potatoes, such as russets, peeled and cut into 1-inch chunks**	¼ **cup low-fat buttermilk**
1 **cup water**	2 **tablespoons thinly sliced scallions**
½ **cup defatted chicken broth**	⅛ **teaspoon freshly ground pepper, preferably white**
2 **garlic cloves, unpeeled**	**Large pinch of salt**

In a medium saucepan, combine the potatoes, water, broth, and garlic. Cover and bring to a boil over high heat. Reduce the heat to medium-low and simmer for 12 to 15 minutes, or until the potatoes are fork-tender.

Just before the potatoes are done, place the buttermilk in a small, heavy saucepan and warm it over low heat.

Drain the potatoes well; discard the garlic cloves. Return the potatoes to the pan and mash them with a potato masher or in a food processor.

Stir the warmed buttermilk, scallions, pepper, and salt into the potatoes and serve.

---

provides one-third of the Daily Value for vitamin C. All that for zero fat and cholesterol. Sweet potatoes provide comparable nutrition, with an added bonus: a bounty of beta-carotene. Beta-carotene is converted to vitamin A by the body and is considered a powerful weapon in fighting off diseases like cancer.

When barely processed (such as when baked whole), potatoes retain their stellar qualities. Unfortunately, Americans prefer their potatoes highly processed as french fries and potato puffs or smothered in high-fat sauces and toppings. Processed potatoes lose their vitamin C, and unless you practice portion control, they pack on pounds.

It all boils down to this: In their freshest forms, white potatoes and sweet potatoes are innocent of all the fattening charges leveled against them. As long as you don't eat them too often in their high-fat versions—scalloped, au gratin, or fried, for example—potatoes can most certainly be part of your successful slimming plan.

Shopping Smarts

Resist the urge to stock up on frozen potatoes, dehydrated packaged products, canned potatoes, and chips. Whenever possible, use whole raw potatoes. Here's what to look for.

White potatoes. Choose only the best. That means looking for spuds that are clean, firm, smooth, and regular in shape. Pass up any with wrinkles, sprouts, cracks, soft dark areas, or green spots. Pick a variety for different uses. Long whites are good all-purpose potatoes with a waxy texture. Round whites and reds are good for boiling. Russets are the perfect baking potatoes. Store your potatoes in a cool, dark, well-ventilated place, where they'll last for several weeks. Don't keep them in the fridge, and don't store them near onions or they'll go bad faster.

Sweet potatoes. These potatoes should be firm, with bright, uniformly colored skin. There are two main types: moist and dry. The moist ones have orange skin and flesh and are usually called yams, although they aren't true yams. The dry sweet potatoes have yellowish-tan skin and yellow flesh that's much drier and crumbly when cooked. Store both kinds unwrapped in a cool, dry, dark place for up to a week. Because sweet potatoes are high in beta-carotene, they deserve weekly appearances on your table.

Processed products. Instant mashed potatoes, scalloped and au gratin potato mixes, and ready-to-cook hash browns are certainly convenient. If you prepare them without added butter or margarine, they're actually low in fat. Their main drawbacks are low fiber, high sodium, and no vitamin C. Think of them as stand-ins for when you don't have time to prepare fresh potatoes. Treat potato chips—even the fat-free ones—as just that: treats. They don't count as a vegetable!

Lean Menu-Makers

Relegated to the role of side dish, potatoes are often given short shrift by dieters. But baked, boiled, or mashed potatoes can be low-fat fillers, actually helping you to avoid overeating higher-calorie foods. They go with just about any type of meat, poultry, and seafood. And potatoes can be meals in themselves. Here are some super supper solutions.

- Grill potatoes to accompany burgers. Wrap them in foil and grill whole. Or slice and mix with peppers, onions, mushrooms, and herbs; wrap in foil and toss on the grill. Sweet potatoes work just as well as white.

- Serve up roast chicken, turkey tenders, or meat loaf with great low-fat mashed potatoes. Add one or two peeled garlic cloves to the pot when cooking the potatoes. Mash the garlic along with the potatoes. Leave out the butter or margarine and replace it with creamy, buttery-tasting low-fat buttermilk. (Or use nonfat sour cream, fat-free milk, or evaporated fat-free milk instead of the buttermilk.) For even more flavor, boil the potatoes in nonfat chicken or beef broth.

- Make quick, homemade warm potato salad for a picnic. Microwave sliced potatoes until tender and toss with fat-free Italian dressing and chopped scallions.

- Another picnic special: Toss sliced or cubed cooked potatoes with fat-free mayonnaise and chopped hard-boiled eggs (use only the whites for zero cholesterol and less fat). Add diced vegetables, such as onions, red and green bell peppers, and celery.

- Instead of preparing candied sweet potatoes, serve roast turkey or lean ham with mashed baked sweet potatoes mixed with crushed pineapple. Other ideas: Mash sweet potatoes with orange juice, sprinkle with a smattering of brown sugar, and bake at 350°F until warm. Or layer mashed sweet potatoes on top of pineapple rings and bake until the pineapple softens.

- Make a meal out of a potato. Scoop the flesh out of one large baked spud, leaving the skin as a shell. Mix with 1/2 cup low-fat cottage cheese, 1/2 cup chopped steamed vegetables, and fresh or dried herbs. Spoon into the potato skin and sprinkle with one tablespoon of reduced-fat Cheddar cheese. Heat in an oven or microwave until the cheese melts.

- For a lean vegetarian entrée, halve a baked potato and top it with one cup of meatless chili. Add a large green salad with fat-free dressing or a fruit salad to complete the meal.

- Create your own "pouch potato" meals. Cube a medium potato and mix with three ounces of lean meat or poultry. Add one cup of diced or thinly sliced vegetables. Moisten with low-fat gravy, broth, soy sauce, or other reduced-fat flavoring. Wrap tightly in a large sheet of foil. Place on a baking sheet and bake at 450°F for 35 minutes.

Weight-Friendly Substitutions

Here's how to pep up potatoes without blowing your calorie budget.

- Top baked potatoes with one tablespoon of light sour cream instead of butter and save 80 calories and eight grams of fat. Or sprinkle spuds with butter-flavored flakes.

- Mix plain nonfat yogurt, chopped cucumbers, dried dill, salt, and pepper for a terrific tuber topper. Other ideas: soy sauce and sesame seeds; sautéed mushrooms and onions; fat-free cottage cheese mixed with chives; salsa and nonfat sour cream.

- Opt for a medium baked potato with one tablespoon of low-fat sour cream instead of 20 french fries—you save 35 calories and 5.5 grams of fat.

- Cube sweet and white potatoes and toss with a little olive oil. Roast at 400°F for about 20 minutes, or until tender.

- Make your own potato chips. Slice white or sweet potatoes into very thin rounds and toss with a drizzle of canola oil. Place in a single layer on a baking sheet and bake at 400°F until crispy, about 10 minutes.

- Use cubed sweet potatoes as a stand-in for some of the beef in traditional beef stew and soup recipes.

- Snack on sweet potatoes instead of potato chips or fries. Keep baked sweet potatoes in the refrigerator. Peel and slice for a sweet, fiber-packed snack or sandwich companion.

New Foods to Try

If you think Peruvian Purple, Yukon Gold, and Red Cloud are next fall's fashion colors, you haven't been hanging out in the produce aisle. They're names of potatoes you should try. Potatoes now come in wonderful new shades and shapes, so you can serve them often but not feel like you're eating the same thing all the time. Yukon Gold, Yellow Finn, and Daisy Gold are marked by moist yellow flesh that boasts a buttery flavor. They're great mashed, baked, or roasted. Look for other interesting types like All-Blue, Purple Chief, Rose Finn Apple, and Russian Banana. "New" potatoes are simply spuds of any type picked small. They're excellent boiled or roasted whole.

Dining Out

You already know that a baked potato is a smarter choice than restaurant fries, scalloped potatoes, potatoes au gratin, or mashed potatoes. To jazz up a baked potato, pick sour cream over butter. Sour cream contains 30 calories and 3 grams of fat per tablespoon versus butter's 100 calories and 11 grams of fat. Naturally, the calorie advantage will evaporate if you use a heavy hand with that sour cream. Even better, calorie-wise, are salsa and lemon juice.

When adding any fat to spuds, avoid mixing it in with the potato pulp—its flavor disappears, and you end up needing more of it. Instead, mash the pulp first, then layer with a small amount of topping for flavor with less fat.

Ordering a potato can help you avoid ordering a big entrée. You can easily pair a large baked potato with shrimp cocktail and a green salad with low-fat dressing for a lean, yet satisfying meal.

Avoid any menu item whose description combines the words "loaded" and "stuffed" in the same sentence as potato. A large spud with chili and cheese has 482 calories and 22 grams of fat. As for potato skins, if you must indulge, share them with several dining companions.

When it comes to salad bar potato salad, just walk on by. Without a doubt, it's concocted with copious quantities of full-fat mayonnaise. Likewise, skip the chips and fries that come with sandwiches. Ask for a green salad or pretzels instead.

Salad Dressings

For many women, the mention of salad conjures up one of two images: First is a pale palette of iceberg lettuce, tasteless tomatoes, and a limp sliver of cucumber, graced with a spritz of lemon juice, which leaves you famished. The other is a heaping plate of cheese chunks, hard-cooked eggs, and bacon bits piled on an obligatory leaf or two of Romaine lettuce, then generously bathed in a blue cheese or creamy dressing.

Neither of these salads is likely to help you lose weight.

Surprised? You shouldn't be. The first salad is low in calories, to be sure. But it's also low in flavor, so it may not satisfy your appetite. Salad number two is really a one-course meal that may be high in calories and fat. And it just may fool you into thinking you're eating light.

That said, salads have great potential for being naturally low in fat and calories—if you stick to vegetables, fruits, grain products, and other lean or low-fat ingredients. After all, vegetables and fruits have little or no fat. Besides their nutrients, they can supply fair amounts of fiber, which fills you up without adding calories.

When it comes to "dressing up" a salad, though, you need to proceed carefully. In a study of women 19 to 50 years old, salad dressings were their primary source of dietary fat.

Here's how to scout out figure-friendly dressings.

Shopping Smarts

When time is short or if you're all thumbs in the kitchen, the quickest way to put your salad on a diet is to stock up on bottled reduced-fat or fat-free dressings. If you have a few minutes, make your own fresh, more flavorful versions. To create a little salad magic on short notice, just keep a variety of vinegars, oils, and seasonings as well as yogurt or low-fat buttermilk on hand. Either way, here's what to look for.

Prepared salad dressings. Nearly every supermarket has shelves full of reduced-fat, low-fat, and fat-free salad dressings, from old standards like Thousand Island to all sorts of exotic herbed concoctions. Because manufacturers may use various starches and stabilizers as fat replacers, these dressings aren't entirely calorie-free. And with so much variety, the amount of calories in these products varies. To find those with the fewest calories, you'll still want to check out the Nutrition Facts on the food label, and you'll have to experiment to find which ones you like best.

You might also look for packaged salad dressing mixes at the store. Just add vinegar and oil, using less oil and more vinegar.

Vinegars. Vinegar has practically no calories and can be paired with any oil—in proportions you control—plus a number of savory herbs and flavorings. Start with the basics: cider vinegar, red wine vinegar, and white vinegar. Try dark, sweet balsamic vinegar for a unique, strong flavor that is great on greens. When you're following a recipe for an oil-and-vinegar vinaigrette, cut back on the oil and use more vinegar instead.

Oils. All oils have about the same about of fat and calories—14 grams of fat and 125 calories per tablespoon. The difference is the amount of saturated fat, not total fat. Olive oil is high in monounsaturated fat, which can actually help lower your total cholesterol count. Don't assume that "light" olive oil has fewer calories—it's simply lighter in flavor and color, not fat.

To get the most flavor from the least amount of oil on salads, choose stronger-flavored oils, such as extra-virgin olive oil, sesame oil, walnut or other nut oils, or herb-infused oils.

Seasonings. To keep your tastebuds stimulated, don't stop with oil and vinegar. Boost the flavor of homemade dressings with fresh herbs from the grocery store or your garden. Tarragon, oregano, basil, and parsley are basics. Keep fresh or minced, jarred garlic on hand, too.

Lean Menu-Makers

Switching to reduced-fat, low-fat, or fat-free dressing helps put a lid on calories. But with a few nutrient-dense add-ons, you can also pump up the nutritional value of these standard salads.

Coleslaw

- Combine standard slaw mix (grated cabbage, onions, peppers, and carrots) with dried cranberries, chopped apples, and fat-free poppy seed dressing.

Best and Worst Salad Dressings

You can dress your salad without any fat by tossing it with a bit of lemon or pineapple juice or a dash of balsamic or flavored vinegar. Or if it's something creamy you're craving, you might want to check out one of the reduced-fat, low-fat, or fat-free bottled varieties of such favorites as ranch or Italian. Look for salad dressings that have three grams of fat or fewer and 40 calories or fewer per serving. Just be aware that the serving size listed on the label is often quite small, so measure the amount you put on your salad carefully. Here's how some popular dressings measure up.

Best Choices

Salad Dressing	Portion	Calories	Grams of Fat
Balsamic vinegar	1 Tbsp.	10	0.0
Fat-free mayonnaise	1 Tbsp.	10	0.0
Fat-free Italian	2 Tbsp.	15	0.0
Low-fat mayonnaise	1 Tbsp.	25	1.0
Fat-free French	2 Tbsp.	30	0.0
Fat-free vinaigrette	2 Tbsp.	35	0.0
Low-fat raspberry vinaigrette	2 Tbsp.	35	1.5
Fat-free ranch	2 Tbsp.	40	0.0
Low-fat blue cheese	2 Tbsp.	40	1.5

Worst Choices

Salad Dressing	Portion	Calories	Grams of Fat
Blue cheese	2 Tbsp.	170	17.0
Ranch	2 Tbsp.	160	17.0
Sweet-and-sour	2 Tbsp.	160	13.0
Honey-dijon	2 Tbsp.	150	15.0
Thousand Island	2 Tbsp.	140	12.0
French	2 Tbsp.	120	12.0
Russian	2 Tbsp.	110	6.0
Regular mayonnaise	1 Tbsp.	100	11.0
Italian	2 Tbsp.	100	10.0
Caesar dressing	2 Tbsp.	100	9.0

- Stir together broccoli slaw mix, chopped red bell pepper, and reduced-fat honey-dijon dressing.

Potato salad

- Combine cooked potatoes with cooked green beans, chopped pimiento, and reduced-fat creamy dill dressing.
- Combine cooked potatoes with lean ham, chopped green onions, and reduced-fat honey-dijon dressing.

Three-bean salad

- Toss canned, drained beans (green beans, pinto beans, and cannellini beans) with chopped yellow bell pepper, halved cherry tomatoes, and fat-free red wine vinaigrette.
- Toss canned, drained beans (black beans, kidney beans, and chickpeas) with chopped onion, canned (drained) corn, chopped celery, and reduced-fat bacon-tomato dressing.

Other makeovers

- Marinate boneless chicken breasts in honey-dijon dressing, shrimp in raspberry vinaigrette, or salmon steaks in creamy dill dressing.
- Add Russian dressing to crabmeat salad.
- Brush Italian dressing on a crusty baguette.
- Dip asparagus, bell pepper rings, and zucchini sticks in ranch dressing or poppy seed dressing.

Weight-Friendly Substitutions

Using a reduced-fat, low-fat, or fat-free dressing from your supermarket is one way to cut fat and calories. Using less oil and more vinegar in vinaigrette dressings is another. Here are some other suggestions.

In place of high-fat dressings

- Fill a spray bottle with a full-flavored oil to lightly spritz your greens. You'll end up using much less oil.
- Skip the oil entirely, and just dress your greens with balsamic vinegar. Or try an herb- or berry-flavored vinegar that you can buy at the store or make yourself.

- Toss salads with a splash of juice or a mixture of juices—orange, tangerine, lemon, lime, pineapple, or tomato juice all work well—and freshly ground pepper.
- For a creamy, homemade dressing for tossed salad, slaw, potato salad, or chicken salad, use plain fat-free yogurt thinned with low-fat buttermilk, and add minced fresh herbs, such as chives, tarragon, or dill.
- Puree low-fat cottage cheese in a blender. Add fat-free milk or low-fat buttermilk, and flavor with fresh herbs, Parmesan cheese, and pepper.

To dress up dressing

- Toss any dressing with minced herbs (such as tarragon, sage, thyme, parsley, basil, chervil, chives, or garlic), curry, poppy or celery seed, or capers.
- Add a few teaspoons of plain or fruit yogurt to herbed vinegar for a creamy version of vinaigrette.
- Blend a flavorful mustard or horseradish into vinaigrette or thinned yogurt.

No-fat ways to dress a salad

- Grate a little orange, lime, or lemon peel or some fresh ginger over fresh greens, fruit salad, and poultry or seafood salad.
- In garden salads, toss in some distinctively flavored greens such as watercress, endive, arugula, radicchio, or frisée (available at supermarkets with extensive produce sections).
- For pasta or garden salads, toss in chopped sun-dried tomatoes or chopped hot chile peppers.
- Toss green salads with edible flowers (purchased in the produce department, not at the florist).

Dining Out

Many weight-conscious women automatically order salad when they dine out, figuring it's bound to be lower in calories than burgers, steak sandwiches, fried fish, and other higher-fat menu choices. Or they opt for a tour of the salad bar. If you opt for high-calorie add-ons, however, a

Make It *Better*

Creamy Blue Cheese Dressing

MAKES 8 SERVINGS

OR 1 CUP

Per 2 tablespoons

26 calories

1 gram of fat

(37 percent of

calories from fat)

A lot of women think blue cheese dressing is off-limits when they're trying to lose weight. Au contraire! Blue cheese is so flavorful that by pairing a small amount with fat-free cottage cheese, you can save 144 calories and 16 grams of fat. To make over other creamy dressings, substitute pureed, fat-free cottage cheese or yogurt for sour cream or other high-fat ingredients and flavor with garlic and herbs.

1   **cup fat-free cottage cheese**

2   **tablespoons crumbled blue cheese**

2   **tablespoons fat-free milk**

1   **clove garlic, minced**

In a blender or food processor, blend or process the cottage cheese, blue cheese, milk, and garlic on low speed for 20 seconds. (The blue cheese will still be chunky.) To store, cover tightly and refrigerate for up to 1 week.

salad from the salad bar can weigh in at more than 1,000 calories. Same goes if you order a taco salad, which is loaded with sour cream, guacamole dressing, and cheese and comes in a deep-fried shell.

To keep a restaurant salad from turning into a surprise calorie-fest, remember these tips.

When you order from the menu

- Order salad dressing on the side. Then add just a small amount before you enjoy the salad.

- Ask for a fat-free or a lower-fat dressing. If one isn't available, ask for vinegar and oil served separately so you can mix your own.

- Enjoy an appetizer salad as your main dish. Complement it with a cup of low-fat soup and a freshly baked roll.

- Caesar salad, some spinach salads, antipasto, and salads mixed with mayonnaise are made with higher-fat dressing or bacon fat. To cut the calories in half, split the salad with someone else or eat only half.

When you visit a salad bar

- Go light with the ladle, and look for the lower-fat dressing options. Otherwise, you can easily end up with more dressing than you realize—sometimes as much as a quarter-cup.

- Build your salad with lower-fat ingredients, such as broccoli, bell pepper, sliced mushrooms, tomatoes, and cucumbers. You might not even miss the dressing if you omit it!

- Skip salads that are already mixed with high-fat dressings, such as creamy slaw, creamy potato salad, and vegetables in heavy oil-and-vinegar marinades. Or have just a taste.

Snacks

It's every dieter's dream: snack and lose weight. Pure fantasy? Not necessarily. Oh, sure, munching chocolate bars morning, noon, and night won't bring you closer to your goals. But there's a lot more to snack on than candy—and it's stuff your belly, butt, and thighs will thank you for.

Smart snacks pack valuable nutrients along with satisfaction and comfort—vitamins A and C, fiber, and more. For example, you can increase folate with nuts, calcium with frozen yogurt, and fiber with fig bars. Make the right choices, and you can really nibble those excess pounds away.

Best and Worst Snacks

Approach snacks like meals—choose foods with the least amount of fat and the most valuable nutrition. Obviously, nutrient-dense, naturally fat-free vegetables and fruits are smart snacks anytime. Otherwise, try to choose crackers, cookies, and other snacks with no more than three grams of fat in a 100-calorie serving. The exceptions: soy nuts and yucca chips. As snack foods go, they're incredibly nutrient-dense, redeeming their fat and calorie contents.

Best Choices			
Snack Food	Portion	Calories	Grams of Fat
Tomato juice	½ cup	20	0.0
Baby carrots with 1 Tbsp. fat-free ranch dip	5 carrots	45	0.0
Air-popped popcorn	3 cups	90	0.0
Cereal bar	1 bar	92	3.0
Baked tortilla chips	13 chips (1 oz.)	110	1.0
Baked potato chips	11 chips (1 oz.)	110	1.5
Yucca chips	15–16 chips (1 oz.)	130	6.0
Roasted soy nuts	⅓ cup (1 oz.)	150	7.0

Worst Choices			
Snack Food	Portion	Calories	Grams of Fat
Jumbo candy bar	1 bar (7 oz.)	1,000	60.0
Regular microwave popcorn	1 bag (about 12 cups)	480	36.0
Premium ice cream	½ cup	220	15.0
Macadamia nuts	1 oz.	203	21.7
Potato chips	15–16 chips (1 oz.)	150	10.0
Banana chips	10–12 chips (1 oz.)	147	9.5
Jumbo chocolate chip cookie	1 cookie (about 3 in.)	140	7.0

Make It *Better*

Chewy Oatmeal Cookies

MAKES 36 COOKIES

Per cookie

76 calories

1.7 grams of fat

(20 percent of

calories from fat)

If your gang is clamoring for homemade cookies, you can indulge them (and yourself) without guilt. If you like, substitute ⅓ cup miniature semisweet chocolate chips for ⅓ cup of the raisins. The calories and fat per cookie will increase slightly to 81 calories and 2.1 grams of fat.

1½ **cups all-purpose flour**	1 **egg**
1 **teaspoon ground cinnamon**	⅓ **cup fat-free milk**
¾ **teaspoon baking soda**	1 **tablespoon light corn syrup**
¼ **teaspoon salt**	1 **teaspoon vanilla**
¼ **cup margarine or unsalted butter, at room temperature**	1½ **cups quick-cooking rolled oats**
½ **cup sugar**	⅔ **cup raisins**
½ **cup packed light brown sugar**	

Preheat the oven to 375°F. Coat 2 baking sheets with nonstick spray.

In a medium bowl, combine the flour, cinnamon, baking soda, and salt. Mix well.

In a large bowl, combine the margarine or butter, sugar, and brown sugar. Using an electric mixer, beat on medium speed until blended. Add the egg and beat for 2 to 3 minutes, or until light and fluffy. Add the milk, corn syrup, and vanilla. Beat until blended.

Reduce the speed to low and gradually add the flour mixture, beating until just combined. Stir in the oats and raisins.

Drop the dough by level tablespoons onto the prepared baking sheets. Bake 1 sheet at a time for 8 to 10 minutes, or until lightly browned. Transfer the cookies to a wire rack to cool.

Shopping Smarts

To find nutrient-dense snacks, read more than just the information about fat and calories on the label. Look for fiber, calcium, iron, and other vitamins and minerals. Take Rice Krispie Treat Bars, for example. These convenient treats rack up only 90 calories and two grams of fat apiece, but their real benefit is their vitamin and mineral fortification. They offer far more nutrition than a doughnut or sugar cookies.

Consider the "crunch factor" when choosing snacks. Crunchy foods like baby carrots, apple slices, daikon radishes (which are milder than regular radishes), cucumbers, and pickles take longer to eat than soft snack cakes, for instance. And they tend to be satisfying, so you may eat less of them. Here are other noteworthy noshes.

Cereal bars. These tend to be a better choice than granola bars because they're lower in fat and higher in nutrients. Many one-ounce granola bars contain 128 calories and 5.8 grams of fat, while many cereal bars might have 92 calories and 0 grams of fat. What really sets them apart, though, is the fact that cereal bars are fortified with between 10 and 50 percent of your Daily Value for many vitamins and minerals.

String cheese. This mozzarella-like cheese offers a helping of calcium without a lot of fat—as long as you don't eat the whole package. Look for the kind that's portion-controlled in sticks of three-quarter ounces.

Nuts. They're filled with fiber, iron, and all kinds of trace minerals and immunity-enhancing nutrients. Their biggest drawback, of course, is fat (even though it's heart-smart unsaturated fat). But if you learn to eat just a handful to satisfy that snack urge, you can reap their nutritional benefits. Remember that one ounce is considered a serving, and that's roughly one-quarter cup. Soy nuts are surprisingly low in fat compared to other nuts. One ounce has 7 grams of fat compared with 14 grams for peanuts. An even better idea: chestnuts. Five chestnuts have only 103 calories and 1 gram of fat.

Popcorn. Air-popped popcorn has only 30 calories and no fat in one cup. Microwave popcorn is a whole other animal. Eat a bag of it, and you've put away 33 grams or more of fat—over half your daily allowance. If you can't resist microwave popcorn, look for light or low-fat types. Even then, take a good look at the label. The entire bag contains roughly three servings, so if you're downing it by yourself, you could get as much as 330 calories and 15 grams of fat.

Chips. Save half the calories and all the fat by eating fat-free potato chips. (Regular chips pack 150 calories and 10 grams of fat in a one-ounce, 15-chip serving; fat-free chips have 75 calories and 0 gram of fat.) Low-fat tortilla chips have 90 calories and 1 gram of fat in a serving, compared with 142 calories and 7.4 grams of fat for regular.

Lean Menu-Makers

Here's how to improve the nutritional profile of some of your favorite snacks.

- Turn candy or a cookie into a nutrient-filled mini-meal by combining it with a glass of juice or a piece of fresh fruit.
- Dip fresh apple slices in fat-free caramel sauce.
- Stir a spoonful of crunchy, vitamin E–rich wheat germ into a carton of fat-free yogurt.
- Turn an ordinary glass of skim milk into a powerhouse of nutrition. Mix fat-free dairy milk or soy milk with a packet of Carnation Instant Breakfast.
- Satisfy chocolate cravings with fat-free chocolate pudding. Make your own from instant pudding mix and fat-free milk or buy four-ounce snack packs.
- Spruce up rice cakes with a thin layer of peanut butter, soy nut butter, or fat-free apple butter.
- Jazz up air-popped popcorn with a splash of Tabasco sauce.
- Give cake frosting a calcium kick. Mix a container of fat-free whipped topping with a container of fruit-flavored or vanilla yogurt.

Weight-Friendly Substitutions

Smart substitutions may just mean finding a new version of a favorite high-fat food. Baked fat-free chips instead of regular. Chocolate caramel popcorn cakes rather than caramels. Cinnamon streusel rice cakes instead of cinnamon streusel coffee cake. Oreo cereal in place of Oreo cookies (it's fortified with extra vitamins and minerals that the cookies don't have). Other smart swaps:

- Soy nut butter instead of peanut butter. It's lower in fat and contains cancer-fighting isoflavones.

- Vegetable cocktail, tomato, grapefruit, or orange juice instead of empty-calorie soda.
- Reduced-fat Chex Mix, which you can make from a recipe on the cereal box, instead of high-fat nut mixes.

New Foods to Try

A snack can be defined any way you want. Think beyond chips, doughnuts, and candy bars.

Dried fruit. Try cranberries, blueberries, and orange-flavor prunes in addition to the old standby dried apricots, peaches, and pears. They're naturally sweet and chock-full of fiber and vitamins.

Fresh fruit. Get out of the bananas and oranges rut. Try other fruits like mangoes, papayas, ugli fruit (a tangerine-grapefruit hybrid from Jamaica), champagne grapes, figs, Asian pears, and interesting apple varieties like Fuji, Royal Gala, Jonagold, and Braeburn.

Soup. Choose canned and instant soups that are high in fiber, like black bean, minestrone, lentil, and split pea. Pop into the microwave for an instant snack.

Cereal. It's not just breakfast food. And even when sugar-coated, it is much more nutrient-dense than cake, candy, and cookies. Eat bite-size cereal right out of the box. You can even find convenient snack-size bags of cereal like Post Snack-Abouts.

Soy power bars. Choose ones that remind you of a decadent treat, like GeniSoy Soy Protein Bars in peanut butter fudge or apple spice yogurt. They're not only extremely satisfying but also filled with protein, fiber, and lots of vitamins.

Cracker Jacks. Sweet, crunchy caramel corn with only 120 calories and two grams of fat in a half-cup!

Yucca chips. Made from a starchy tropical root vegetable, these crispy chips have more than twice the fiber of regular potato chips—as well as 40 percent less fat. Available in flavors like barbecue, garlic, cilantro, and picante 'n cream cheese, they're a terrific snack.

Office Snacks

Your good intentions needn't be left at home when you head to work. Just take along portable snacks like the following.

Desk drawer delights. Stock up on light microwave popcorn, low-fat crackers, rice cakes, low-fat cookies, dried fruit, soy nuts, reduced-fat peanuts, or cereal bars.

For the office fridge. Keep a stash of yogurt, baby carrots or cut-up vegetables, salad in a bag with low-fat dressing, skim milk, low-fat chocolate milk, hummus, and low-fat cream cheese spreads. (Travel tip: These snacks work great in the car; pack them in an insulated bag or cooler with ice packs.)

Soups and Chowders

Hearty or delicate, piping hot or refreshingly chilled, chunky or smooth, creamy or clear, soup can serve as the prelude to a nutritious meal—or as its centerpiece. Take minestrone: Chock-full of vegetables and pasta, minestrone (Italian for "big soup") is a hearty main dish for a wintry day. In contrast, chilled gazpacho—based on tomatoes, peppers, and cucumbers—is a refreshing starter in peak-summer heat. Both are low in fat and a super way to work in the three to five servings of vegetables a day that all women need. And they're just some of the many low-fat, nutrient-rich soups you can put on your table.

Because soup is sipped, not chewed, it takes time to eat, which is a benefit for women who tend to overeat at mealtime. Studies suggest that people who start their meals with soup eat less food and consume fewer calories than those who do not.

Best and Worst Soups

Depending on their ingredients, soups can be the source of many nutrients. When selecting soups to buy or prepare, your best choices are low-fat versions with three grams of fat or fewer per serving.

Best Choices

Soup	Portion	Calories	Grams of Fat
Miso soup	1 cup	35	0.0
Gazpacho soup	1 cup	56	0.2
Vegetable soup	1 cup	90	2.0
Minestrone	1 cup	120	2.0
Bean soup, made without bacon	1 cup	130	0.5
Chicken soup, made with defatted broth	1 cup	160	3.0

Worst Choices

Soup	Portion	Calories	Grams of Fat
Potato soup, made with cream	1 cup	220	14.0
New England clam chowder	1 cup	200	13.0
Chicken soup, made with regular broth	1 cup	175	6.0
Bean soup, made with bacon	1 cup	172	6.0
Cream of mushroom soup	1 cup	170	13.0
Cheese soup	1 cup	156	10.5
Borscht, topped with sour cream	1 cup	152	5.0
Bisque, made with cream	1 cup	120	5.0

Make It *Better*

Hearty Seafood Chowder

MAKES 4 SERVINGS

Per serving

252 calories

4.1 grams of fat

(15 percent of

calories from fat)

Thanks to the use of defatted chicken stock and evaporated fat-free milk, this authentic-tasting seafood chowder graces you with nearly 9 fewer grams of fat per serving than conventional chowder made with butter and cream.

12 **shucked chowder clams**	1 **bay leaf**
5 **cups defatted chicken stock**	½ **teaspoon dried oregano**
2 **large baking potatoes, peeled and diced**	¼ **teaspoon dried tarragon**
1 **large onion, diced**	¼ **teaspoon ground black pepper**
1 **carrot, diced**	8 **ounces cod, cut into 1" pieces**
1 **stalk celery, diced**	1 **cup evaporated fat-free milk**
1 **tablespoon minced fresh parsley**	

In a 3-quart saucepan, combine the clams and 2 cups of the stock. Bring to a boil over high heat. Reduce the heat to medium and simmer for 3 minutes. Remove the clams with a slotted spoon and set aside.

Add the potatoes, onion, carrot, celery, parsley, bay leaf, oregano, tarragon, pepper, and remaining 3 cups of stock to the saucepan. Bring to a boil, then cook over medium heat for 15 minutes, or until the vegetables are softened. Remove and discard the bay leaf.

Ladle about half of the vegetables and about 1 cup of the liquid into a blender. Blend until smooth. Return to the saucepan. Add the cod and simmer for 5 minutes, or until the cod is cooked through.

Chop the clams finely and add to the saucepan. Stir in the milk and heat briefly.

Soup is versatile—the ultimate mix-and-match food. Depending on the ingredients, soups supply various amounts of valuable nutrients. Vegetable soup can be loaded with vitamins A and C, folate, and potassium. Hearty soups made with rice, pasta, or other grains—chicken with rice, beef noodle, or turkey barley, for example—contribute complex carbohydrates, plus some fiber (if made with whole grains). Soups like chowder that are made with milk fortify your diet with calcium. And soup can be a great way to extend poultry, meat, and fish, yet get the protein, iron, and B vitamins you need for the day. Finally, bean soups, such as split pea or lentil soups, are satisfying ways to add meatless dishes to your menu.

To build your soup repertoire, know the lingo. *Broth*—flavorful liquid that's strained from cooking vegetables, meat, or poultry in water—is low in fat, especially when chilled and skimmed of fat. *Consommé* is simply concentrated broth. *Chowder* is a thick, chunky soup made with milk or cream, or thickened with a flour-butter mixture. *Bisque* is a rich, thick soup typically made with a base of seafood, vegetables, butter, and cream. (But don't worry—you can easily "de-fat" chowder and other rich, creamy homemade soups or shop for low-fat varieties.)

Shopping Smarts

If you're like most women, you probably rely on canned soups for fast "heat and eat" meals. Supermarket shelves are stocked with every variety of soup you can think of—and some you probably haven't. Think beyond old standbys like tomato and chicken noodle. For further versatility, you can combine two prepared soups, or fortify them with a variety of mix-ins.

To find soups with the least amount of fat and calories, read the Nutrition Facts labels. Clear soups are usually lower in fat and calories than creamy soups. You'll also find low-fat and fat-free versions of cream of mushroom, cream of celery, and other higher-fat soups. Very often, the heartier the soup, the more nutrients you get.

Whether you make soup from scratch or buy prepared soups, these health-smart tips can help you stock a soup-ready kitchen.

Canned broth. Stock your pantry with vegetable broth and fat-free beef and chicken broth—they serve as the base for all kinds of flavorful homemade soups. If you're sodium sensitive (or cooking for someone who is), buy broth with the lowest sodium content. Or make your own broth without added salt, then chill and skim off the fat.

Ready-to-eat soups or condensed soups. Ready-to-eat soups simply need to be heated. With condensed soup, some of the water is re-moved, so you need to reconstitute them before heating. For more flavor and nutrients, use milk, broth, vegetable juice, or water left over from cooking vegetables instead of plain water when you heat them.

Dehydrated soups. Most are low in fat. To prepare, just add hot liquid, perhaps low-sodium broth.

Soup Up Your Soup

With a little creativity and a few simple items from the supermarket, you can add homemade flavor and a nutritional boost to low-fat soups. Here's what to look for.

- Canned stewed Mexican-flavored tomatoes, diced tomatoes flavored with Italian herbs, or plain, diced tomatoes. Add to corn chowder for a chunky texture.
- Pre-cut veggies (frozen, canned, or fresh, including stir-fry medleys) or cooked leftovers. Add to potato soup or other extra-chunky soups.
- Canned beans, such as black, cannellini (white kidney), kidney (red), or chickpeas. To reduce the sodium content, rinse the beans under running water before adding them to the soup. Mix them into vegetable noodle soup.
- Firm tofu (smooth, creamy white soybean curd sold in blocks in the produce section). The firm variety keeps its shape when sliced. Add to chicken noodle or vegetable soup.
- Canned crabmeat, clams, or diced chicken. Add to tomato soup.
- Tortellini (fresh or dried), Chinese noodles, no-yolk egg noodles, or small pasta shapes, such as orzo, pastina, and couscous. These are especially good in turkey vegetable soup.
- Brown rice or barley. Mix into reduced-fat cream of mushroom soup.
- Sun-dried tomatoes or dried or canned mushrooms. Dried varieties pack more flavor. Try them in onion or bean soup.
- From your freezer: Diced cooked skinless poultry, lean ground beef, seafood, leftover

cooked meat, soy patties (to crumble for soup). Add them to vegetable soup for a hearty main-dish soup.

To further enhance low-fat soups, garnish them with these easy toppings.

- Chopped chives, cilantro, or parsley. These are colorful ways to spice up low-fat chowder.
- A dollop of plain, fat-free yogurt. Add for some extra calcium on split pea or black bean soup.
- A few shreds of cheese or a sprinkle of Parmesan. Cheese gives body to turkey barley soup or minestrone.

Lean Menu-Makers

Paired with a salad or sandwich, soup rounds out a meal without rounding out your hips or waistline. Serve a cup of soup as an appetizer, or a fruit soup as dessert. (In Japan, soup is served for breakfast.) Consider these accompaniments for your favorite soups.

Chicken soup

- Pita bread pocket stuffed with vegetables and tangerine segments on the side
- A pumpernickel bagel with fat-free cream cheese, and an apple
- Chilled fruit salad and matzo crackers
- Pear halves filled with fat-free cottage cheese, and rye crackers

Tomato soup

- Grilled chicken and spinach salad with low-fat dressing and breadsticks
- Toasted low-fat Monterey Jack sandwich and bell pepper sticks
- Tuna-sprout wrap (in a tortilla) and apple slices

Vegetable soup

- Turkey sandwich on pita bread and fresh berries
- Bean burrito and mango slices
- Small crusty whole-wheat "bread bowl" (made from a hollowed-out whole-wheat roll), topped with low-fat Cheddar cheese

Weight-Friendly Substitutions

If you're trying to slim down, you don't have to throw out your family's favorite recipes for chowder, potato, or other creamy soups or thick stews. You can lower the fat and boost the nutrients with these simple tricks.

Cream-based soup

- Replace the cream with a calcium-rich alternative such as fat-free evaporated milk, low-fat buttermilk, or low-fat milk fortified with nonfat dry milk.
- For cold fruit soups, blend in nonfat yogurt (plain or fruit).

Thick, hearty soup or stew

- Add starchy, raw vegetables, such as grated potatoes, yams, or parsnips. Simmer until thickened. In a hurry? Mix in potato flakes or leftover mashed potatoes instead. When the vegetables in your soup are thoroughly cooked, puree half or all the veggies, then stir the puree into the soup. (One cup of pureed vegetables thickens three to four cups of broth.) Or blend in a small can of tomato paste. Simmer vegetable, chicken, or beef soup with rice, barley, oatmeal, or pasta, or try adding cooked, mashed beans (perhaps kidney, pinto, black, or cannellini beans).

Dining Out

For lunch or a light dinner, ordering soup as an appetizer plus a salad with bread or crackers may be all you need.

Restaurant menus usually offer at least two choices of soup. Before ordering, ask about the ingredients. Keep in mind that soup prepared without cream, cream cheese, sour cream, egg yolks, cheese, butter, or oil is usually lower in fat. And remember that clear soups are generally lower in fat than cream soups. For example, thick, creamy New England clam chowder averages about 13 grams of fat per cup, compared with 3.4 grams of fat for the same amount of tomato-based Manhattan clam chowder. If you must have a richer cream soup, order a cup instead of a bowl. And if you ladle soup from the soup and salad bar, take one ladle, not two.

Tacos, Tortilla Fillings, and Wraps

Long before wraps became trendy, consumers were tucking all kinds of foods inside tortilla shells. Now you can have even more fun thinking of adventuresome flavor combinations that match your goals for weight-conscious eating. Best of all, tortillas and wraps are a satisfying way to work meatless meals into your menu without hearing any complaints from the meat-lovers in your household.

Although we think of tacos as crisp tortilla shells, a taco is really any rolled and stuffed corn tortilla, whether it's soft or crisp. As a handheld wrapping for various fillings, tortillas are just another form of sandwich bread. The basic difference is the flour—corn flour (masa) or wheat flour. Corn tortillas are somewhat lower in calories and fat. A one-ounce (eight-inch) soft corn tortilla has

Best and Worst Tacos, Tortilla Fillings, and Wraps

For calorie-savvy choices, start with soft tortillas. They're generally lower in fat than taco shells, which are fried to make them crisp. Oven-baked tortilla chips have less fat than regular tortilla chips, too. For the stuffings, you can concoct a hearty filling with all kinds of low-fat and fat-free ingredients. Read the labels to compare.

Best Choices			
Item, filling, or topping	Portion	Calories	Grams of Fat
Salsa	2 Tbsp.	10	0.0
Fat-free sour cream	2 Tbsp.	20	0.0
Corn tortilla	1 tortilla (1 oz.)	70	0.6
Fat-free refried beans	½ cup	100	0.0
Baked tortilla chips	13 chips (1 oz.)	110	1.0
Flour tortilla	1 tortilla (1¼ oz.)	115	3.4

Worst Choices			
Item, filling, or topping	Portion	Calories	Grams of Fat
Taco salad	1 large salad (21 oz.)	905	61.0
Soft ground beef taco	1 taco	226	9.7
Soft chicken taco	1 taco	183	5.1
Regular tortilla chips	13 chips (1 oz.)	140	8.0
Refried beans made with lard	½ cup	140	3.0
Taco shells	2 shells (1 oz.)	120	5.0
Guacamole	2 Tbsp.	60	5.0
Sour cream	2 Tbsp.	60	5.0

about one gram of fat and 70 calories, compared to slightly more than three grams of fat and 115 calories in an eight-inch wheat tortilla, which weighs slightly more. Taco shells are another story: Fry corn tortillas to a crisp, and two five-inch shells—a one-ounce serving—go up to about six grams of fat and 120 calories.

If you're making your own tortilla dishes, you can control calories and fat by tucking in plenty of vegetables; lean meat, poultry, and fish; and even

Make It *Better*

Chicken Quesadillas

MAKES 4 SERVINGS

Per serving

401 calories

5.7 grams of fat

(13 percent of

calories from fat)

To enhance the color and flavor of these quesadillas, sprinkle them with an assortment of condiments, such as chopped red bell peppers, onions, tomatoes, and radishes. Altogether, this trimmed-down version of a Mexican favorite has 504 fewer calories and 55 fewer grams of fat than a taco salad.

¼ cup lime juice

2 tablespoons chopped cilantro

1 serrano chili pepper, seeded and finely chopped (wear rubber gloves when handling)

4 boneless, skinless chicken breast halves (4 ounces each)

1 red bell pepper, seeded and thinly sliced

1 green bell pepper, seeded and thinly sliced

1 cup scallions sliced into 1" lengths

1 cup thinly sliced mushrooms

½ cup jalapeño jelly

8 flour tortillas, 8" in diameter

Preheat the oven to 400°F. In a shallow bowl, combine the lime juice, cilantro, chili pepper, and chicken. Cover and marinate for 15 minutes. Remove the chicken from the marinade and cook for 6 to 8 minutes over a charcoal fire or in a stovetop skillet, turning once, or until the chicken is cooked through. Thinly slice the chicken on a diagonal.

Coat a large nonstick frying pan with nonstick spray. Add the red pepper, green pepper, scallions, and mushrooms and cook over medium heat until the scallions are golden and the vegetables are tender. Add the jalapeño jelly and cook until the jelly melts.

Coat a baking sheet with nonstick spray. Combine the chicken with the vegetables. Divide among the tortillas. Place the tortillas on the prepared baking sheet and bake for 5 minutes.

fruit. You can also make filling mixtures with beans and rice. And tortillas can be moistened with salsas and other low-fat sauces and spreads.

Whether you prefer Tex-Mex flavors or want to take your tastebuds beyond the border, here's how to fit tortillas and wraps into a weight-conscious eating plan for breakfast, lunch, dinner, and snacks.

Shopping Smarts

Wrap up quick, nutrition-minded meals today—starting with the tortillas, wraps, fillings, sauces, and seasonings you buy.

Tortillas. You can buy soft wheat and corn tortillas in various sizes, keep them on hand in your refrigerator or freezer, and use them to suit your needs when you and your family are hungry but time for dinner is short. The 8- and 10-inch tortillas are fine for handheld wraps; use the smaller size if tortillas are to be stuffed, rolled, and baked, or layered and stacked. As you compare Nutrition Facts labels, pay attention to the size; tortillas with more calories and fat just may be bigger or weigh more.

Choose between wheat and corn tortillas, depending on their use.

- Wheat tortillas. These are pliable, yet sturdy, so they're best for wraps, but they work well for anything.

- Corn tortillas. Since they often break when they're folded, use corn tortillas for baked recipes. You'll need to soften them in sauce, such as tomato sauce or low-fat creamy soup, before filling. Since they're fried, taco shells supply considerable amounts of fat and calories. They're not your best bet if you want less of both.

Fillings. For quick and satisfying tacos, wraps, and other filled tortillas that help you reach your calorie target, stock your kitchen with a variety of these ingredients.

- Canned beans. Refried beans are great in burritos; just add salsa. Look for the fat-free varieties. Drained kidney beans, chickpeas, black beans, and other canned beans make great filling "combos" with ground meat or veggies for

Mexican dishes or international wraps with Greek, Asian, or Italian ingredients.

- Lean ground turkey or lean ground beef, boneless chicken breast, and lean stir-fry beef or pork for your freezer. Cook these items first with a zesty seasoning, then use them for fajitas (stir-fried marinated chicken or meat and vegetables served in a warm flour tortilla), enchiladas (corn tortillas stuffed with beans, cheese, chicken, or meat and a sauce), burritos (flour tortillas that are folded then rolled to enclose the savory filling), or quesadillas (filled flour tortillas that are folded in half and then browned under a broiler). Or layer tortillas with a filling of shredded lean meat or poultry for a tostada.

- Canned crabmeat or tuna. Combined with rice, crabmeat or tuna is great for Asian-style wraps.

- Chopped frozen vegetables. Mix them into vegetarian tortilla wrap fillings, or combine them with meat, chicken, or seafood fillings.

- Cheese. For fewer calories, look for low-fat or fat-free varieties. Monterey Jack or jalapeño cheese is typical in many Mexican tortilla dishes. You can also find low-fat blends of shredded Mexican cheeses. Almost any brick cheese will do.

Savory sauces of all kinds. Try tomato salsas with stir-fried meat, fruit salsas with stir-fried chicken, barbecue sauce with canned beans, picante sauce with chopped vegetables, and chutneys with cooked seafood.

Seasonings. Experiment with taco seasoning for Mexican fillings or barbecue wraps; ginger, soy sauce, and green onion for a California wrap; oregano, basil, and garlic for an Italian herb wrap; or most any combination of herbs and spices.

Frozen tortilla dishes. When time is even shorter, keep some prepared tortilla dishes on hand. You'll find low-fat versions of burritos, enchiladas, and more in the freezer case. Check the Nutrition Facts label to compare the fat and calorie contents.

Lean Menu-Makers

Tortillas are a great resource if you want to eat lean *and* wrap up what you need in your diet. For a hearty main dish or nutritious snack, fill them with a mixture of lean and low-fat ingredients from a variety of sources, focusing on grain products, beans, vegetables, lean meats or dairy, and even fruit. (Helpful hint: Warm the tortillas so they're easier to roll.) Start with these quick-to-make ideas.

Breakfast tortillas

- Fill a soft tortilla with scrambled eggs, chopped tomato, and shredded low-fat cheese. Serve with sliced oranges.
- Layer a tortilla with lox (thinly sliced smoked salmon), fat-free cream cheese, capers, and dill, then roll. Serve with pineapple juice.
- Line the shell with lettuce, then wrap with a mixture of low-fat cottage cheese, chopped fruit, and mint. Serve with tomato juice.

Quick lunch or light dinner options

- Spread tortillas with mustard, then wrap up an HLT (lean ham, lettuce, and tomato) tortilla. Serve with pineapple spears.
- Spread tortillas with hummus, then wrap with turkey slices, bell pepper sticks, and sprouts. Serve with grapes.
- Combine cooked rice, grilled or boiled shrimp, chopped mango, and cilantro (a form of parsley), then wrap. Serve with bell pepper sticks.

Oven-baked tortillas

- For spinach quesadillas, sprinkle tortillas with shredded low-fat cheese and frozen spinach that has been thawed and drained; fold, and bake. Serve with sliced papaya.
- For barbecued chicken enchiladas, dip tortillas in tomato sauce, then fill with barbecued chicken, roll, top with barbecue sauce and shredded low-fat cheese, and bake. Serve with rice and beans.

Weight-Friendly Substitutions

If stuffed soft tortillas are popular at your house, you've probably already thought of substituting fat-free cheese and sour cream for the full-fat versions. Here's what else you can do to enjoy your favorite combos while keeping calories and fat down.

- Use soft corn tortillas instead of crisp taco shells.
- Substitute salsa and yogurt cheese for guacamole and regular sour cream. (Make yogurt cheese by draining gelatin-free yogurt overnight until it is a thick consistency.)
- Use lean meat, skinless chicken, or seafood in tortilla fillings.
- Use refried beans without fat, or mash your own using any type of canned beans.

You can also bulk up tortillas with lower-fat fillings. Figure about 1 to 1¼ cups of filler for a 10-inch tortilla. Try mixing in any of the following with chopped meat, poultry, and seafood.

- Chopped broccoli, zucchini, tomato, or bell pepper, or grated carrots in cooked or raw fillings; add sprouts, sliced artichokes, or chopped lettuce for salad-type fillings
- Chopped fresh or dried fruit for a sweet spark of flavor
- Cooked rice, wild rice, bulgur, couscous, or orzo; canned beans of all kinds; or diced potatoes

Dining Out

Heading to a Mexican restaurant? When you're trying to slim down, skip high-fat tortilla dishes. Both chimichangas and flautas are fried, and fat from other ingredients, such as ground beef, cheese, guacamole, and sour cream, add up. Fajitas, with stir-fried lean meat or boneless chicken and veggies, can be lower in calories. For any wrapped-up Mexican tortilla, ask that any high-fat toppings be served on the side so you control the amount you eat. Or skip the high-fat toppings and ask for extra salsa. Beware of taco salads served in a crispy tortilla bowl with high-fat dressing—they can have more fat and calories than a double patty hamburger at a fast-food chain.

Try ordering wraps, which are featured at a growing number of fast-food shops and restaurants. Look for those made with lower-fat ingredients—don't be shy about asking how they're made. Some restaurants may offer nutrition information to help you make your choices.

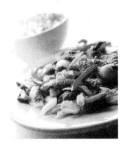

Menu Magic

To jump-start your shape-up efforts, follow this one-week meal plan. Using the food selections nutritionists rate as best, plus the "Make It Better" recipes, you'll eat well and love it.

Designed by Kim Galeaz, R.D, a registered dietitian and food and nutrition consultant in Indianapolis, this menu offers three tasty meals a day, plus snacks, for about 1,600 calories and 44 grams of fat (25 percent of total calories from fat) or less per day.

"This meal plan supplies lots of flavor and variety (so you don't get bored) and fiber (so you feel satisfied and full, and don't overeat)," says Galeaz. "It also keeps you fueled all day long, to maintain energy as you exercise regularly to lose weight and tone up. There's even plenty of room for extras, like fats, sweets, and treats."

With this menu, you can start banishing your belly, butt, and thighs today while perking up classic family recipes and introducing exciting new foods into your menu. Break out of the rut of eating the same breakfast morning after morning, packing the same three lunch meals week in and week out, or cooking the same four family recipes over and over. Then use what you've learned to expand your weekly menu, using shopping, meal planning, and cooking strategies for eating lean.

"Have fun with flavors and foods," says Galeaz. "Be creative and adventurous."

For more menu plans, be sure to visit our Web site at www.banishbbt.com.

Monday

Breakfast

¾ cup Three-Grain Granola (see page 34) with ½ cup fat-free milk

1 cup fresh grapefruit juice

Snack

1 banana

Lunch

½ whole-wheat pita pocket stuffed with 1 ounce lean deli honey ham

6 slices Fuji apple

1 ounce reduced-fat sharp Cheddar cheese, sliced

1 teaspoon light mayonnaise

1 cup green and red pepper strips

Snack

1 Chewy Oatmeal Cookie (see page 98)

1 cup fat-free milk

Dinner

1½ cups angel hair pasta topped with 1 cup commercial pasta sauce

1 cup steamed zucchini and summer squash

1 soft breadstick

Snack

1 cup fat-free white chocolate raspberry yogurt

Daily Tally
1,625 calories,
20 grams of fat,
11 percent of calories from fat

Tuesday

Breakfast

1 cup vanilla fortified soy milk mixed with 1 packet mocha instant breakfast powder

½ blueberry bagel

1 tablespoon light cream cheese

Snack

1 tangelo

Lunch

California-Style Turkey Burger on crusty roll (see page 32) with shredded lettuce and 2 slices tomato

1 cup broccoli coleslaw mixed with 2 tablespoons low-fat coleslaw dressing

Snack

1 fresh pear

¼ cup roasted salted soy nuts

Dinner

1 bowl Hearty Seafood Chowder (see page 102)

3 ounces orange roughy, broiled with lemon juice and oregano

1 cup bow-tie pasta

1 cup fresh steamed asparagus spears

Snack

1 cup low-fat chocolate milk

Daily Tally
1,652 calories
32 grams of fat
17 percent of calories from fat

Wednesday

Breakfast

1 fast-food English muffin and egg sandwich

1 cup fat-free milk

Snack

1 cup vegetable juice

4 whole-grain crackers

Lunch

Deli sandwich made with 2 slices hearty multi-grain bread, 1 ounce reduced-fat Swiss cheese, 1 ounce reduced-fat Cheddar cheese, ¼ cup alfalfa sprouts, and 1 teaspoon spicy mustard

Tossed green salad made with 1 cup fresh spinach leaves, ½ cup romaine lettuce, and 1 tablespoon chopped walnuts, and topped with a sprinkling of balsamic vinegar and a squeeze of fresh lemon

¾ cup chopped fresh mango cubes

Snack

¼ cup low-fat spinach dip with 1 mini pita bread, cut into wedges

Dinner

Beef stir-fry made with 3 ounces lean sirloin steak strips and 1 cup Chinese stir-fry vegetables

1 cup brown rice

1 fortune cookie

1 cup honeydew melon cubes

Snack

1 slice New York Cheesecake (see page 54)

Daily Tally
1,618 calories
44 grams of fat
24 percent of calories from fat

Thursday

Breakfast

1 cup lemon nonfat yogurt mixed with 1 tablespoon wheat germ

1 cup fresh strawberries, sliced

Snack

1 Good-for-Your-Waistline Muffin (see page 25)

Lunch

One 3-ounce veggie burger on poppyseed kaiser roll with ¼ cup fresh spinach leaves and 2 slices tomato

12 baby carrots

1 cup fat-free milk

Snack

1 cup black bean soup

4 whole-grain crackers

Dinner

1 serving Oven-Fried Chicken (see page 41)

1 serving Buttermilk Mashed Potatoes (see page 90)

1 cup fresh broccoli spears, steamed

1 whole-wheat dinner roll

Snack

1 cup fresh red grapes

Daily Tally
1,640 calories
26 grams of fat
14 percent of calories from fat

Friday

Breakfast

2 slices cinnamon swirl bread, toasted and topped with 1 tablespoon peanut butter

1 cup cantaloupe chunks

Snack

1 cup low-fat chocolate milk

Lunch

3 ounces Albacore tuna, water packed and drained, served over 2 cups mixed fresh spinach leaves, arugula, and red-leaf lettuce, with ¼ cup sun-dried tomatoes

1 serving Creamy Blue Cheese Dressing (see page 96)

1 cup fresh pineapple slices

Snack

4 chocolate graham cracker squares

1 cup fat-free milk

Dinner

1 serving Very Veggie Pizza (see page 88)

2 soft breadsticks dipped in ½ cup low-fat marinara sauce

Snack

½ cup low-fat strawberry frozen yogurt drizzled with 1 teaspoon chocolate syrup

Daily Tally
1,610 calories
29 grams of fat
16 percent of calories from fat

Saturday

Breakfast

1 Basil and Mushroom Omelette (see page 56)

1 wheat English muffin

1 teaspoon light margarine

1 cup fresh orange juice

Snack

1 cup Key lime nonfat yogurt

Lunch

3 ounces broiled shrimp kabobs made with ½ a carrot and ¼ of a bell pepper

1½ cups red peppers and zucchini slices, roasted on the grill

½ cup couscous

Snack

1 cup fat-free milk

1 kiwifruit

Dinner

1 serving Chicken Quesadillas (see page 106)

14 baked tortilla chips

¼ cup hot salsa

Snack

½ cup fresh raspberries

2 fat-free mint creme cookies

Daily Tally
1,621 calories
27 grams of fat
15 percent of calories from fatt

Sunday

Breakfast

1 sesame seed bagel, toasted and topped with 1 tablespoon apple butter

1 cup fat-free milk

Snack

½ cup fresh blueberries

1 piece string cheese (¾ oz.)

Lunch

1 serving Beef and Spinach Lasagna (see page 84)

1½ cups tossed spinach leaves and romaine lettuce with 4 cherry tomatoes and 2 tablespoons fat-free Italian dressing

1 slice Italian bread sprayed with olive oil vegetable spray and a sprinkling of garlic powder

Snack

¼ cup dried cherries

Dinner

3 ounces lean boneless pork loin (baked, broiled, or grilled) served with Thigh-Friendly Mushroom Gravy (see page 72)

1 baked sweet potato, sprinkled with cinnamon

½ cup steamed fresh green beans

1 whole-wheat dinner roll

Snack

6 ounces light cranberry juice cocktail

Daily Tally
1,650 calories
27 grams of fat
15 percent of calories from fat

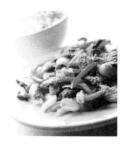

The Best and Worst Cooking Techniques

Plain grilled chicken breast, steamed vegetables, and boiled white rice. You could live on a steady diet of it. But would you want to? How many days in a row could you choke down this healthy meal before a big-time binge grabbed you by the arm—and made you do things you wouldn't tell your best friend?

It's a simple fact. All the austere low-fat cooking in the world won't put you any closer to your weight goal if the food lacks appeal.

Research shows that it's the very sparseness of diet plans that dooms them to failure. They simply do not satisfy in the long run, leading you to throw in the towel again and again. There is hope, however. "Flavorful reduced-fat cooking techniques can help get you off the diet roller coaster for good," says Elizabeth Ward, R.D., a registered dietitian and nutrition consultant in Stoneham, Massachusetts, spokesperson for the American Dietetic Association, and author of *Pregnancy Nutrition: Good Health for You and Your Baby*, among other publications.

That's the message for 52-year-old Sarah. You met her earlier, in chapter two. She's the mother of four grown children who spares no high-fat ingredients in her cooking, despite the fact that she and her spouse must lose weight.

In Sarah's Kitchen

Sarah knows weight loss is imperative but finds it hard to change her cooking habits after all these years. She's typical of many women her age who've been losing, and gaining back, the same unwanted pounds for years.

A quick look around Sarah's kitchen tells the story of her battle of the bulge.

Pantry panic. Her cupboard shelves strain under the weight of packaged noodle, potato, and rice dishes, which Sarah prepares with butter and full-fat milk. Cans of gravy and fat-laden biscuit and stuffing mixes pair up with the meat and potatoes she and her husband consume more often than not. Creamy canned condensed soups are the basis for easy casseroles Sarah concocts on busy weeknights. Cheesy pasta sauces, including Alfredo, make for quick entrées.

Vegetable shortening is on hand for frying chicken and making moist, flaky baked goods. You don't even want to hear about the gallon jug of oil hogging space on the bottom shelf.

Sarah stocks the makings of sweet stuff, including chopped nuts and chocolate chips, which are just as easily eaten as snacks as they are added to recipes. Fat-filled brownie and cake mixes make an appearance, too. (Don't forget the frosting!)

Freezer folly. Sarah fills her freezer with beef and pork, including fatty sirloin, ribs, and sausage. There's lots of ground chuck for casseroles and meat sauces. Cheese and meat ravioli serve as quick fare on busy weeknights. The vegetables in residence come with their own butter sauce. Sarah's nod to lower-fat dinners: breaded chicken cutlets and fish fillets. When she's feeling really virtuous, she relies on low-calorie frozen dinners.

Refrigerator reality check. Down below, the refrigerator contents don't bode much better for weight loss. There's reduced-fat milk, but it's 2 percent rather than fat-free. Nondairy creamer shows up for coffee, but it's hardly fat-free, so Sarah may as well use the half-and-half she keeps on hand for sauces and sweets. Hard cheeses (including Cheddar), cream cheese, and sour cream crowd the shelves to help Sarah serve up the sauces, casseroles, and baked goods she and her spouse so often enjoy. On the plus side, Sarah sometimes totes low-fat cottage cheese and fruit for lunch, so both are plentiful here.

There's no shortage of eggs in this kitchen, because fried eggs with bacon is her husband's favorite breakfast. Sarah also needs plenty of eggs to concoct sauces and baked goodies. She buys butter for sautéing veggies, flavoring rice, making sauces, and baking her weekly batch of muffins.

Vegetables do overflow their bin. But all too often, Sarah doesn't get around to them until they're past their prime. So she sautés them in butter to make them palatable—or blankets them with cheese sauce. Like most busy cooks, Sarah relies on convenience vegetables, such as shredded carrots, bagged salad greens, and coleslaw mix. Ideally, they're a smart way to boost vegetable consumption. But if you smother them with full-fat salad dressing (and Sarah does), you cancel out their low-fat, low-calorie benefits.

Countertop confusion. A quick glance at Sarah's countertop reveals a deep-fat fryer she has used for years. No wonder weight loss has been so elusive! Frying is sheer folly when weight control is the goal. Eight ounces of fried fish contains about 175 calories more than the same amount broiled. Ounce for ounce, fried chicken breast with skin contains 1½ times the calories of skinless grilled or broiled breast—and triple the fat.

Cooking Light Lessons

Believe it or not, Sarah isn't a lost cause. In spite of her kitchen's fat traps, she needn't totally revamp her diet. Some artful substitutions—of both ingredients and cooking methods—will go a long way toward getting her on track. You don't have to incorporate all of the fat-slashing techniques that follow into your cooking repertoire. But the more you use, the greater your calorie—and fat—savings. Consider this: Eating 100 fewer calories a day can result in more than 10 pounds lost in a year's time, provided you don't eat more of other foods or decrease your activity level. What does that mean in tabletop terms? Something as painless as cutting one tablespoon of butter or margarine from your daily diet. (Use a little less on your toast, on your baked potato, in the sauté pan—you won't even miss it!)

Baking

So many different kinds of foods can be baked that this cooking method offers the greatest opportunity for calorie cutting.

Main-dish misery. They're convenient. They're comfort foods. They're caloric killers. Casseroles prepared with the traditional meat, cream, cheese, and butter can bust your calorie budget. Check out chicken pot pie: It easily has 400 to 500 calories per serving for a frozen entrée. Homemade can top that. The good news? There are dozens of ways to lighten up such family favorites.

- For meat and poultry casseroles, use no more than three ounces of meat per serving and remove visible fat before cooking. When browning ground meat, drain off the fat that collects in the skillet. Then get rid of even more fat by transferring the meat to a colander and rinsing it with warm water. Better yet, start with lean ground beef (92 percent lean or better) or substitute ground turkey or chicken breast. (Be aware that meat labeled just "ground turkey" or "ground chicken" may contain fattier dark meat as well as skin.) Finally, replace some meat with cooked rice, couscous, or beans, or with low-fat cottage cheese.

- Ground turkey or chicken breast can also stand in for some or all of the hamburger in meat loaf. Increase fiber (and reduce grams of fat per serving) by extending the meat with rolled oats and shredded veggies, including carrots and zucchini.

- Lighten up comfort foods like chicken fricassee, macaroni and cheese, croquettes, and chicken à la king with low-fat versions of milk, evaporated milk, sour cream, cream cheese, or yogurt. For lasagna and eggplant parmigiana, use reduced-fat mozzarella, Cheddar, ricotta, or other cheese. (Further lighten eggplant dishes by baking the slices instead of frying them before assembling the casserole.)

- When using fat-free cheese, shred it finely to promote even melting. Keep in mind that fat-free cheese tends to turn rubbery and tough when exposed to direct heat—so reduced-fat cheese may be a better option for casserole and pizza toppings.

- Substitute half of the fattier feta cheese that recipes sometimes call for with nonfat cottage cheese. Make your own nonfat substitute for sour cream by pureeing one cup of fat-free cottage cheese with one tablespoon of lemon juice in a food processor until perfectly smooth.

- Lighten quiche, croquettes, lasagna, and meat loaf by replacing some or all of the eggs with fat-free egg substitute or egg whites (use one-quarter cup of egg substitute or two whites for every whole egg). Leave the crust off the quiche.

- Prepare low-calorie sauces for casseroles by thickening fat-free broth or fat-free milk with cornstarch or arrowroot. Or use low-fat versions of condensed soups like cream of chicken, mushroom, celery, or broccoli.

Sumptuous seafood. Baking is best for lower-fat fish, such as cod, grouper, haddock, halibut, snapper, and sole. But be quick about it: Lean fish loses moisture faster than its fattier cousins like salmon, swordfish, and bluefish. One good no-fat technique is to wrap the fish in foil or parchment paper, which essentially steams it. Another is to lightly coat the fish with flour, then bake it in a covered dish with a little fat-free broth or wine and your choice of herbs. These techniques are also suitable for scallops, shrimp, and oysters.

Poultry preparation. Dredge skinless, boneless pieces (breasts are leanest) in a little flour seasoned with ground pepper. Then bake in a shallow pan with fat-free broth or wine, chopped fresh herbs (or crumbled dried ones), and minced garlic.

Vegetables and fruit. Whole baked white and sweet potatoes are perennial favorites—and much lower in fat than their scalloped and candied cousins. Instead of smothering them with butter, use nonfat sour cream or yogurt and chopped chives. For low-fat fries, cut potatoes into wedges, mist with nonstick spray, and bake in a single layer until tender and browned.

Onions, carrots, peppers, turnips, and winter squash also do well when baked, whether whole or in pieces. Baked raisin-stuffed apples and pears can double as healthy side dishes for pork and poultry as well as desserts.

Sweet stuff. You can trim down your favorite muffin and quick bread recipes by eliminating some fat and sugar. Start with one of the following suggestions. If that works to your satisfaction, incorporate another. (Don't try them all at once, or you might end up with inedible baked goods.)

- You can often replace half of the fat in a recipe with pureed fruit. Applesauce, apple butter (which contains no butter), and pureed prunes work great. For variety, try mashed cooked peaches, pears, or sweet potatoes. Low-fat or fat-free buttermilk is also an option. When dealing with cake and brownie mixes, follow the fat-cutting directions on the box.

- Low-fat or nonfat milk and buttermilk are suitable whole-milk substitutes. A combination of equal portions of 1 percent milk and evaporated fat-free milk can stand in for light cream.

- Nuts contain an amazing amount of calories and fat (although it's basically unsaturated fat). Cutting half a cup of walnuts from a quick bread or muffin recipe saves you 385 calories and 37 grams of fat. When you do use nuts, give them a flavor boost by toasting them first (at 350°F for five minutes); then chop them finely for better dispersal. And choose ones with distinctive flavor (black walnuts pack more punch than standard English walnuts, for instance).

- Let raisins or other dried fruit (such as cranberries, cherries, blueberries, apricots, and peaches) stand in for all or some of the nuts in quick breads and muffins.

- Opt for miniature chocolate chips in cookies and breads. Their smaller size distributes the chocolate flavor better—which also means you can use less.

- Cut back on the amount of sugar in recipes. For every half-cup you eliminate, you save 387 calories. A smidgen of ground cinnamon or nutmeg or a teaspoon of vanilla extract helps to compensate for the lost sweetness.

- Leave the top crust off fruit pies. Prepare pumpkin or squash pie without a crust.

- Using one-quarter cup of fat-free egg substitute in place of an egg saves about 50 calories; using two egg whites for every whole egg saves about 42 calories.

- Reduced-fat sour cream and cream cheese can easily replace their full-fat counterparts in coffee cakes and cheesecakes.

- Grease baking pans with nonstick spray instead of butter, margarine, or shortening.

Roasting

Roasting is another form of baking and is typically reserved for large pieces of meat and vegetables. The beauty of roasting is its simplicity. You place food, such as a whole chicken or turkey, in the oven and don't fuss with it until it's nearly done.

Simply succulent. For extra flavor, marinate meat, especially lower-fat cuts (such as top round or top sirloin), before cooking and baste it as it roasts. Broth, wine, juice, and low-fat vinegar-based salad dressings work well for both applications. Trim meat calories by slicing off visible fat before cooking. Roast meat and poultry on a rack in a roasting pan to allow fat to drip off; that way, it's not reabsorbed. Always roast poultry with the skin on to preserve moisture, but remove it before eating for a big fat savings.

Vegetable magic. Roasting vegetables brings out their sweet, mellow flavors. Nearly any vegetable tastes great when roasted, even artichokes, asparagus, green beans, eggplant, cauliflower, broccoli, and winter squash.

Lay out large chunks of vegetables in a single layer on a baking tray. Mist the vegetables with nonstick spray. Bake at 375° to 425°F until nicely browned, stirring the vegetables occasionally as they cook.

Roasted bell peppers are excellent in salads and as side dishes. In sandwiches, they make mayonnaise unnecessary. Bake whole peppers at about 450°F until the skin blackens. It takes about 10 minutes on each side, but you need to check them every few minutes. (Alternately, you can broil them, turning the peppers every five minutes.) Let cool. Then halve, peel, remove the seeds, and slice.

Roasted garlic is a creamy substitute for butter on bread and baked potatoes and pairs well with roasted meat. Trim the tip of a garlic bulb to expose the cloves and wrap in foil. Roast at 375°F until the bulb softens, about 30 minutes. Cool slightly, then squeeze out the garlic.

Braising

This slow, moist cooking method is perfect for the leanest cuts of meat, including rump and bottom round, and for hard vegetables like carrots and rutabagas. Long, gentle cooking in a small amount of liquid turns sinewy meats into succulent treats and gives vegetables an extra measure of flavor.

The secret to successful braising is to just simmer—not boil—the food. An oven set at 325° to 350°F is ideal, but you can also braise on the stove top. Either way, a pot with a tight-fitting lid, such as a Dutch oven or a casserole, is essential.

Maximum flavor. The choice of liquid is key here. Water will suffice, but you enhance flavor better with fat-free broth, wine, fruit juice, or beer. You need enough liquid to cover about a third of the food. Kick the flavor up a notch with herbs and spices.

Sear heaven. Braised meats are at their best when first seared in a hot skillet. Searing browns the meat's surface, sealing in moisture. Searing also cooks off surface fat, which you should discard before continuing with the recipe.

A cooling break. After braising meat, allow it to cool in its liquid in the refrigerator for a few

Smart Seasonings

When food tastes great, there's no need to smother it with high-fat sauces. That's where herbs and spices come in. To get the most from them, keep these tips in mind.

Spice rack savvy. Chances are, many jars have been on your spice rack for years—and their flavor deteriorated long ago. Although replacing them is costly, it pays in the long run.

If you really want to keep your aromatics fresh, write the date of purchase on the bottom of each jar and discard any that are more than a year old.

A good basic set of herbs includes dried basil, bay leaves, chili powder, dill, oregano, paprika, rosemary, and thyme. Useful spices include ground cinnamon, cloves, ginger, and nutmeg. When you're feeling more adventurous, experiment with less familiar flavor enhancers like cumin, mint, sage, Cajun spice mix, Chinese five-spice powder, and curry.

The perfect pepper-upper. Purchase peppercorns whole and grind as needed to preserve their punch. Black peppercorns are all you really need, but a mixture of red, green, white, and black will provide incomparable seasoning.

Fresh as a daisy. Dried herbs keep longer, but you can't beat the taste of fresh. Wash them when you bring them home, then dry gently with paper towels and store in the refrigerator. To use, chop with a sharp knife or snip with kitchen shears. Keep fresh garlic on hand as well as fresh ginger (store the garlic in a cool, dry place and the ginger in the refrigerator).

While you're at it. Make sure you have on hand a variety of vinegars, including balsamic, raspberry, red wine, rice, and malt. Vinegar's acidity tenderizes meat while adding flavor. Really flavorful vinegars can actually let you cut calories in traditional vinaigrette salad dressings. Use one-quarter to one-half the usual oil and make up the difference with vinegar. Pour the dressing into a water bottle with a spray attachment and mist salads and vegetables lightly. (Herbs will clog the sprayer, so add them directly to the food.)

Extra-virgin olive oil is worth the splurge. Usually it's used as a condiment for drizzling over fish, pasta, salads, or fresh vegetables. Because it's expensive, you may want to forgo using it as a cooking oil. Yes, it's 100 percent fat. But its flavor is so intense that you don't need to use much. Ditto for walnut oil and dark sesame oil.

Don't forget dehydrated sun-dried tomatoes to perk up pizzas and pasta dishes. Avoid tomatoes packed in oil, however. They're more costly and contain extra calories from fat.

Lemon and lime juice easily take the place of butter and margarine on steamed vegetables and add some zip to fish and baked chicken. Fresh-squeezed is best, but bottled or frozen will do.

Finally, don't be too quick to banish salt from your table. Sometimes a light shake is all it takes to make low-fat food more palatable.

---

hours. This has a couple of benefits. First, the flavors blend and actually intensify as the food stands. Second, fat that has been rendered into the liquid rises to the top and hardens. Skim off that fat and say goodbye to 100 calories for every tablespoon you throw away. To reheat, return to the oven with hot liquid until the meat is hot, then serve.

Vegging out. Whole potatoes, sweet potatoes, carrots, onions, leeks, and more can be braised, alone or along with meat. One pitfall to braising vegetables is that vitamins can leach into the cooking liquid. So use that liquid—either by turning it into a sauce thickened with cornstarch or by saving it to make soup.

Broiling and Grilling

Only the direction of the heat differentiates these low-fat cooking methods. When you broil, high heat sears the surface of food from the top; when you grill, heat cooks from the bottom. Either way, no fat is required, and natural flavors are preserved. Use specialty wood chips, such as mesquite, when grilling to further enhance the food's appeal.

Melting calories away. Both grilling and broiling help keep calories from meat and poultry to a minimum. As the meat cooks, fat within it liquefies and drips into the broiler pan or into the fire. That's fat you won't be eating!

To enhance flavor and tenderness, marinate meat and poultry before cooking. Acidic liquids like vinegar, fruit juice, and wine do a great job, especially on tough cuts like London broil, flank steak, and skirt steak. More flavor means less high-fat sauce is required to please your palette.

Fish tales. The firmer the fish, the better it stands up to broiling and grilling. Tuna and swordfish steaks are exceptionally suited to these cooking methods. To prevent sticking, brush the grill or broiling rack with a bit of olive or canola oil or spritz it with nonstick spray before adding the fish.

Perfect produce. Most vegetables do best when grilled in pierced foil packets. The foil keeps them from falling through the grids but still allows them to soak up that wonderful smoky flavor. Remember that denser vegetables take longer to cook, so either cut them small or keep them separate from the tender veggies.

You can place vegetables directly on the grill if they're large enough (brush the grill with oil to prevent sticking). Ears of corn, for instance, can be grilled right in their husks. They'll be so sweet you won't even need butter. Kabobs are also perfect for direct grilling. Skewer cherry tomatoes, chunks of bell pepper, and whole mushrooms for colorful vegetable kabobs. Add small pieces of meat, chicken, or shrimp for a meal on a stick. For meatless burgers, grill portobello mushroom caps and stack them on buns with reduced-fat cheese and tomato slices.

Fruit, including pineapple chunks and sliced peaches, pears, and plums, may also be skewered and broiled or grilled. Or wrap larger pieces in foil and grill until soft. Either way, you have the makings of a sweet and refreshing appetizer, side dish, or dessert.

Microwaving

The beauty of microwaving is that you don't need a trace of added fat to seal in flavors and nutrients.

The basics. Cooking time varies depending on a food's moisture content, how much you are cooking, the size of your dish, and the power of your microwave, so keep checking on foods. You may remove foods when they are not quite done, since they continue to cook for a few minutes after they come out. If your oven doesn't have a carousel, rotate food so that it heats evenly.

Microwave mania. Vegetables and fruits are well-suited to low-fat microwave cookery. Whole potatoes and sweet potatoes, which normally take upward of an hour to bake, can be microwaved in minutes. Pierce them with a fork first to allow steam to escape.

Chop other vegetables, such as broccoli, cauliflower, carrots, and green beans, into uniform pieces. Place in a microwave-safe dish with about half an inch of water, fat-free broth, or wine. Cover with a piece of pierced plastic wrap. Cook on high power until just crisp-tender.

Cored whole, halved, or sliced fruits (especially apples and pears) can be microwaved successfully. Pop in some fruit while you're eating dinner, and your fat-free dessert will be ready when you are.

Fuss-free fare. Fish and chicken retain their tenderness when prepared in a microwave. Uniformity counts, however. Tuck under the thin ends of a fish or chicken fillet to ensure even cooking

She Did It!

Cindi Trimmed the Fat and Trimmed Her Weight

Cindi Arvanites, 45, had been dieting on and off since high school.

"I could lose the weight when I changed my eating habits for a short period of time," says this full-time working mom from Peabody, Massachusetts. "But I would always gain it back—and then some."

Nearly two years ago, Cindi finally got fed up. She began cutting calories by eliminating cream from her coffee and replacing full-fat salad dressings with lower-fat versions. Almost immediately, she noticed a flatter belly. Cindi liked what she saw and wanted more. So she and husband Peter set out to trim their favorite home-cooked fare.

"In many cases, we eliminate fatty ingredients entirely or substitute lower-fat ones," she says. For example, 2 percent or fat-free milk thickened with flour replaces cream in sauces, and fat-free milk subs for whole in most recipes.

Poultry and leaner cuts of meat like pork tenderloin dominate the dinner table. Fish makes an appearance once a week. Meatless meals, such as pasta with a vegetable sauce, are standard fare.

Cindi and Peter make their own pizza with prepared dough, tomato sauce, and a smattering of low-fat mozzarella cheese. They continue to cook up family favorites, including chop suey and stuffed peppers, but they use ground turkey breast and 95-percent lean hamburger to cut fat.

There are some ingredients you just can't eliminate, says Cindi. "When a recipe calls for butter, we use just enough for a hint of flavor."

For the most part, however, she relies heavily on low-calorie flavor boosters instead of added fat. "Spices, balsamic vinegar, and fat-free chicken broth work wonders!" she notes.

After months of dietary moderation, Cindi added exercise to her routine. "I ride my stationary bike faithfully five times a week for up to 30 minutes," she says. "Biking has really reduced my thighs and hips."

After seven months, Cindi's weight loss topped 20 pounds. Best of all, her new habits have stuck.

"This is the first time I have lost weight and kept it off," she says. "It works because I don't feel deprived."

---

and moistness. Place in a dish with a half-inch of fat-free broth or wine and chopped or dried herbs. Cover and microwave until just cooked through. Let stand a few minutes to finish cooking.

Microwaves don't brown meat, but you can cook ground beef, chicken breast, or turkey breast to use in lasagna, chili, hamburger casseroles, and spaghetti sauce. Crumble the meat into a glass bowl and microwave until no longer pink (stop and stir every two minutes). Drain the meat before using.

Miscellaneous morsels. Invest in a microwave container for popcorn. Like air-popping, microwaving is a low-fat way to prepare this healthy snack (just don't add butter when serving). You can also scramble eggs in the microwave instead of frying them. Simply beat eggs or egg substitute with a bit of water, cover, and cook for a minute or until just set.

Steaming

Steaming is a straightforward cooking method that, like microwaving, preserves taste and nutrients without added fat. It's an inexpensive technique, too, requiring only a collapsible steamer insert or a rack. (If you get into steaming big time, you can invest in an electric steamer or stovetop steamer pot.)

Gathering steam. Most every vegetable is suitable for steaming. Cook veggies only until crisp-tender for fullest flavor. Poultry, fish, and shellfish work well, too. Forgo the traditional water for flavorful fat-free broth, wine, beer, or fruit juice. Add seasonings like herbs, spices, and garlic to the liquid. Use a pan that's big enough for the steam to circulate, and cover it with a tight lid. To steam fish, poultry, or vegetables in the oven, wrap them tightly in foil or parchment and bake at a high temperature (about 450°F) about 20 minutes, or until the food is tender.

Stir-Frying and Stir-Steaming

The two techniques of stir-frying and stir-steaming are identical, using a small amount of either oil or liquid to quickly cook foods. By combining bite-size pieces of meat, poultry, or seafood with lots of low-calorie vegetables, you can make a little protein go a long way. And because foods cook so fast, they retain both flavor and nutrients.

Great beginnings. Cutting is the first step in stir-frying and stir-steaming. Having sharp knives on hand makes these reduced-fat techniques faster and easier. Prepare all your ingredients, including seasonings such as garlic and fresh ginger, before starting to cook. Make sure your meat and vegetables are cut small so they cook fast. If desired, marinate the meat in a little low-salt soy sauce for more flavor.

Next, get out a large nonstick skillet or wok. A wok is helpful because it radiates heat quickly and evenly. Its rounded bottom and tall sides allow you to move food around fast without tossing it out of the pan. Coat the pan lightly with nonstick spray or a few pumps from a plastic bottle filled with canola, corn, or peanut oil (these oils won't burn under high heat). Heat the pan well. Forgoing the two tablespoons of oil typically used in stir-frying saves 240 calories right off the bat.

Stir-steaming is simply stir-frying without the fat. Add a few tablespoons of water, fat-free broth, juice, wine, or beer to the hot pan before starting to cook your meat and vegetables.

A quick job. Once the pan is hot, add the meat, poultry, or seafood, limiting the amount to three ounces per serving. When it's almost cooked, add chopped garlic or pungent fresh chopped ginger and toss.

Add chopped vegetables near the end to preserve their crispness. Try combos of bell peppers, pea pods, broccoli, carrots, onions, mushrooms, cauliflower, and asparagus. Cook until just crisp-tender. (It pays to steam denser veggies such as broccoli and carrots ahead of time so they're done at the same time as the tender ones.)

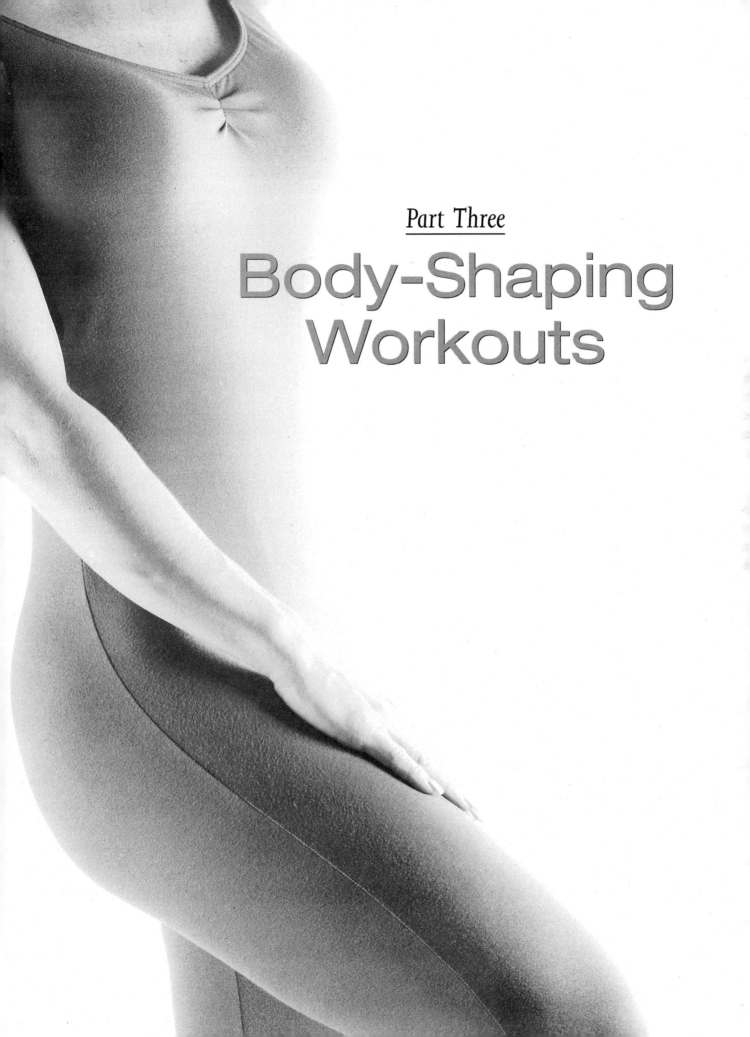

Part Three

Body-Shaping Workouts

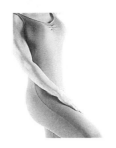

Slim Your Waist and Flatten Your Tummy

Dawn MacInnes's waistline was AWOL. As a teenager and in her twenties, Dawn was extremely active and had a tiny waist—19 to 21 inches. But as she got older, her life changed—and so did her waistline, expanding to 28 inches. Now in her early forties, she has two children, ages 5 and 9.

"I had my first child at 31, and the second in my midthirties," says Dawn, who is a nurse and sales representative for a medical technology company. "I was also working full-time, sitting in an office. Then we relocated from the East Coast to Indiana. Until we got settled in our house, we ate all of our meals at hotels and in restaurants. On the job, I was in my car a lot and ate on the road. Between relocating, traveling, and commuting, my diet went to pot.

"The weight I gained settled in areas where it had never settled before—my upper thighs and middle," Dawn says. "My skirts and jeans were tight. At first, I blamed it on the clothes dryer. But then I got out of denial and realized that I had to do something or I'd have to buy all new clothes. And I'd be as big as a house by the time I reached 50."

Previously, Dawn had tried walking to lose weight, but it didn't trim her waist the way she wanted. So she consulted Marjorie Albohm, an exercise physiologist, certified athletic trainer, and director of sports medicine at Kendrick Memorial Hospital in Mooresville, Indiana. "Marjorie gave me an extensive set of abdominal exercises targeted toward the middle, including curl-ups, crunches, side bends, hip raises, and pelvic tilts. I do my ab exercises faithfully—as many as I can do in 30 minutes three or four days a week, either in the morning or evening. Plus, I walk for a half-hour most afternoons, either outside or on a treadmill."

Within three months, Dawn had regained her trim waistline of 22 inches.

"The results are incredible," she says. "I started to notice improvement in just a month. My waistbands started to feel comfortable. I tried on my jeans, and they fit again. My skirts weren't tight. In fact, they're a little loose now."

Belly Be Gone

When it comes to bemoaning an expanding waistline, Dawn has lots of company. In a survey of more than 500 women conducted for this book, two-thirds of the women—67 percent—cited their bellies as trouble zones. Among the same women, 40 percent cited their waists as problem areas.

Your abdominal muscles confine your internal organs like a snug girdle. But pregnancy can present a challenge to these muscles.

As a baby grows within the womb, the surrounding abdominal muscles—especially the lower abs—stretch . . . and stretch . . . and stretch. With each passing month, the muscle fibers lose strength and elasticity. If you have a second or third baby, the process repeats itself. If you have a cesarean delivery, in which the muscles are surgically separated, the muscles become weaker still, losing their ability to expand and contract. When you add them up, these changes mean that your muscles lose their tone. The result is a post-pregnancy belly bulge.

Even if you've never been pregnant, your tummy can protrude, especially when you approach menopause. Researchers aren't sure why, but the drop in female sex hormones that heralds menopause prompts fat to accumulate over your abs. If you're overweight all over, your abs may be temporarily obscured by an extra layer of fat.

Four Weeks to Tighter Abs

Anything that you can do to tighten your abdominal muscles will help hold in your stomach and other organs. Your abs consist of four muscles, all of which shape your torso.

- The rectus abdominus (upper and lower), a vertical muscle that runs from your rib cage to your pubic bone
- The transverse abdominus, the deepest ab, which runs horizontally across your torso
- The external oblique, a broad, thin muscle that runs diagonally from your ribs to your hip
- The internal oblique muscle, which runs along the front and sides of your torso

The upper and lower abs and the obliques are "helper" muscles: You can press them into service as needed. If you're lying on your back on the beach and you reach forward to apply sunscreen to your knees, you're working your upper abs. If you're lying on the floor watching TV and you raise your legs, you're working your lower abs. If you're standing at the office photocopier and you bend to the right or left, you're working your obliques.

The trouble is, we don't routinely tax our abs very much during the course of a day. If we worked them harder, or more often, or both, they would tighten up and get stronger, and our tummies wouldn't protrude.

To slim your waist and a tummy distended by pregnancy, overweight, or hormonal changes, you need a program of exercises that deliberately works the abs—especially the upper and lower abs and the obliques—as well as a weight-loss regimen to lose excess fat. Working the abs as you go about your daily duties helps, too. The torso-

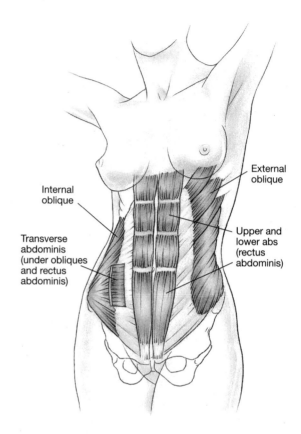

Internal oblique

External oblique

Transverse abdominis (under obliques and rectus abdominis)

Upper and lower abs (rectus abdominis)

To slim your waist and flatten your stomach, you need to work the upper and lower abs and the oblique muscles in the abdominal area.

shaping workouts that follow show you how. They're recommended by Albohm and are the same workouts that she prescribed for Dawn MacInnes.

"Like Dawn, you may see results in as little as four weeks," says Albohm, who works with women ranging from rank beginners who've never broken a sweat to highly trained fitness enthusiasts and everyone in between.

"The abdominal muscles are wonderful muscle groups to work on because they respond very quickly to exercise," says Albohm. "Compared to your buttocks, thighs, or other muscle groups, the abs get stronger pretty quickly."

The workouts that follow produce results because they use the principle of overload. That is, the only way to tone and strengthen a muscle is to boost the effort by increasing either duration (by doing more repetitions) or intensity (by doing the same number of reps but adding weights to make the exercise harder). If you're new to exercise, start at the beginner level. If you are able to complete the designated program with relative ease for three consecutive workout sessions, then it's time to progress to the next level.

"You'll feel results in about two weeks," says Albohm. "By four weeks, you should see some tightening or slight changes in contour. And by six weeks, you'll look and feel toned. If you don't, you're not doing the exercises correctly."

Women who have had children are eager to regain their pre-pregnancy shapes, Albohm notes, but this may take more effort. "Because the abs stretch to support the size of a fetus, it's hard for your tummy to return to its pre-pregnancy level. By working your abs, though, you can tighten the muscles that have been stretched and regain muscle tone."

Maximum Results with Minimum Effort

To make sure you get the results you're after, Albohm suggests doing these torso-shaping workouts in front of a mirror so you can check your position. "If you've never exercised before, you may have no idea what position your head, neck, shoulders, and back are in, or how far off the floor you are."

Here are some other tips from Albohm for getting the fastest results with the least effort.

Work all the abs. If you're trying to regain muscle tone after pregnancy, you will probably want to focus more on the lower abs. But don't neglect the others. As a rule, you should work the upper and lower abs and the obliques equally.

Flex those knees. If you don't, you're likely to use your hip muscles, not your abs, which will defeat the purpose of the exercise. As you advance, you may be doing straight-leg raises.

Flatten your back. You should flatten your back against the floor to protect your lower-back

muscles against strain. You'll probably want to use an exercise mat, but a carpeted floor or large, folded towel may work just as well.

Start easy. Three to 10 repetitions is the maximum for beginners.

Use slow, controlled movements. Use slow, steady movements and hold each position for a count of two, suggests Albohm. If you experience pain or discomfort when performing an exercise, stop and substitute another version, she advises. If pain persists, see your physician.

Be consistent. "Next to performing the exercises correctly, exercising regularly is key," says Albohm. The beginner, intermediate, and experienced workouts outlined on the following pages should be done three or four times a week. Use the everyday version that's shown with some of the exercises to work the same muscles in your daily life.

Combine ab work with diet and aerobics. "You can't say, 'I want to take three inches off my waist,' do 500 ab exercises and nothing else, and expect it to work—it won't," says Albohm. If you ignore aerobic exercise—and a sensible diet—your belly will show it.

Combining aerobics with ab workouts helps in two ways: The combination burns calories, which helps get rid of excess weight all over, including the abdomen, and it gives your abs a little boost.

"The fact that you're supporting your body as you move forces the muscles to contract," explains Albohm. "If you deliberately contract your abs during aerobic exercise, you'll benefit even more."

Be patient. "Don't expect results overnight. If you're a beginner, start at the beginner level. When working at one level becomes easy and effortless, move on to the next," says Albohm.

If you would like to see demonstrations of how to perform these and other exercises for slimming your waist and flattening your tummy, visit our Web site at www.banishbbt.com.

Curl-Ups 1

Muscles Worked
Upper abs

Performance Hints

- Use your abs to do the work. Don't pull yourself up with your arms.

- Keep your back flat on the floor.

Intensity

Beginner: 1 set of 3 to 10 reps, 3 days per week

Intermediate: 2 sets of 10 reps, 3 days per week

Experienced: 3 or 4 sets of 10 reps, 3 or 4 days per week

Everyday Version for Upper Abs

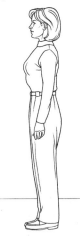

While standing, contract your upper abdominals by inhaling sharply and holding in your abdominal muscles. Breathing normally, hold for 6 to 8 seconds, then release.

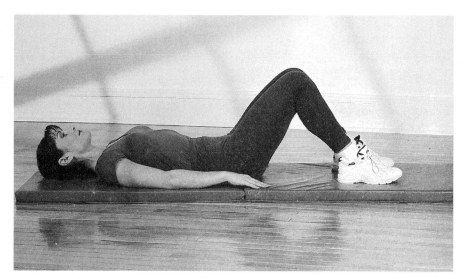

Lie on your back with your pelvis tilted to flatten your back against the floor, arms at your sides, knees bent at approximately a 90-degree angle, and your feet flat on the floor, as shown.

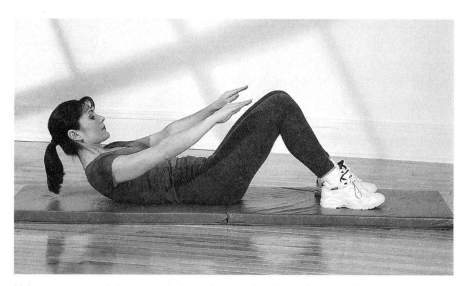

Using your upper abdominal muscles, raise your head and shoulders from the floor, as shown. Your arms should be extended out in front. Hold for 2 seconds. Then lower your shoulders to the floor in a slow, controlled motion, touching your shoulders lightly on the floor. Repeat.

Curl-Ups 2

Muscles Worked
Upper abs

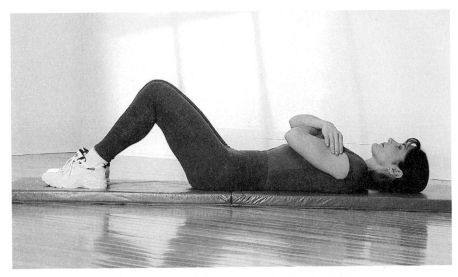

Lie on your back with your pelvis tilted to flatten your back, arms folded across your chest, knees bent approximately 90 degrees, and your feet flat on the floor, as shown.

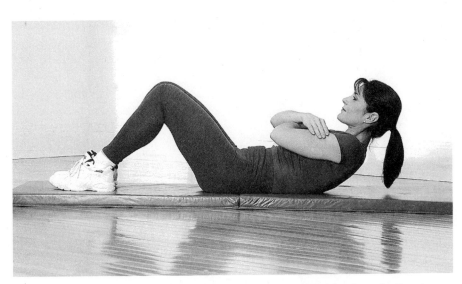

Using your upper abdominal muscles, raise your head and shoulders from the floor toward your knees, as shown. Hold for 2 seconds. Then lower your upper body in a slow, controlled motion, touching your shoulders lightly on the floor. Repeat.

Performance Hints

- Keep your feet and lower back flat on the floor.
- Don't rock, using the momentum to pull yourself up.
- Don't strain your head or neck when rising.

Intensity

Beginner: 1 set of 3 to 10 reps, 3 days per week

Intermediate: 2 sets of 10 reps, 3 days per week

Experienced: 3 or 4 sets of 10 reps, 3 or 4 days per week

Variation

To increase intensity further, you can hold a 1-pound dumbbell on your chest while performing this curl-up. To further increase intensity, add up to 3 pounds.

Curl-Ups 3

Muscles Worked
Upper abs

Performance Hints

- Don't pull your head and neck upward when lifting your shoulders.
- To prevent neck strain, keep your chin forward and your eyes focused toward the ceiling.
- Keep your elbows out to your sides so you can barely see them.

Intensity

Beginner: 1 set of 3 to 10 reps, 3 days per week

Intermediate: 2 sets of 10 reps, 3 days per week

Experienced: 3 or 4 sets of 10 reps, 3 or 4 days per week

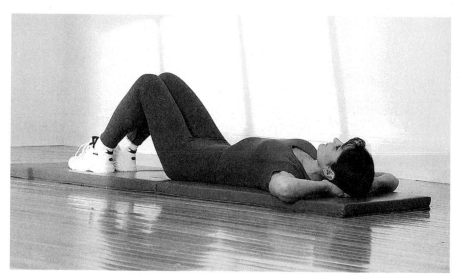

Lie on your back with your pelvis tilted to flatten your back, your knees bent at approximately 90 degrees, and your hands clasped behind your head. Your elbows should be out to your sides, and your feet flat on the floor, as shown.

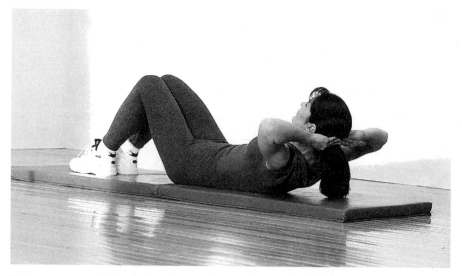

Using your upper abdominals, raise your head and shoulders off the floor. Hold for 2 seconds. Then lower your upper body to the floor in a slow, controlled motion, touching your shoulders lightly on the floor. Repeat.

Knee-Up Crunches

Muscles Worked
Upper abs

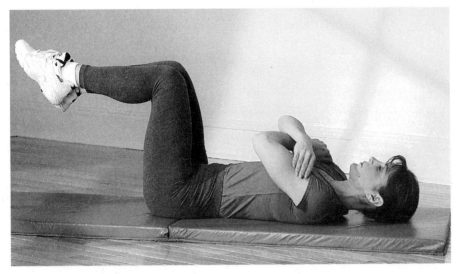

Lie on your back with your legs raised so that your thighs are perpendicular to your body and your calves and feet are parallel to the floor. Fold your arms across your chest, as shown.

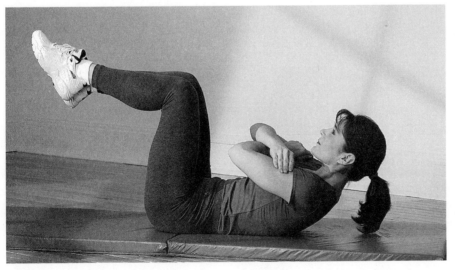

Using the muscles of your upper abs, raise your shoulders and upper back off the floor in a forward curling motion. Hold for 2 seconds. Then slowly lower your shoulders to the starting position, lightly touching them to the floor. Repeat.

Performance Hints

- Make sure that your shoulders lift off the floor.
- Don't use momentum to perform the move.
- Keep the small of your back pressed against the floor.

Intensity

Beginner: 1 set of 3 to 10 reps, 3 days per week

Intermediate: 2 sets of 10 reps, 3 days per week

Experienced: 3 or 4 sets of 10 reps, 3 or 4 days per week

Variation

To increase intensity further, you can hold a 1-pound dumbbell on your chest while performing this crunch. To further increase intensity, use 2 pounds.

Everyday Version for Upper Abs

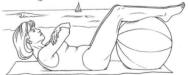

You can simulate this exercise while lying on the beach or your living room floor with your legs propped up by a beach ball, as shown.

Crunches with Knees Up, Spread

Muscles Worked
Upper abs

Performance Hints

- Keep the movement slow and controlled.
- Don't pull your head or neck with your hands as you go up.
- Don't rest your shoulders on the floor at the bottom of the movement.

Intensity Level

Beginner: 1 set of 3 to 10 reps, 3 days per week

Intermediate: 2 sets of 10 reps, 3 days per week

Experienced: 3 or 4 sets of 10 reps, 3 or 4 days per week

Everyday Version for Upper Abs

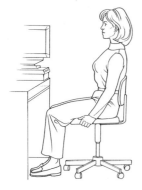

While sitting at your desk, contract your upper abdominals by inhaling sharply and pulling in your abdominal area. Breathing normally, hold for 6 to 8 seconds, then relax. Repeat.

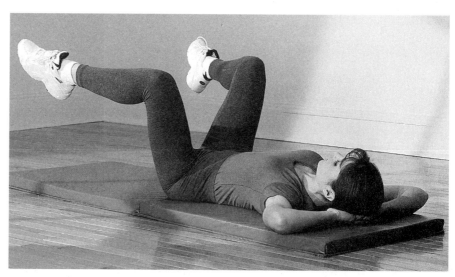

Lying on your back, raise your legs so your thighs are perpendicular to your body, with your calves and feet raised and parallel to the floor, and your hands behind your head with your elbows extended. Spread your legs as shown.

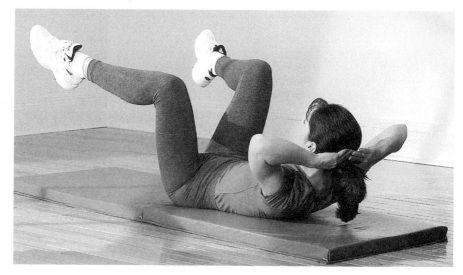

Using your upper abs, raise your shoulders and upper back off the floor in a slow, controlled forward curling motion. Hold for 2 seconds. Then lower your shoulders to the starting position, lightly touching them to the floor. Repeat.

Inclined Board Crunches

Muscles Worked
Upper abs

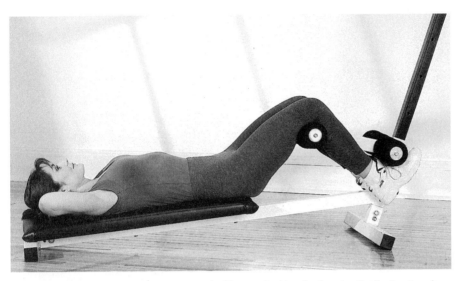

Lie flat on your back on an inclined board with your feet hooked under the footrest and your hands behind your head, with your elbows extended, as shown.

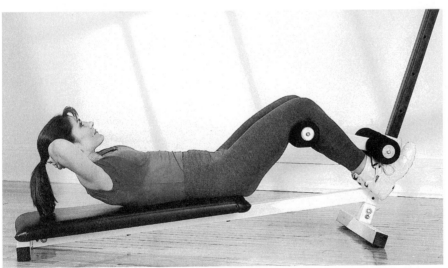

Using your upper abs, raise your head and shoulders off the bench in a forward curling motion. Hold for 2 seconds. Then lower your shoulders in a slow, controlled motion to the starting position, lightly touching them to the bench. Repeat.

Performance Hints

- Don't use your hands to pull up on your head and neck.
- Don't relax at the bottom of the movement.

Intensity

Beginner: 1 set of 3 to 10 reps, 3 days per week

Intermediate: 2 sets of 10 reps, 3 days per week

Experienced: 3 or 4 sets of 10 reps, 3 or 4 days per week

Variation

You can increase the intensity by increasing the angle of the bench.

Everyday Version for Upper Abs

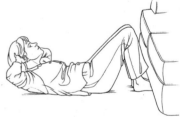

You can simulate this exercise by performing it with your feet hooked underneath a very heavy, secure piece of furniture, as shown.

Hip Raises

Muscles Worked
Lower abs

Performance Hints

- Do not use your arms or shoulders to assist in the lift.
- Do not rock your hips backward.
- Do not let your legs fall backward toward your head.

Intensity

Beginner: 1 set of 3 to 10 reps, 3 days per week

Intermediate: 2 sets of 10 reps, 3 days per week

Experienced: 3 or 4 sets of 10 reps, 3 or 4 days per week

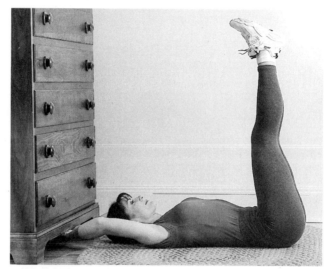

Lie on your back with your legs extended upward, toes pointed, and your arms extended overhead. Hold on to a heavy, secure piece of furniture such as the bottom of a desk, dresser, or couch.

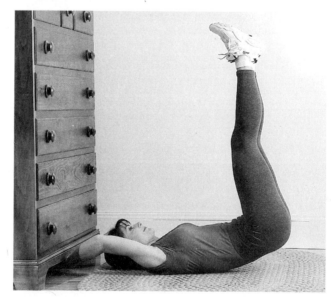

Using your lower abdominal muscles, raise your hips off the floor and lift your legs, knees slightly flexed, straight in the air, as shown. Hold for 2 seconds. Then lower your legs, touching your hips lightly on the floor; repeat.

Modified Knee Raises

Muscles Worked
Lower abs

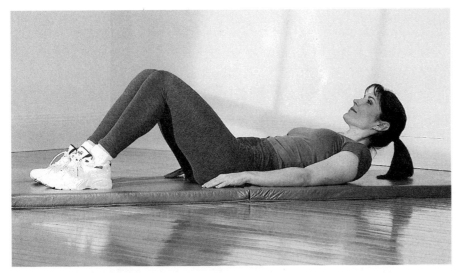

Lie on your back with your pelvis tilted to flatten your back and your knees bent. Your arms should be extended next to your body with your hands palms down, your head up, and your shoulder blades slightly off the floor, as shown.

Performance Hints

- Keep the opposite foot on the floor.
- Do not raise your head and neck too far off the floor; your shoulder blades should be only slightly off the floor.

Intensity

Beginner: 1 set of 3 to 10 reps, 3 days per week

Intermediate: 2 sets of 10 reps, 3 days per week

Experienced: 3 or 4 sets of 10 reps, 3 or 4 days per week

Using your lower abdominals, raise one leg at a time toward your chest in a slow, controlled motion, as shown. Hold for 2 seconds. Then lower your leg slowly until your heel lightly touches the floor. Repeat with the opposite leg.

Pelvic Tilts

Muscles Worked
Lower abs

Performance Hint

- Don't raise your head and neck off the floor.

Intensity

Beginner: 1 set of 3 to 10 reps, 3 days per week

Intermediate: 2 sets of 10 reps, 3 days per week

Experienced: 3 or 4 sets of 10 reps, 3 or 4 days per week

Everyday Version for Lower Abs

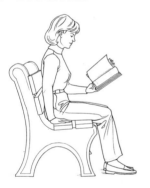

While sitting, perform the same exercise by slightly tilting your pelvis up and contracting your lower abdominals and slightly pushing your lower back flat. Hold for 8 to 10 seconds, then release.

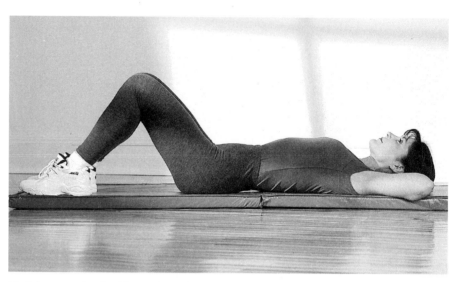

Lie flat on your back with your knees bent at approximately a 90-degree angle and your hands behind your head, elbows extended to your sides, and your head on the floor, as shown.

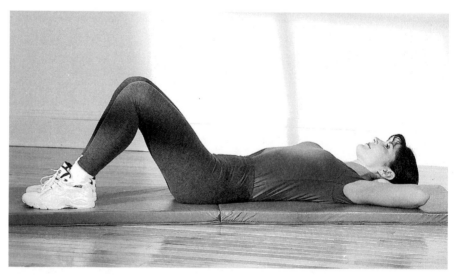

Lift your pelvis up and toward your rib cage, tightening your lower abdominal muscles and gently "pushing" back into the floor. Hold for 2 seconds. Relax and let your pelvis rotate back to its normal position. Repeat the exercise in a slow, controlled manner.

Reverse Curls

Muscles Worked
Lower abs

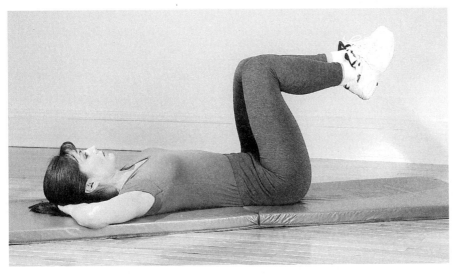

Lie flat on your back with your head flat on the floor, your hands behind your head supporting your neck, and your elbows out. Raise your legs so that your thighs are perpendicular to your body, as shown, and your calves and feet are parallel to the floor.

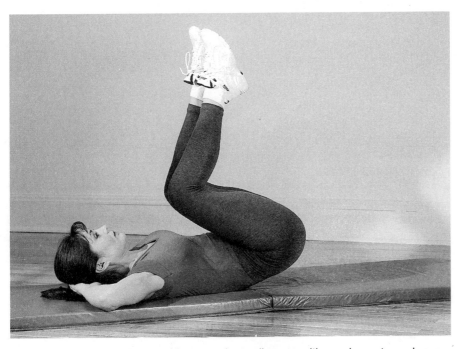

Using your lower abs, raise your hips toward your rib cage, with your knees toward your forehead, as shown. Hold for a count of 2. Then lower your hips in a slow, controlled motion, keeping your abs contracted until your hips contact the floor. Repeat.

Performance Hints

- Don't rock or use momentum to perform the curl.
- Don't rest your hips on the floor at the bottom of the curl.
- Keep constant tension on your abs during the exercise.

Intensity

Beginner: 1 set of 3 to 10 reps, 3 days per week

Intermediate: 2 sets of 10 reps, 3 days per week

Experienced: 3 or 4 sets of 10 reps, 3 or 4 days per week

Variation

To increase intensity, you may straighten your lower legs slightly as you perform the exercise.

Single-Knee Lifts

Muscles Worked

Upper and lower abs

Performance Hints

- When rising, don't pull on your head and neck with your arms.
- Raise your torso and knees together in an equidistant curling motion.
- Don't use momentum to rock upward.

Intensity

Beginner: 1 set of 3 to 10 reps on each side, 3 days per week

Intermediate: 2 sets of 10 reps on each side, 3 days per week

Experienced: 3 or 4 sets of 10 reps on each side, 3 or 4 days per week

Everyday Version for Upper and Lower Abs

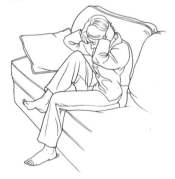

While sitting, place your hands behind your head. With one foot flat on the floor, bring the opposite knee up to meet your torso. Contract your upper abdominals as you crunch forward to meet your raised knee; hold for 8 to 10 seconds. Return your upper body and leg in a slow, controlled motion. Repeat with the opposite leg. Repeat the exercise using your lower abdominals.

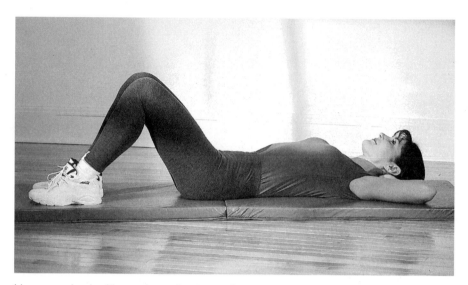

Lie on your back with your knees bent, your feet on the floor, and your pelvis tilted to flatten your back. Your hands should be behind your head, and your elbows extended, as shown.

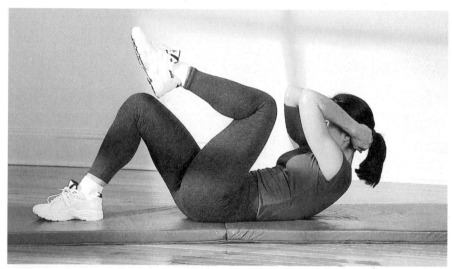

Using your upper and lower abs, simultaneously raise one knee and your torso, bringing both elbows to the knee. Hold for 2 seconds. Then lower your upper body and leg in a slow, controlled motion. Repeat on the opposite side.

Diagonal Curl-Ups 1

Muscles Worked
Obliques

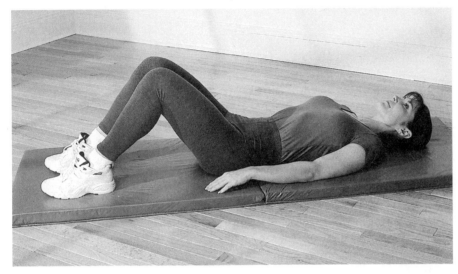

Lie on your back with your feet flat on the floor, your knees bent at approximately a 90-degree angle, your pelvis tilted to flatten your back, and your arms straight at your sides, as shown.

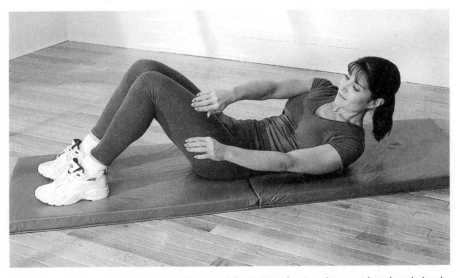

Extend your arms, as shown, and use your oblique muscles to raise your head and shoulders, rotating to one side as your shoulders lift off the floor. Hold for 2 seconds. Then lower your shoulders in a slow, controlled motion, touching them lightly to the floor. Repeat the exercise on the opposite side.

Performance Hints

- Don't use your arms to pull up your shoulders.
- As you rotate your torso, use a slow, controlled motion and keep your oblique muscles contracted.
- Don't use momentum to alternate from side to side.

Intensity

Beginner: 1 set of 3 to 10 reps on each side, 3 days per week

Intermediate: 2 sets of 10 reps on each side, 3 days per week

Experienced: 3 or 4 sets of 10 reps on each side, 3 or 4 days per week

Everyday Version for Obliques

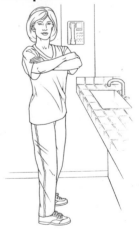

While standing at your kitchen counter or a photocopier, rotate your upper body one quarter turn in a slow, controlled motion. Fold your arms and contract your abdominal muscles while turning. Hold for 6 to 8 seconds, then repeat the exercise to the opposite side.

Diagonal Curl-Ups 2

Muscles Worked
Obliques

Performance Hints

- Keep your feet flat on the floor.
- Don't use momentum when rotating from side to side.
- Don't over-rotate.

Intensity

Beginner: 1 set of 3 to 10 reps on each side, 3 days per week

Intermediate: 2 sets of 10 reps on each side, 3 days per week

Experienced: 3 or 4 sets of 10 reps on each side, 3 or 4 days per week

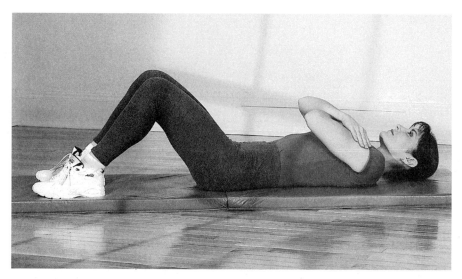

Lie on your back with your pelvis tilted to flatten your back against the floor, your knees bent at approximately a 90-degree angle, your feet flat on the floor, and your arms folded across your chest, as shown.

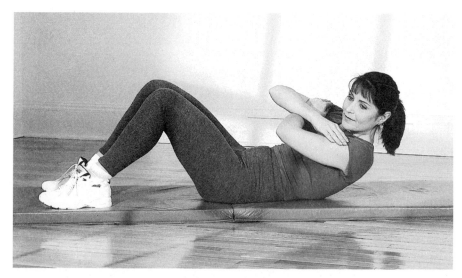

Use your oblique muscles to raise your head and shoulders from the floor, rotating to one side as your shoulders lift off the floor. Hold for 2 seconds. Lower your shoulders in a slow, controlled motion, touching them lightly to the floor. Repeat the exercise in the opposite direction.

Diagonal Curl-Ups 3

Muscles Worked
Obliques

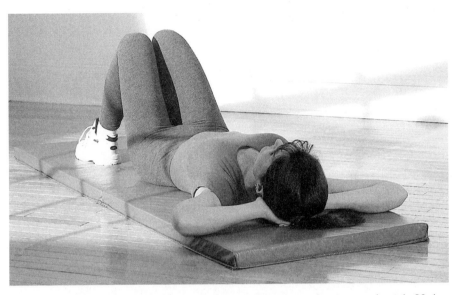

Lie on your back with your feet flat on the floor and your knees bent approximately 90 degrees, with your pelvis tilted to flatten your back. Your hands should be clasped behind your head with your elbows out to your sides, as shown.

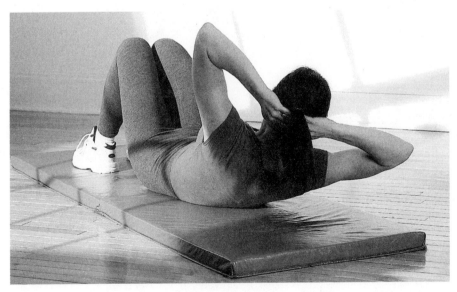

Use your oblique muscles to raise your head and shoulders, rotating to one side as your shoulders lift off the floor. Hold for 2 seconds. Then lower your shoulders in a slow, controlled motion, touching them lightly to the floor. Repeat the exercise in the opposite direction.

Performance Hints

- Don't pull on your head and neck.
- Don't over-rotate.
- Don't use momentum when alternating sides.

Intensity

Beginner: 1 set of 3 to 10 reps on each side, 3 days per week

Intermediate: 2 sets of 10 reps on each side, 3 days per week

Experienced: 3 or 4 sets of 10 reps on each side, 3 or 4 days per week

Side Crunches

Muscles Worked
Obliques

Performance Hints

- Make sure your upper body is lifted off the floor, not just your head and neck.
- Don't pull on your head and neck with your hand.
- Feel the muscle contraction in the oblique area.

Intensity

Beginner: 1 set of 3 to 10 reps on each side, 3 days per week

Intermediate: 2 sets of 10 reps on each side, 3 days per week

Experienced: 3 or 4 sets of 10 reps on each side, 3 or 4 days per week

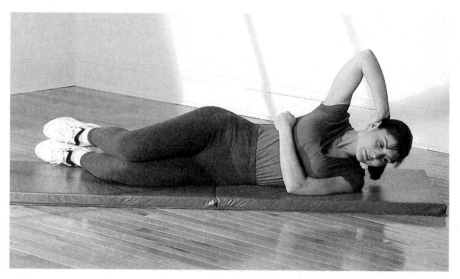

Lie on your left hip, with your knees bent so your thighs are almost perpendicular to your body. Place your right hand behind your head, elbow extended, and your left hand on top of your right side, as shown.

Everyday Version for Obliques

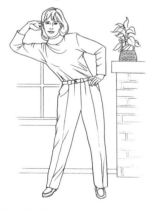

Stand with your feet comfortably apart. Place your right arm behind your head with your elbow extended out, and the other arm on your hip. Using your oblique muscles, flex your trunk to the right side, as shown. Hold for 6 to 8 seconds, then relax. Repeat on the opposite side.

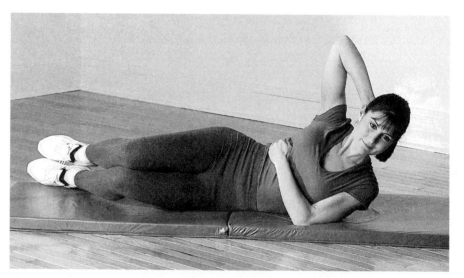

Using your oblique muscles in a crunchlike motion, lift your upper body off the floor and up over your hip, bringing your rib cage toward your hip. Hold for 2 seconds. Then lower your body in a slow, controlled motion, slightly touching the floor. Repeat the movement to the same side until you have completed your repetitions. Then perform the same exercise on the opposite side.

Side Bends

Muscles Worked
Obliques

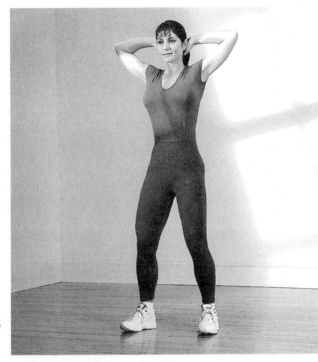

Stand with your knees slightly bent, feet shoulder-width apart, hands behind your head, and elbows extended out, as shown.

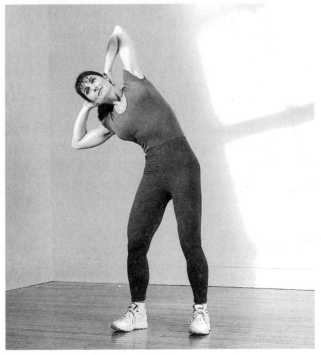

Using your oblique muscles, bend to your right side in a slow, controlled movement, bringing your right elbow toward your right knee. Return to the starting position and repeat the movement to the same side until you have completed your repetitions. Perform the same exercise on the opposite side.

Performance Hints

- Perform the movement in a slow and controlled manner throughout a full range of motion.
- Don't use momentum when performing repetitions.
- Don't lean forward as you bend.

Intensity

Beginner: 1 set of 3 to 10 reps on each side, 3 days per week

Intermediate: 2 sets of 10 reps on each side, 3 days per week

Experienced: 3 or 4 sets of 10 reps on each side, 3 or 4 days per week

Everyday Version for Obliques

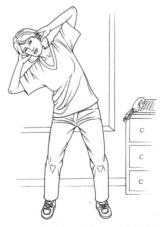

Stand with your feet comfortably apart in a quarter-squat position with your hands behind your head and your elbows extended out. Using your oblique muscles, bend to one side approximately 25 to 30 degrees. Hold for 6 to 8 seconds, then relax. Repeat on the opposite side.

Side Jackknives

Muscles Worked
Obliques

Performance Hints

- Lift both your upper and lower body an equal distance.
- Perform the exercise in a slow, controlled motion; don't use momentum.
- Make sure you lift your upper body off the floor, not just your head.

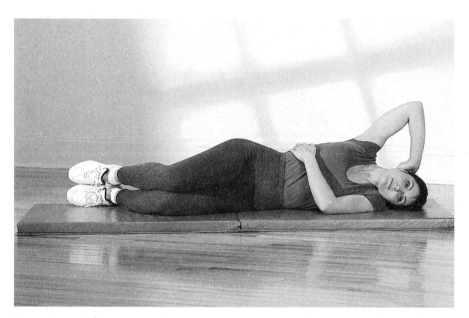

Lie on your left side with your legs together, your knees bent, and your thighs almost perpendicular to your body. Your left arm should be close to your body for support, with your left hand on your waist. Your right hand should be on the side of your head, with elbow bent, as shown.

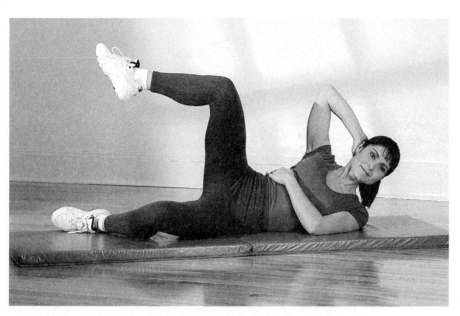

Using your oblique muscles, raise your top leg while simultaneously raising your head, shoulders, and torso, as shown. Hold for 2 seconds. Then lower in a controlled motion. After completing your repetitions, repeat on the opposite side.

Intensity

Beginner: 1 set of 3 to 10 reps on each side, 3 days per week

Intermediate: 2 sets of 10 reps on each side, 3 days per week

Experienced: 3 or 4 sets of 10 reps on each side, 3 or 4 days per week

30-Day Beginner Program

Week I	Week II
Do Exercises Shown 3 Days This Week	**Do Exercises Shown 3 Days This Week**

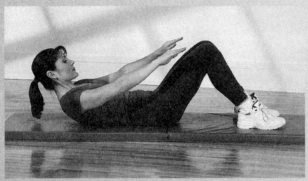

Curl-Ups 1 (page 126)

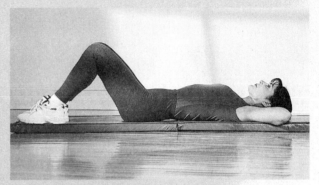

Pelvic Tilts (page 134)

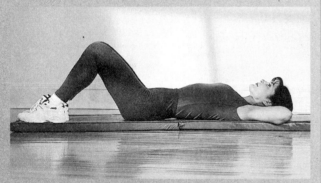

Pelvic Tilts (page 134)

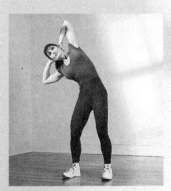

Side Bends (page 141)

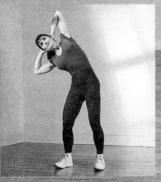

Side Bends (page 141)

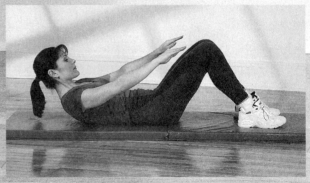

Curl-Ups 1 (page 126)

Week III

**Do Exercises Shown
3 Days This Week**

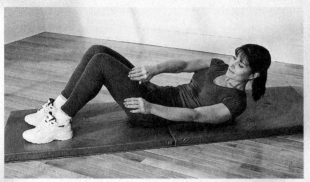

Diagonal Curl-Ups 1 (page 137)

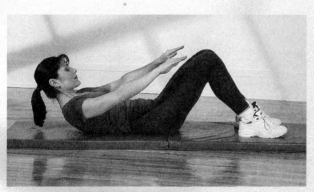

Curl-Ups 1 (page 126)

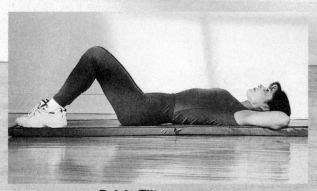

Pelvic Tilts (page 134)

Week IV

**Do Exercises Shown
3 Days This Week**

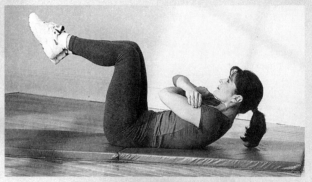

Knee-Up Crunches (page 129)

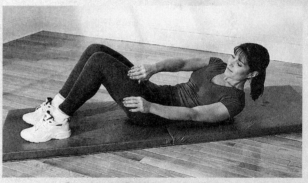

Diagonal Curl-Ups 1 (page 137)

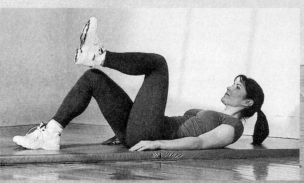

Modified Knee Raises (page 133)

30-Day Intermediate Program

Week I	**Week II**
Do Exercises Shown 3 Days This Week	Do Exercises Shown 3 Days This Week

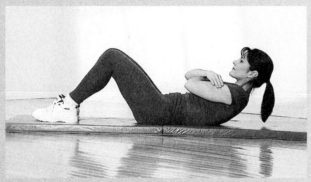

Curl-Ups 2 (page 127)

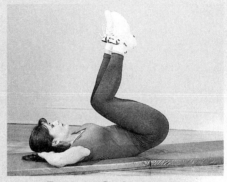

Reverse Curls (page 135)

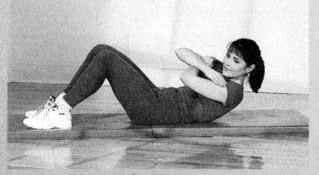

Diagonal Curl-Ups 2 (page 138)

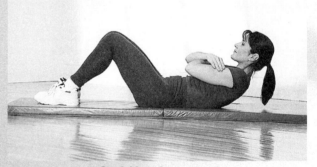

Curl-Ups 2 (page 127)

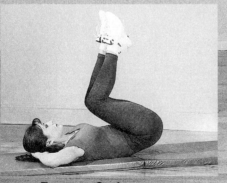

Reverse Curls (page 135)

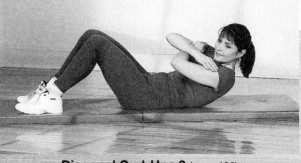

Diagonal Curl-Ups 2 (page 138)

Week III

**Do Exercises Shown
3 Days This Week**

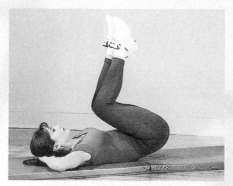

Reverse Curls (page 135)

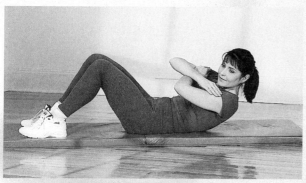

Diagonal Curl-Ups 2 (page 138)

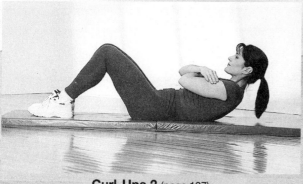

Curl-Ups 2 (page 127)

Week IV

**Do Exercises Shown
3 Days This Week**

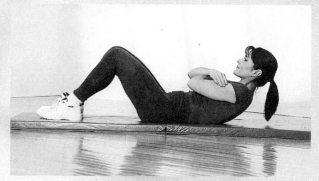

Curl-Ups 2 (page 127)

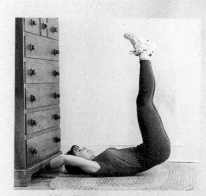

Hip Raises (page 132)

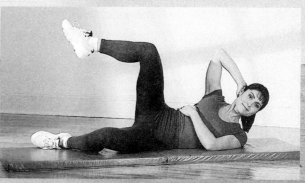

Side Jackknives (page 142)

30-Day Experienced Program

Week I

**Do Exercises Shown
3 or 4 Days This Week**

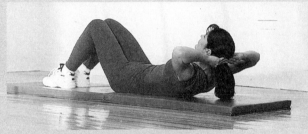

Curl-Ups 3 (page 128)

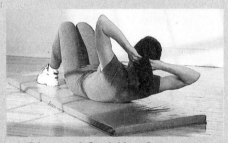

Diagonal Curl-Ups 3 (page 139)

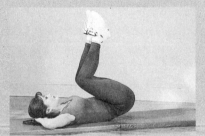

Reverse Curls (page 135)

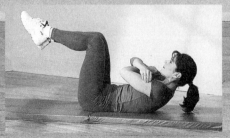

Knee-Up Crunches (page 129)

Week II

**Do Exercises Shown
3 or 4 Days This Week**

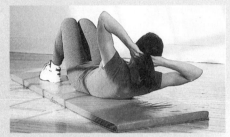

Diagonal Curl-Ups 3 (page 139)

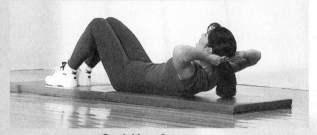

Curl-Ups 3 (page 128)

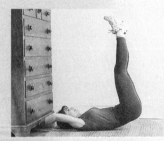

Hip Raises (page 132)

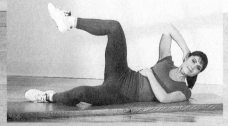

Side Jackknives (page 142)

Week III

**Do Exercises Shown
3 or 4 Days This Week**

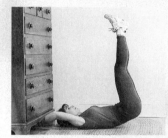

Hip Raises (page 132)

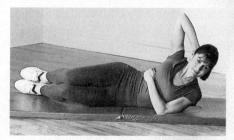

Side Crunches (page 140)

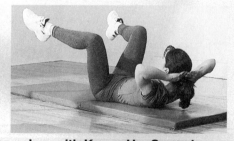

Crunches with Knees Up, Spread (page 130)

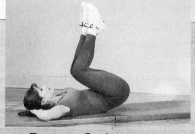

Reverse Curls (page 135)

Week IV

**Do Exercises Shown
3 or 4 Days This Week**

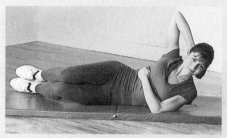

Side Crunches (page 140)

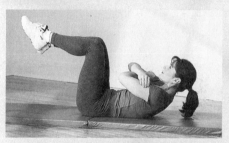

Knee-Up Crunches (page 129)

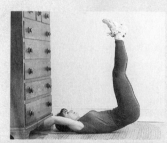

Hip Raises (page 132)

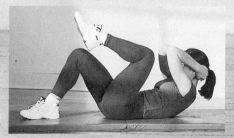

Single-Knee Lifts (page 136)

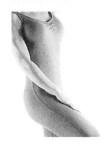

Workouts for Your Hips, Thighs, and Buttocks

By many women's standards, Carrie Givens wasn't what you would call overweight. Before she had children, she weighed a mere 100 pounds. Even at the age of 43, the petite (five-foot-one-inch) mother of three weighed just 117 pounds. Problem was, the extra pounds seemed to have accumulated in her hips and thighs.

"I was definitely pear-shaped," says Carrie, an art teacher in Alliance, Ohio, whose three daughters are now 13, 15, and 19. "I felt frumpy, especially when I tried to find jeans that fit and looked good."

Like many pear-shaped women, Carrie discovered that finding jeans and slacks to fit her proportions was difficult, if not impossible. "I'd find a pair that fit in the hips, but the waist would be too big. If I found a pair that fit in the waist, I couldn't get them over my thighs. I'd try on 20 pairs of jeans, but I still couldn't find a pair that looked stylish and felt comfortable."

Carrie blamed her heavy hips and thighs on heredity, having children, and age. She tried to lose weight—either by cutting out certain foods entirely, not eating altogether, or following "diets" she improvised. She also tried running and swimming, but she wasn't very consistent.

Carrie just couldn't seem to trim her hips and thighs—until she started to work out with weights.

"My sister owns and operates a fitness center, and she encouraged me to try weight training," says Carrie. "I started to work out, doing leg raises, curls, extensions, and especially lunges three days a week. I lost inches on my hips and thighs, but especially my thighs."

In addition, Carrie spends time on a step machine, for 5 to 15 minutes a session, or she does a 40-minute aerobic class to warm up. And she's more consistent about aerobic exercise. "I run, bike, and take aerobics classes. But the weight training has made the most significant difference in my thighs," she says.

Carrie also follows a more structured low-fat diet, which includes lots of fruits, vegetables, cereal, and soy milk. For protein, she eats fish and tofu, and a little red meat.

With her exercise and diet plan, Carrie finally got the results she hoped for. After six months of working out with weights, she weighs 110 pounds. But to Carrie, the important thing is that she lost fat and gained muscle (and more energy). And she finally found jeans that fit and look good.

Thinner, Shapelier Hips and Thighs

Carrie is the classic pear shape, and her quest for thinner hips and thighs is shared by many women, young and not-so-young. In a survey of 500 women conducted for this book, nearly half said they wished they had slimmer thighs, and over 40 percent said they were dissatisfied with their hips. A fair number—25 percent—also said they regarded their backsides as a trouble zone.

It's not that these women want to look like guys, with narrow hips, a flat butt, and wide shoulders. Any physiology teacher will tell you that, by nature's design, women are programmed to have wider lower bodies than men. We need wider pelvic bones for childbearing and to support a growing fetus—and sturdy thighs and generous backsides to support us while we carry the growing fetus for nine months. Add a genetically programmed layer of fat, and you have your mom's hips, thighs, and buttocks.

In some women, like Carrie, this pearlike physique is more exaggerated than in others, even if they're only a few pounds overweight. This makes it hard to find even "relaxed-fit" jeans that are comfortable, and it makes women self-conscious about wearing swimsuits.

"Most women, however, even if they're not overly pear-shaped, will gain weight in their hips and thighs before they gain it anywhere else," points out Marjorie Albohm, an exercise physiologist, certified athletic trainer, and director of sports medicine at Kendrick Memorial Hospital in Mooresville, Indiana. "Men accumulate fat in the abdominal area, and women accumulate fat in the hip and thigh area—that's a fact. All you have to do is look at lots of men and women the next time you are in a crowd or go to the mall. That's how fat is distributed between the genders."

Heavier hips, thighs, and buttocks are more a factor of gender than age. "Whether they're 20 or 40, women still have 10 to 15 percent more body fat than men, even if they work out," says Albohm. As for the myth that pregnancy "stretches" your pelvis and widens your hips, that's just not so, says Albohm. "If women have bigger hips after pregnancy, they've simply gained weight, period."

Nor is sitting at a desk in itself responsible for wider hips and a broader backside—the so-called secretary spread.

"Sitting itself doesn't necessarily determine where fat is deposited," says Albohm. "Our sedentary lifestyle in general does that. Your muscles would be far more toned if you were active—working on a farm, climbing up and down ladders, and so forth. Those are the exercises that tone the muscles in your hips and thighs."

Done correctly, cutting dietary fat and calories can help you lose weight overall, and that can certainly help "shrink" your hips, thighs, and buttocks to some degree. So can aerobic exercise that burns excess body fat and calories as you work your heart and lungs, like walking, jogging, biking, or taking aerobics classes. Purposeful exercise can make up for the kind of sedentary lifestyle that packs pounds on overall, including the hips and thighs. But to see a real difference in your lower body, says Albohm, you have to do what Carrie did—add resistance training to the mix.

Muscles Meant to Be Worked

The muscles that form the hips, thighs, and buttocks include:

- The gluteal muscles (small, medium, and large muscles that form the buttocks)

- The quadriceps (the muscles on the front of the thighs)

- The hamstrings (the muscles on the back of the thighs)

- The abductors (the outer thighs)

- The adductors (the inner thighs)

In some women, the thigh muscles are long and lean; in others, they're shorter and broader. "So again, genetics is a primary factor in the size and shape of your thighs," says Albohm. But so is use (or lack thereof).

The gluteals, quadriceps, and hamstrings are the "worker" muscles—the ones you'd use if you led a life of running, jumping, climbing, and lifting heavy objects. The adductors, in particular, suffer from neglect.

Albohm compares flabby thighs to flabby upper arms. "Women don't use their triceps—the underside of the upper arm—in any day-to-day activity, so the triceps tend to get flabby," she points out. "The same thing happens to your inner thighs."

The same principle applies to your abductors, the outer thigh muscles. "You use your quads, hamstrings, and gluteals to move back and forth and up and down, but you don't move sideways very much," explains Albohm. "But work the inner and outer thigh muscles three days a week, and you'll see a difference."

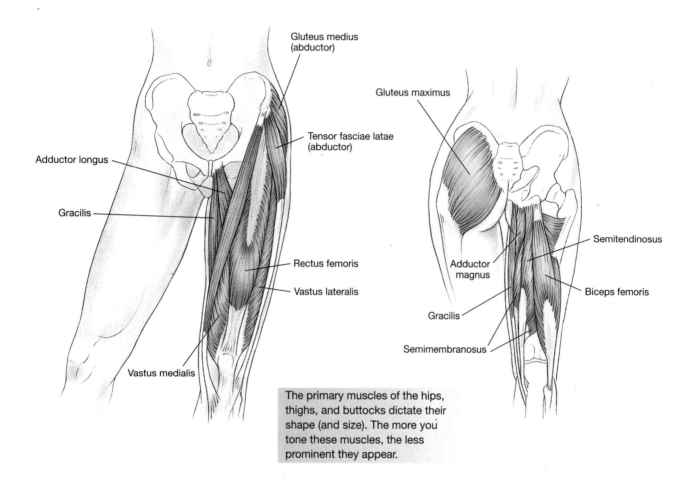

Gluteus medius
(abductor)

Gluteus maximus

Tensor fasciae latae
(abductor)

Adductor longus

Gracilis

Semitendinosus

Rectus femoris

Adductor
magnus

Vastus lateralis

Biceps femoris

Gracilis

Vastus medialis

Semimembranosus

The primary muscles of the hips,
thighs, and buttocks dictate their
shape (and size). The more you
tone these muscles, the less
prominent they appear.

To tone and trim your hips, thighs, and buttocks, "you need a total-body workout with special emphasis on the muscle groups that you want to tone," says Albohm, who designs workout programs specifically for women who want to do something about the weight they carry on their hips and thighs. "Your goal is to change the circumference of this area." Combined with some kind of consistent aerobic exercise—and eating habits that subtract pounds—the workouts that follow can help you reach your goal, she says. If you're just starting to exercise, start with the beginner exercises. If you are able to complete a designated program with relative ease for three consecutive workout sessions, then it's time to proceed to the next level.

You can expect to see some change in as little as 30 days, says Albohm.

Working Smart

As with any exercise, there's a right and a wrong way to go about working your hips, thighs, and buttocks.

Easy does it—at first. Start with the beginner program until you get used to the movements, says Albohm. If you decide to add ankle weights to work your inner and outer thigh muscles, start with light weights and only a few reps. Don't exceed five pounds—you completely change the leverage on your joints.

Do the exercise correctly to avoid injury. If you arch your back while you're doing the hip extension, for example, you could strain your back. And don't cheat—complete the full range of motion.

Make yourself comfortable. For some of the exercises that are done on the floor, you'll probably want to use an exercise mat. If you don't have a mat, a carpeted floor or large, folded towel may work just as well. But if you experience pain or discomfort when performing an exercise, stop and substitute another version, advises Albohm. If pain persists, see your physician.

Keep your movements tight and controlled. Don't swing your way through the exercise or let your muscles go slack.

Work your whole body. "Despite what you may have heard, if it's strenuous enough—if you walk like you really mean it, for example—aerobic exercise can tone your muscles to some degree," says Albohm. "I do aerobics primarily for the cardiovascular effects, for example. But 20 to 30 percent of my effort carries over to strengthen and tone my muscles."

Step right up. Step aerobics is better for the hips, thighs, and buttocks than regular aerobics, because it involves the quads, adductors, abductors, and gluteals, says Albohm. Stairclimbing machines are good for the quads, hamstrings, and gluteals—you work up and down in a straight line.

If you use a stairclimber, program the machine to vary the resistance and height to give your muscles a thorough workout, recommends Albohm. (The same advice applies if you use an elliptical trainer or recumbent bike.)

Measure your progress. It's a good idea to measure your hips, thighs, and buttocks every month, not every week, says Albohm. "Just be sure to measure at the same spot, in the same way, every time." And don't worry that your hips, thighs, and buttocks will get bigger when you follow this program. "Weight training will make muscles bigger only if it's done for that reason. There is a way to train to enlarge muscles—you have to use very, very heavy weights and very short ranges of motion with few repetitions. These exercises don't do that."

Be consistent. "To get the fastest results in the shortest period of time, do the exercises exactly as shown and make them part of your life," says Albohm. "Pay attention to the everyday versions of the exercises, so you'll be working these muscles every day, even when you don't have time to 'work out.'"

No time to go to the gym because you have to rake leaves? "Clean your gutters for two hours," suggests Albohm. "Climbing up and down the ladder is great for your hamstrings and gluteals."

Leg Extensions

Muscles Worked
Quadriceps (front thighs)

Performance Hints

- Keep the working leg slightly bent throughout the motion.
- Maintain proper upper-body position throughout the exercise.
- Use your thigh muscles, not momentum, to lift your leg.

Intensity

Beginner: 3 to 10 reps with each leg, 3 days per week

Intermediate: 2 sets of 10 reps with each leg, 3 days per week

Experienced: 3 or 4 sets of 10 reps with each leg, 3 days per week. For additional resistance, add a 1- or 2-pound ankle weight to each leg.

Everyday Version for Quadriceps and Gluteals

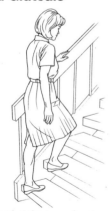

Choose stairs over elevators. If there are many flights of stairs where you work, climb one flight of stairs for 3 weeks; increase the number of flights by 1 every 3 weeks. Or walk up and down the stairs in your home 3 to 5 extra times each day.

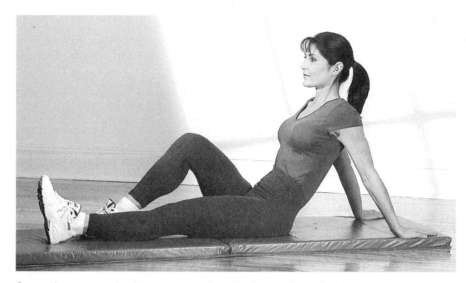

Supporting your trunk with your arms, sit on the floor with one leg extended, the knee slightly bent and foot flexed, as shown. Bend your opposite leg and place your foot flat on the floor.

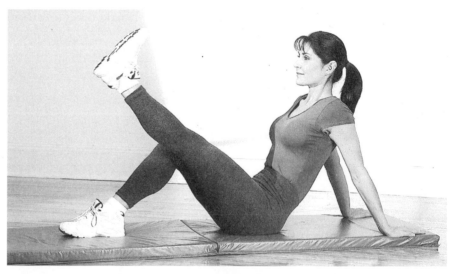

Keeping your knee slightly bent and your foot flexed, lift your leg in a slow and controlled movement until your knee reaches the height of the knee of your bent leg. Return to the starting position. Repeat with the other leg when the set is completed.

Lunges

Muscles Worked
Quadriceps (front thighs), gluteals (buttocks)

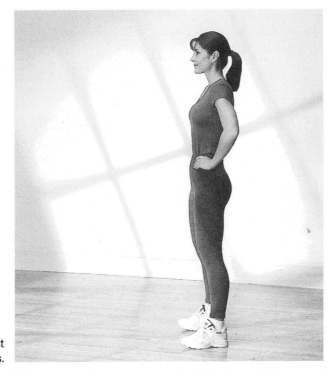

Stand with your feet about 6 inches apart and your toes pointed straight ahead, in their natural position, as shown. For balance, rest your hands on your hips.

Performance Hints

- Keep your torso from leaning forward by looking straight ahead. Checking your position in a mirror may help.
- Do a full stretch with each lunge. Don't shorten the lunge as you do repetitions.
- Don't let your left knee extend beyond your toes.
- You should feel the stretch in your quadriceps.

Intensity

Beginner: 1 set of 3 to 10 reps with each leg, 3 days per week

Intermediate: 2 sets of 10 reps with each leg, 3 days per week

Experienced: 3 sets of 10 reps with each leg, 3 days per week, holding a 1- or 2-pound dumbbell in each hand

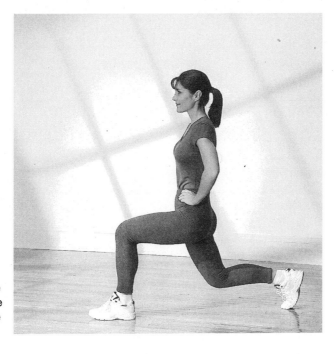

Step forward with your left foot as far as possible, bending your right knee as you do. In a controlled move, continue the lunge until your right knee almost touches the floor, and then slowly return to the starting position. Do one set, then repeat with the opposite leg.

Squats

Muscles Worked

Quadriceps (front thighs), gluteals (buttocks)

Performance Hints

- As you bend, keep your knees in direct line with your feet.
- Don't let your knees extend beyond your toes.
- Don't drop your buttocks lower than parallel to the floor.

Intensity

Beginner: 3 to 10 reps, 3 days per week

Intermediate: 2 sets of 10 reps, 3 days per week

Experienced: 3 sets of 10 reps, 3 days per week

Everyday Version for Quadriceps and Gluteals

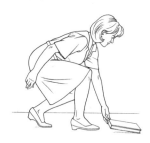

As you go about your daily activities, squat slightly to pick up or lift objects. (This is also safer than bending, because it protects the lower back from muscle injury.)

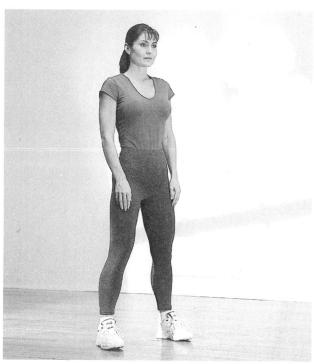

Stand with your feet shoulder-width apart. Tighten your abdomen and stand straight, looking directly ahead, focusing on a point so that your head and back are straight throughout the entire exercise.

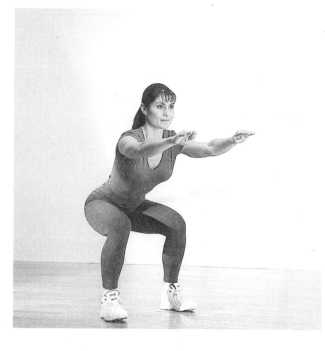

Slowly lower yourself into a squatting position by bending your legs at the knees.

Descend to a position where your thighs are parallel to the ground. Return to the starting position. Repeat.

Wall Squats

Muscles Worked
Quadriceps (front thighs)

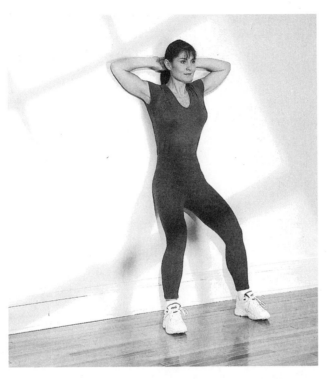

Stand and lean back against a wall, feet shoulder-width apart, toes pointed slightly outward. With your hands behind your head, your trunk straight, and your shoulders back, "walk" your feet forward approximately 18 inches from the wall, or far enough so that your shins remain perpendicular to the floor, as shown.

Performance Hints

- Keep your trunk straight at all times.
- Don't bend your legs any lower than where your thighs are parallel to the floor.
- Use a slow, controlled motion.

Intensity

Beginner: 1 set of 3 to 10 reps, 3 days per week

Intermediate: 2 sets of 10 reps, 3 days per week

Experienced: 3 sets of 10 reps, 3 days per week

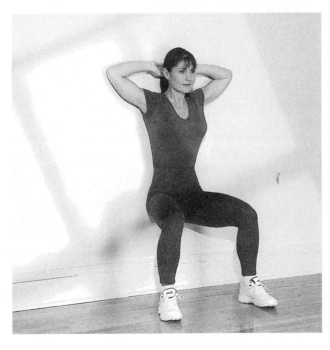

Using the wall to maintain balance, lower yourself in a slow, controlled movement until your thighs are parallel to the floor, as shown. Then return to the starting position and repeat.

Leg Curls

Muscles Worked
Hamstrings (backs of thighs)

Performance Hints

- As you do this exercise, concentrate on your hamstring muscles, tightening them as you raise your heel toward your buttocks.

- Keep the knee of the support leg slightly flexed.

- Use your hamstrings, not momentum, to perform this exercise.

Intensity

Beginner: 1 set of 3 to 10 reps, 3 days per week

Intermediate: 2 sets of 10 reps, 3 days per week

Experienced: 3 sets of 10 reps, 3 days per week. You can increase the effort by adding a 1-pound ankle weight to each leg.

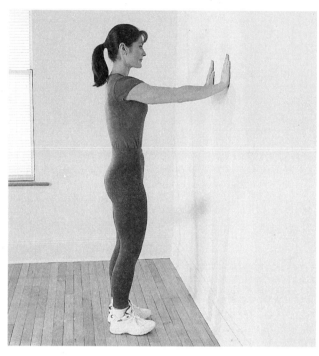

Stand facing a wall with your hands on the wall for balance, and your feet approximately 12 to 15 inches from the wall, as shown.

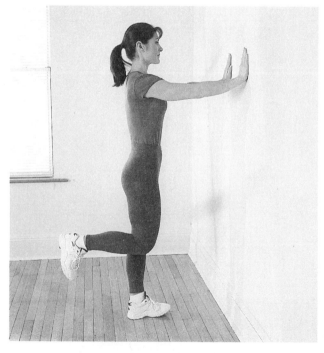

Slowly bend one leg at the knee, raising the heel toward your buttocks in a slow, controlled movement until your lower leg is parallel to the floor. Do one set, then repeat with the opposite leg.

Prone Single-Leg Raises

Muscles Worked

Hamstrings (backs of thighs), gluteals (buttocks)

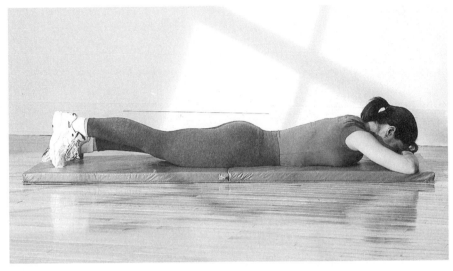

Lie flat on your stomach with your legs extended and your hands folded in front of you, with your forehead resting on your hands.

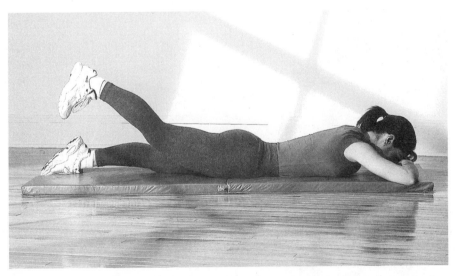

Keeping your leg extended, your foot flexed, and your knee slightly bent, raise one leg in a slow, controlled motion until you feel tightness in the muscles of your buttocks. Return to the starting position. Complete one set, then repeat with the other leg.

Performance Hints

- Don't raise your leg so high that you feel pain in your lower back.
- Squeeze your buttocks as you raise your leg.
- Keep the motion slow and controlled.

Intensity

Beginner: 1 set of 3 to 10 reps with each leg, 3 days per week

Intermediate: 2 sets of 10 reps with each leg, 3 days per week

Experienced: 3 sets of 10 reps with each leg, 3 days per week. To increase intensity further, you can add a 1- or 2-pound ankle weight to each ankle.

Back Leg Extensions

Muscles Worked

Hamstrings (backs of thighs), gluteals (buttocks)

Performance Hints

- Keep your body stationary as you work each leg.
- Don't raise the extended leg so high that you feel pain in your lower back.
- Be sure to tighten your buttocks muscles while performing this exercise.

Intensity

Beginner: 1 set of 3 to 10 reps with each leg, 3 days per week

Intermediate: 2 sets of 10 reps with each leg, 3 days per week

Experienced: 3 sets of 10 reps with each leg, 3 days per week. To increase intensity further, you can add a 1- or 2-pound ankle weight to each ankle.

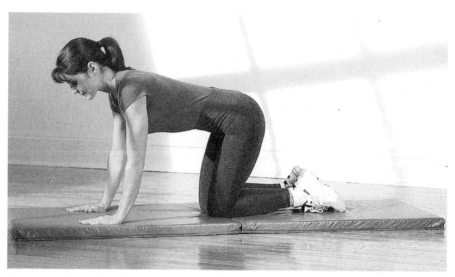

Get down on all fours, with your arms fully extended, elbows locked, and your head and neck aligned with your spine.

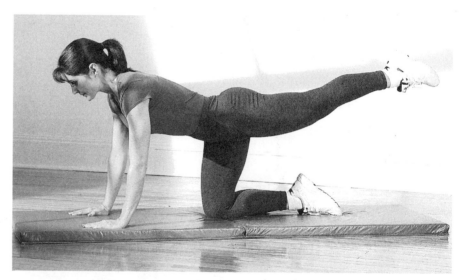

Using your buttocks muscles, extend and raise one leg until your thigh is parallel to the floor. Return to the starting position. Do one set, then repeat with the opposite leg.

Bent-Leg Extensions

Muscles Worked

Hamstrings (backs of thighs), gluteals (buttocks)

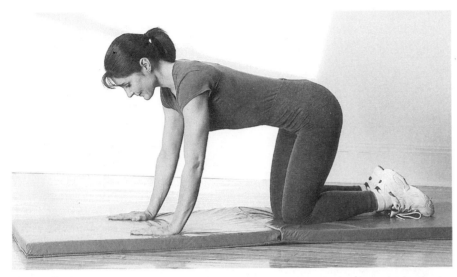

Get down on all fours, with your arms fully extended, elbows locked, and your head and neck aligned with your spine.

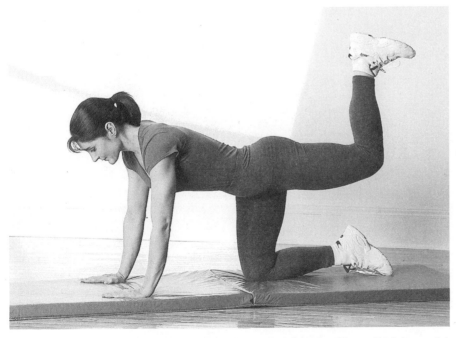

Extend one leg, bent at a 90-degree angle, with your foot flexed, until your thigh is parallel to the ground, as shown. Return to the starting position. Do one set, then repeat with your other leg.

Performance Hints

- Use one slow, continuous controlled motion throughout the exercise.
- Don't extend the leg you're working higher than parallel to the floor.
- Use your buttocks muscles, not momentum, to raise your leg.

Intensity

Beginner: 1 set of 3 to 10 reps with each leg, 3 days per week

Intermediate: 2 sets of 10 reps with each leg, 3 days per week

Experienced: 3 sets of 10 reps with each leg, 3 days per week. You can increase resistance by adding a 1- or 2-pound ankle weight to each leg.

Everyday Version for Gluteals, Hamstrings, and Outer Thighs

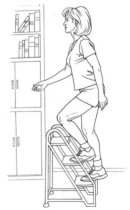

Spend 3 to 5 minutes climbing and descending a stepladder, for 30 seconds at a time, with a 15-second rest between intervals.

Pelvic Lifts

Muscles Worked

Hamstrings (backs of thighs), gluteals (buttocks)

Performance Hints

- Raise your hips only until your back is straight. Don't arch your back.
- Keep your buttocks muscles contracted at all times.
- Use a slow, controlled motion.

Intensity

Beginner: 1 set of 10 reps, 3 days per week

Intermediate: 2 sets of 10 reps, 3 days per week

Experienced: 3 sets of 10 reps, 3 days per week

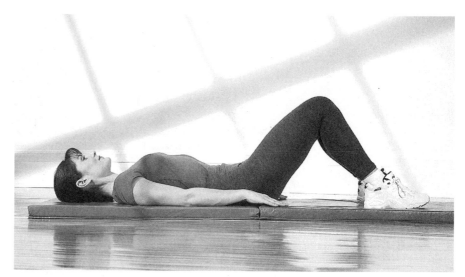

Lie on your back with your knees bent and your feet flat on the floor, with your hands at your sides, palms down.

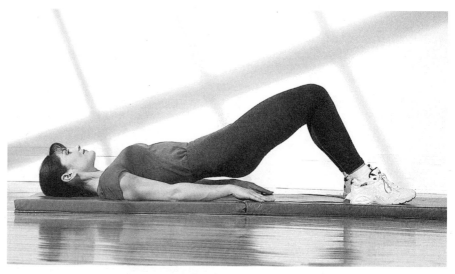

Lift your pelvis toward the ceiling, as shown, squeezing your buttocks, until your back is straight. Repeat.

Bent-Knee Crossovers

Muscles Worked

Gluteals (buttocks), hamstrings (backs of thighs), abductors (outer thighs)

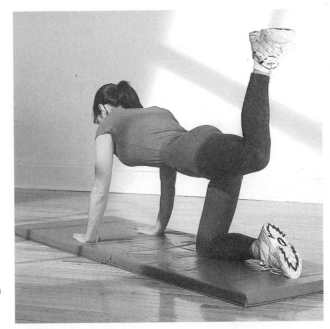

Get down on all fours with your back flat, then bend and raise one leg, as shown.

Performance Hints

- Keep your thigh parallel to the floor at the top of the motion.
- To initiate the exercise, move your foot toward the ceiling.
- Use one slow, controlled movement throughout the exercise.

Intensity

Beginner: 1 set of 3 to 10 reps with each leg, 3 days per week

Intermediate: 2 sets of 10 reps with each leg, 3 days per week

Experienced: 3 sets of 10 reps with each leg, 3 days per week. You can increase the intensity by adding a 1-pound ankle weight to each leg.

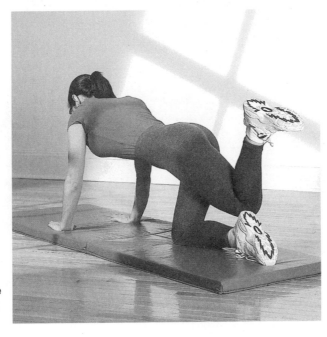

Keeping the raised leg bent at a 90-degree angle throughout the exercise, lift your leg up and back, crossing over the calf of the nonworking leg. Keep your buttocks tight at all times. Return to the starting position. Do one set, then repeat with the other leg.

Side-Lying Straight-Leg Raises

Muscles Worked

Gluteals (buttocks), abductors (outer thighs)

Performance Hints

- Keep your upper leg rotated downward.
- Keep your upper body stable.
- Use a slow, controlled motion.

Intensity

Beginner: 1 set of 3 to 10 reps with each leg, 3 days per week

Intermediate: 2 sets of 10 reps with each leg, 3 days per week

Experienced: 3 sets of 10 reps with each leg, 3 days per week. You can increase resistance by adding a 1- or 2-pound ankle weight to each leg.

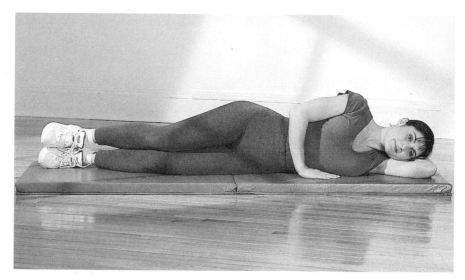

Lie on your side with your legs together, supporting your head with one arm and balancing yourself with the other, as shown.

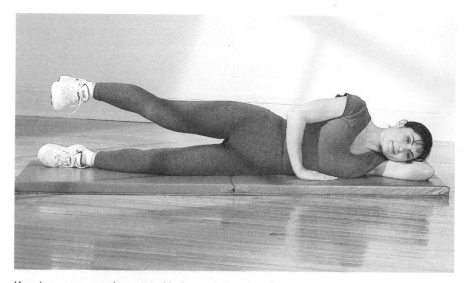

Keeping your upper leg rotated in (toe pointing down) and your foot flexed, raise the top leg in a slow, controlled motion approximately 10 to 12 inches off the floor without moving your torso. Return to the starting position. Do one set, then repeat with the opposite leg.

Standing Abductions

Muscles Worked
Gluteals (buttocks), and abductors (outer thighs)

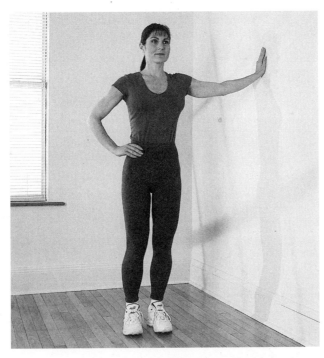

Holding on to a wall for balance, stand with your knees slightly bent, as shown.

Performance Hints

- Use the muscles of your outer thigh and hip to lift your leg.
- Keep the stationary leg slightly flexed.
- Lift the leg in a slow, controlled movement.
- Don't twist your shoulders and chest.

Intensity

Beginner: 1 set of 3 to 10 reps with each leg, 3 days per week

Intermediate: 2 sets of 10 reps with each leg, 3 days per week

Experienced: 3 sets of 10 reps with each leg, 3 days per week. You can increase resistance by adding a 1- or 2-pound ankle weight to each leg.

Everyday Version for Gluteals and Abductors

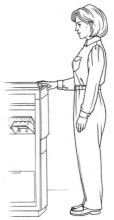

While standing, contract your buttocks, hold for 6 to 8 seconds, and then release. Do for 1 to 3 minutes, 2 to 3 times per day.

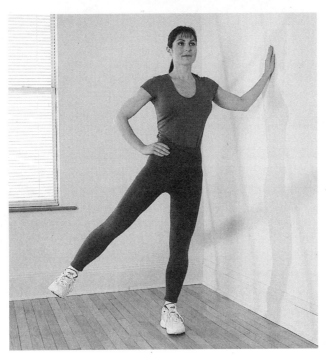

Keeping your knee slightly bent, lift the working leg to the side. Your foot should be flexed. Lift as far as you can without moving your upper torso. Return to the starting position. Do one set, then repeat with the opposite leg.

Seated Abductions

Muscles Worked
Abductors (outer thighs)

Performance Hints

- Keep your knee slightly flexed and your foot flexed throughout the motion.
- Don't move your upper body.

Intensity

Beginner: 1 set of 3 to 10 reps with each leg, 3 days per week

Intermediate: 2 sets of 10 reps with each leg, 3 days per week

Experienced: 3 sets of 10 reps with each leg, 3 days per week. You can increase resistance by adding a 1- or 2-pound ankle weight to each leg.

Everyday Version for Abductors

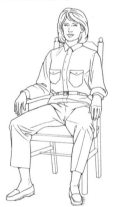

While seated, press your outer thighs against the sides or arms of the chair; hold for 6 to 8 seconds. Repeat for 1 to 3 minutes, 3 times per day.

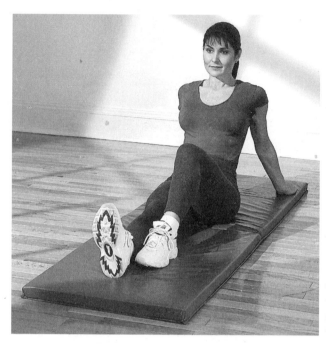

While supporting your upper body with your arms and with your elbows slightly bent, sit on the floor with one leg extended and the knee slightly bent and foot flexed, as shown.

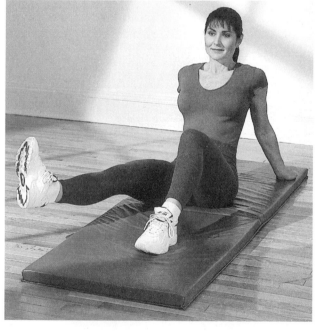

Keeping your knee slightly bent and your foot flexed, move the working leg to the side as far as you can, as shown, without moving your torso. Return to the starting position. Do one set, then repeat with the other leg.

Side-Lying Bent-Leg Raises

Muscles Worked
Abductors (outer thighs)

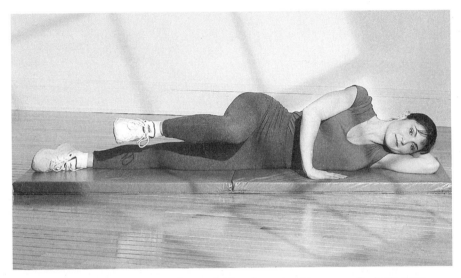

Lie on your side with your bottom leg straight and your top leg perpendicular to your body, with the knee bent at 90 degrees. Support your head with your bottom arm and stabilize your body by placing the palm of the other hand down in front of your chest.

Performance Hints

- Keep the knee of your upper leg bent and your foot flexed throughout the motion.
- Keep your upper body still throughout the exercise.

Intensity

Beginner: 1 set of 3 to 10 reps with each leg, 3 days per week

Intermediate: 2 sets of 10 reps with each leg, 3 days per week

Experienced: 3 sets of 10 reps with each leg, 3 days per week. You can increase resistance by adding a 1- or 2-pound ankle weight to each leg.

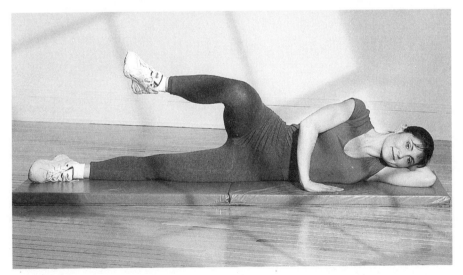

Keeping your top leg perpendicular to your body, raise it up in a slow and controlled motion as high as you can without twisting your torso or compromising your foot position. Return to the starting position and repeat with your other leg when the set is complete.

Fire Hydrants

Muscles Worked

Abductors (outer thighs), adductors (inner thighs), gluteals (buttocks)

Performance Hints

- To keep your back straight and your spine properly aligned, hold your head straight (not raised or lowered).

- Perform this exercise in a slow, controlled, continuous motion.

Intensity

Beginner: 1 set of 3 to 10 reps with each leg, 3 days per week

Intermediate: 2 sets of 10 reps with each leg, 3 days per week

Experienced: 3 sets of 10 reps with each leg, 3 days per week

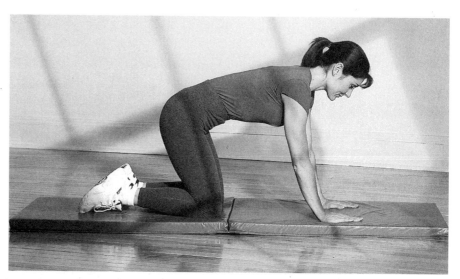

Get down on all fours, with your arms extended, your elbows locked, and your back parallel to the floor.

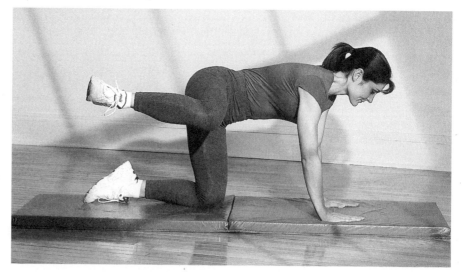

Lift one leg to the side at a 90-degree angle until it is parallel to the floor. Return to the starting position. Do one set, then repeat with the opposite leg.

Inner Leg Raises

Muscles Worked
Adductors (inner thighs)

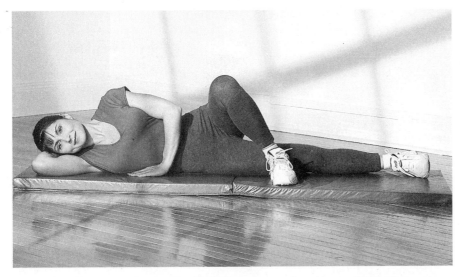

Lie on your side, supporting your head with your arm, and your upper body with your opposite hand, as shown. Bend your top leg and place it in front of your other leg so your foot is flat on the floor and your bottom leg is straight with the knee slightly bent and the foot flexed.

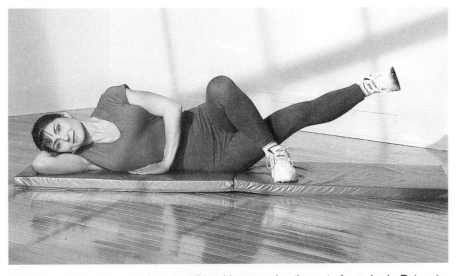

Raise your bottom leg as high as possible without moving the rest of your body. Return to the starting position without touching your foot to the floor. Do one set, then repeat with your other leg.

Performance Hints

- Keep your upper body still.
- Keep your inner thigh facing the ceiling.
- Perform the movement in a slow, controlled manner.

Intensity

Beginner: 1 set of 3 to 10 reps with each leg, 3 days per week

Intermediate: 2 sets of 10 reps with each leg, 3 days per week

Experienced: 3 sets of 10 reps with each leg, 3 days per week. You can increase resistance by adding a 1- or 2-pound ankle weight to each leg.

Everyday Version for Adductors

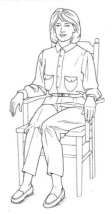

While seated, contract your inner thigh muscles by pushing your knees together; hold for 6 to 8 seconds. Release. Do for 1 to 3 minutes, 3 times per day.

Seated Inner Leg Raises

Muscles Worked
Adductors (inner thighs)

Performance Hints

- Keep the leg you're working 1 inch above the floor at all times.
- Keep your upper torso straight and square to the rest of your body.
- Perform the movement in a slow, controlled motion.

Intensity

Beginner: 1 set of 3 to 10 reps with each leg, 3 days per week

Intermediate: 2 sets of 10 reps with each leg, 3 days per week

Experienced: 3 sets of 10 reps with each leg, 3 days per week. You can increase resistance by adding a 1- or 2-pound ankle weight to each leg.

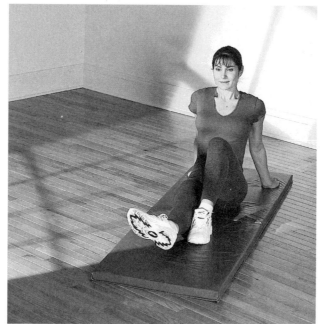

Sit with one leg bent and the foot flat on the floor, leaning back and supporting yourself as shown. Extend the other leg, bending your knee slightly, flexing your foot, and rotating your hip (toes pointed out).

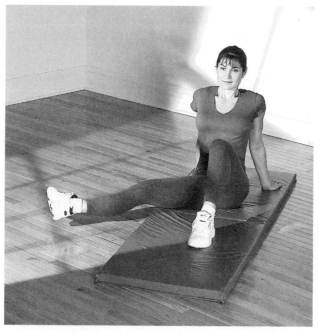

Move the working leg outward as far as you can without losing your balance. Return to the starting position without touching your foot to the floor. Do one set, then repeat with your other leg.

Butterfly Leg Raises

Muscles Worked
Adductors (inner thighs)

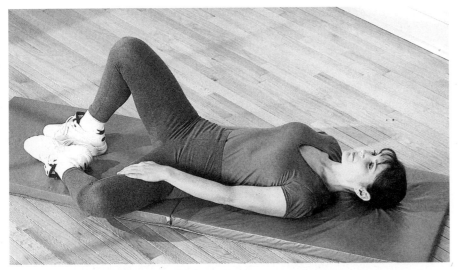

Lie on your back with one leg bent and the foot flat on the floor, and the other leg bent and lowered to the side, as shown. The sole of the foot of the lowered leg should face the side of the other foot.

Performance Hints
- Keep both legs bent throughout the motion.
- Using your hand, provide as much resistance as needed to make the exercise challenging.
- Keep your lower back pressed to the floor.

Intensity

Beginner: 1 set of 3 to 10 reps with each leg, 3 days per week

Intermediate: 2 sets of 10 reps with each leg, 3 days per week

Experienced: 3 sets of 10 reps with each leg, 3 days per week

Keeping your legs bent, raise the lowered knee toward the opposite knee, pressing against the inner thigh with your hand, as shown, for resistance. Return to the starting position. Do one set, then repeat with the other leg.

Single-Leg Pelvic Lifts

Muscles Worked
Gluteals (buttocks) and adductors (inner thighs)

Performance Hints

- Raise your pelvis until your back is straight, but no higher (not arched).
- Keep your buttock muscles contracted at all times.
- Perform this move in a slow, controlled manner.

Intensity

Beginner: 1 set of 10 reps, 3 days per week

Intermediate: 2 sets of 10 reps, 3 days per week

Experienced: 3 sets of 10 reps, 3 days per week. You can increase the intensity by straightening your leg instead of resting it on the other knee.

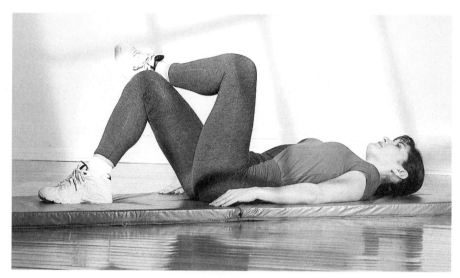

Lie on your back with one knee bent and the foot flat on the floor, with your hands at your sides. Cross the opposite leg over the bent leg, with your ankle resting just above the knee.

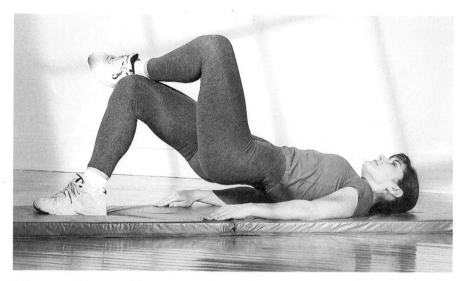

Raise your pelvis toward the ceiling, squeezing the muscles in your buttocks as you lift. Return to the starting position. Do one set, then repeat with the other leg.

Scissors

Muscles Worked
Adductors (inner thighs), abductors (outer thighs)

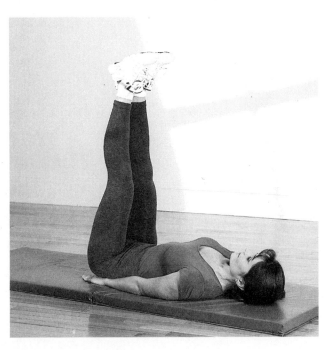

Lie on your back with your head resting on the floor. Place your palms flat on the floor under your buttocks and raise your legs, with your knees slightly bent, almost perpendicular to the floor. Your feet should be slightly flexed with your toes pointed slightly outward.

Performance Hints

- Use your inner and outer thigh muscles, not momentum, to perform the exercise.
- Keep your back flat on the floor.
- As you perform the exercise, maintain muscle tension in your inner and outer thighs.

Intensity

Beginner: 1 set of 10 reps, 3 days per week

Intermediate: 2 sets of 10 reps, 3 days per week

Experienced: 3 sets of 10 reps, 3 days per week. Use rubber tubing attached at your ankles or lower-leg area to increase the intensity.

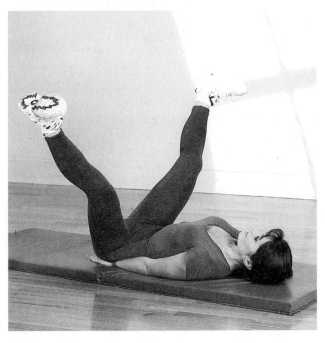

Using a slow, controlled movement, spread your legs as far apart as possible. Return to the starting position. Repeat.

30-Day Beginner Program

Week I

**Do Exercises Shown
3 Days This Week**

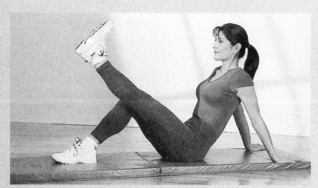

Leg Extensions (page 154)

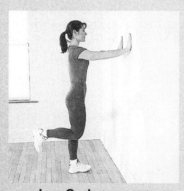

Leg Curls (page 158)

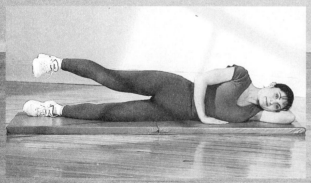

Side-Lying Straight-Leg Raises (page 164)

Week II

**Do Exercises Shown
3 Days This Week**

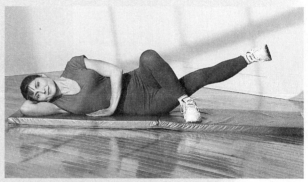

Inner Leg Raises (page 169)

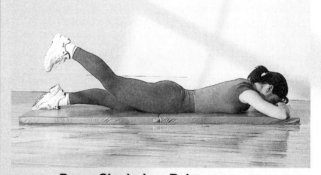

Prone Single-Leg Raises (page 159)

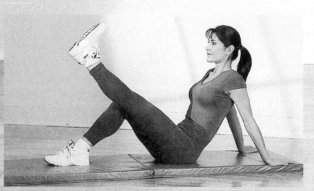

Leg Extensions (page 154)

Week III

**Do Exercises Shown
3 Days This Week**

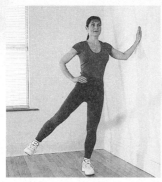

Standing Abductions (page 165)

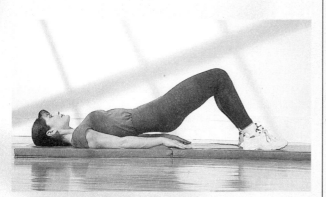

Pelvic Lifts (page 162)

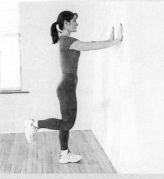

Leg Curls (page 158)

Week IV

**Do Exercises Shown
3 Days This Week**

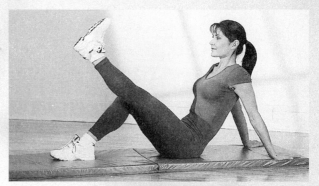

Leg Extensions (page 154)

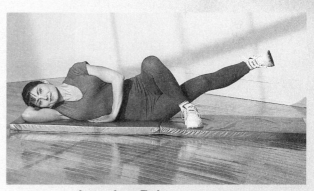

Inner Leg Raises (page 169)

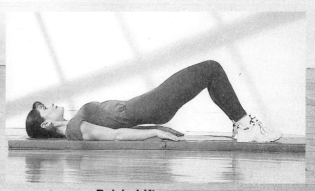

Pelvic Lifts (page 162)

30-Day Intermediate Program

Week I	Week II
Do Exercises Shown 3 Days This Week	**Do Exercises Shown 3 Days This Week**

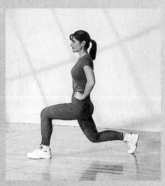

Lunges (page 155)

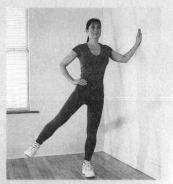

Standing Abductions (page 165)

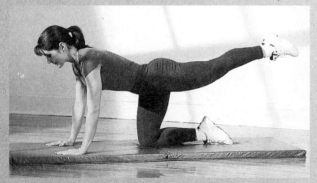

Back Leg Extensions (page 160)

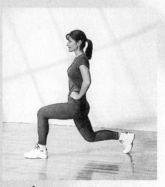

Lunges (page 155)

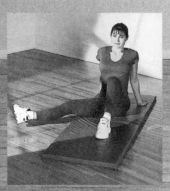

Seated Inner Leg Raises (page 170)

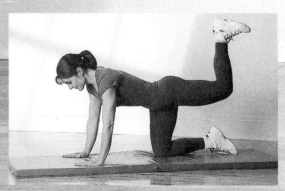

Bent-Leg Extensions (page 161)

Week III

**Do Exercises Shown
3 Days This Week**

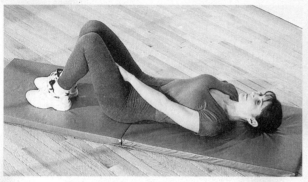

Butterfly Leg Raises (page 171)

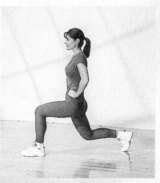

Lunges (page 155)

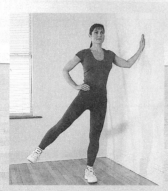

Standing Abductions (page 165)

Week IV

**Do Exercises Shown
3 Days This Week**

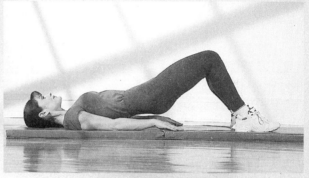

Pelvic Lifts (page 162)

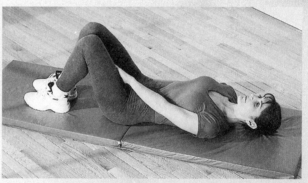

Butterfly Leg Raises (page 171)

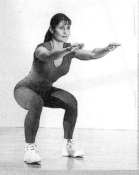

Squats (page 156)

30-Day Experienced Program

Week I	Week II

Week I

**Do Exercises Shown
3 Days This Week**

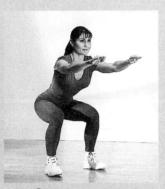

Squats (page 156)

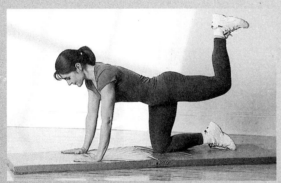

Bent-Leg Extensions (page 161)

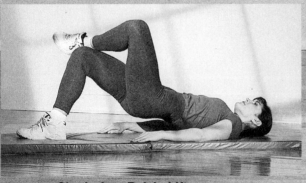

Single-Leg Pelvic Lifts (page 172)

Week II

**Do Exercises Shown
3 Days This Week**

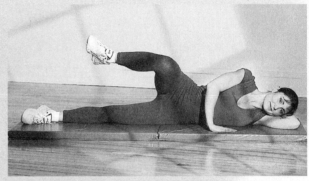

Side-Lying Bent-Leg Raises (page 167)

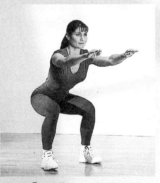

Squats (page 156)

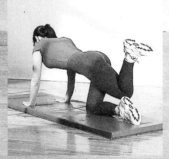

Bent-Knee Crossovers (page 163)

Week III

**Do Exercises Shown
3 Days This Week**

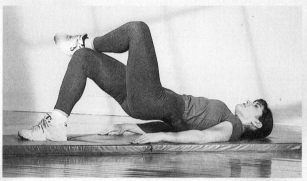

Single-Leg Pelvic Lifts (page 172)

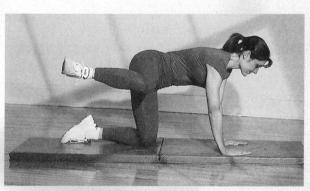

Fire Hydrants (page 168)

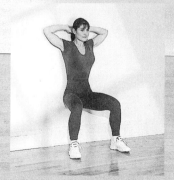

Wall Squats (page 157)

Week IV

**Do Exercises Shown
3 Days This Week**

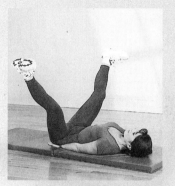

Scissors (page 173)

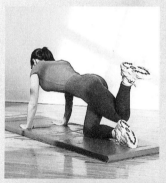

Bent-Knee Crossovers (page 163)

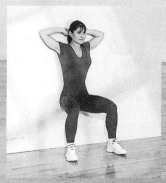

Wall Squats (page 157)

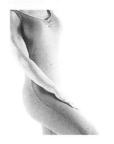

Stretch into Shape

Stretching keeps your muscles flexible, helping to prepare them for exercise and recover from the effort afterward. Skip the stretches, and you won't get nearly the benefits you should from aerobic exercise and resistance training.

"Stretching helps you move freely during aerobic exercise, it enables your muscles to build more strength during weight training, and it helps keep muscles long and lean," says Sharon Willett, a physical therapist and sports trainer at the Virginia Sportsmedicine Institute in Arlington, Virginia.

Stretching increases your range of motion by making your muscles, tendons, and joints more flexible. So the more you stretch, the greater benefit you'll get from your workouts, and the sooner you'll see results.

Contrary to what you may have heard in the past, experts agree you should warm up your muscles before stretching, to avoid tearing "cold" or stiff muscles.

Stretching Prevents Muscle Strain

Lack of flexibility not only slows your progress but also can lead to injury, which can derail even the best-laid exercise routines. And unless you've been athletic all your life, chances are you're not as flexible as you need to be to get the most out of your body-toning workouts.

When you were a baby, you were so flexible that you could probably put your toes in your mouth. When you were a teenager, you could slither under a limbo bar. But as an adult, you probably wouldn't even think of taking a turn when the limbo music begins. As we age, both our muscles and tendons lose their flexibility. If the only exercise we get is flipping through the TV listings at breakneck pace, our muscles flex even less, getting stiffer over the years.

"Aside from the aging process, our habits and daily activities can also cause our muscles and tendons to shorten," says Willett. Even your shoes can inhibit your flexibility. For example, in women, wearing high heels shortens the hamstrings and calves. This won't be a problem when you're sitting still, says Willett. But if you try to do a leg curl or squat, the shortened muscles won't do the job willingly. Try to push a shortened muscle or tendon through too much exercise or range of motion, and you'll develop pain or an injury, such as tendinitis (inflammation of the tendon).

Ironically, it's not only aging and lifestyle that can affect flexibility, but exercise, too. "Weight training and weight-bearing exercise like jogging contract muscles again and again, shortening the muscles and tendons involved," says Willett. "So you have to take the time to stretch out your muscles again after you use them. If you do so, not only will your muscles and tendons retain their elasticity but also they'll be able to get even stronger. An exercise program that includes all three elements (cardiovascular, strength, and flexibility) will keep your muscles and tendons in the best shape possible."

Burn Fat While You Stretch

In addition to keeping you flexible, stretching burns calories and helps you relax.

"Stretching isn't aerobic," concedes Willett. "But you'll burn more calories by stretching than you will by sitting and doing nothing." For a 150-pound woman, 30 minutes of stretching burns 60 to 100 calories—about the same as gentle yoga—compared to 22 calories for sitting still.

As an added incentive, you'll find that stretching is extremely relaxing, especially after a workout. "Stretching will slowly lower your heart rate after an activity," says Willett. "That has a calming effect on most people. Also, the deep breathing and stillness required for stretching are really helpful for releasing tension both in the muscles and in the mind."

The Right Way to Stretch

Experts recommend that you stretch all your muscle groups, rather than just doing the stretches that target your particular trouble spot. All your muscles and tendons work together, so if you ignore one stretch, then you won't get maximum benefit from the others.

As for how to stretch, it should come fairly naturally. We raise our arms when we get out of bed; we wiggle our backs if we feel a muscle ache. All of these motions are really stretches. It's easy. Still, for maximum effectiveness, you need to keep a few rules in mind when you stretch, says Willett.

Warm your muscles. Stretching is not a warmup. Spend at least five minutes doing some form of light aerobic exercise, such as walking, climbing stairs, or cleaning the house. Work hard enough so that you feel warm and you sweat slightly. If you stretch after your workout, your muscles will be warm and supple.

Don't bounce. Pushing your muscles in short, jerky movements tears the muscle fibers. Instead, slowly and evenly move into the stretch until you feel resistance, then back off a little and hold that position.

Hold each stretch for 20 seconds. "Stretches held for at least 20 seconds increase flexibility the most," says Willett. And don't hold your breath. Instead, take two or three deep breaths as you hold the stretch.

Do each stretch two, three, or four times. The real benefits come in increments, with each subsequent stretch.

When (and How Often) to Stretch

Stretching doesn't take much time—as little as 10 minutes should do it. And it's easy to fit into a busy workout schedule—all you need is an exercise mat. As for when to stretch, you have a number of options.

- If you've just begun your exercise program, it's best to stretch each muscle group immediately after an activity in which you've used those muscles, says Willett. So if you're doing squats to tone your butt, for example, stretch the gluteus muscles immediately after the exercise. And if you're working out every day, that means you'll stretch every day.

- If you're comfortable with your routine and never feel sore afterward, says Willett, feel free to do all of your stretches at the end of your workout.

- If it's convenient, you can also stretch without doing other exercise (except warming up). You'll benefit from two half-hour sessions a week even on days when you don't exercise.

"You can even stretch while you watch TV," says Willett. "There's no reason to be formal about it."

Press-Ups

Muscles Stretched
Upper and lower abs

Easier Version: Prop-Up

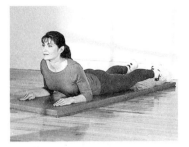

If you're unable to do the regular version because of wrist, arm, or lower-back pain, prop yourself up on your forearms and raise your chest up while keeping your hips on the floor.

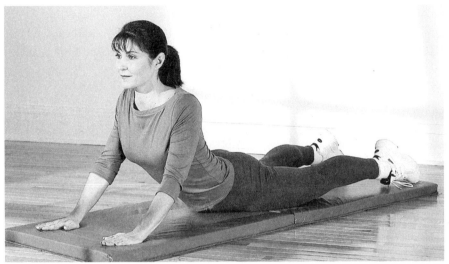

Lie on your stomach with your hands on the floor, directly under your shoulders. Raise your upper body as far as you can by straightening your elbows and arching your back, keeping your hips in contact with the floor. Keep your chest upright so your shoulders are not hunched up by your ears. You should feel the stretch along the front of your body. You can lift your chin, but don't drop your head back. Hold for 20 to 30 seconds. Repeat four times.

Knee Squeezes

Muscles Stretched
Upper, middle, and lower back muscles

**Easier Version:
Single-Knee Squeeze**

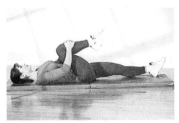

If you're unable to work both knees at the same time, start by bringing one knee up to your chest and holding the stretch for 20 to 30 seconds. Relax and repeat with the opposite knee. Also, you don't have to bring your head up off the floor if it puts too much strain on your neck.

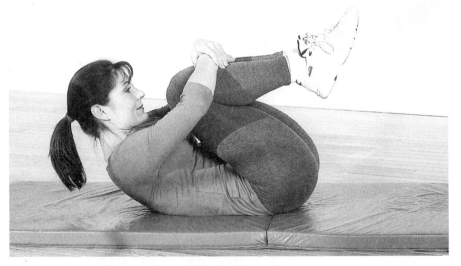

Lie on your back with your legs outstretched. Bend both knees and hold, as shown. Bring them toward your chest until you feel a stretch. Tuck your chin in and slowly bring your head up to meet your knees. Stay relaxed. Hold for 20 to 30 seconds. Repeat four times.

Spinal Twists

Muscles Stretched
Middle and lower back muscles

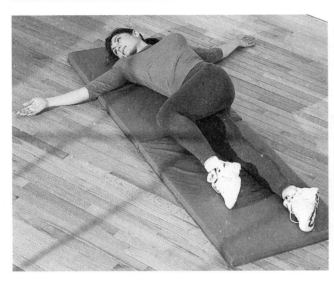

Lie on your back with your arms out to each side (perpendicular to your body). Keeping your shoulders flat on the floor, bend your left knee up toward your chest and slowly bring the bent leg across your body. Turn your head to look at your right hand until you feel a stretch. Hold for 20 to 30 seconds, then repeat to the other side. Do four stretches on each side.

Figure Four Stretches

Muscles Stretched
Gluteus maximus (buttocks)

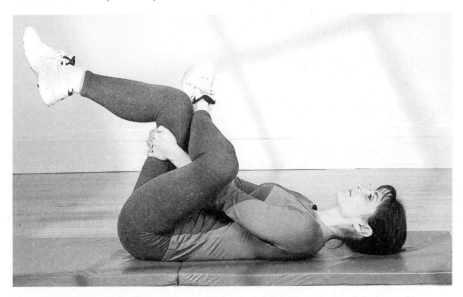

Lie on your back with both knees bent. Cross your left foot over your right knee. Place your hands behind your right knee and slowly bring your knee toward your chest. You should feel the stretch in your left buttock area. Hold for 20 to 30 seconds, then repeat on the opposite side. Stretch each side four times.

Hip Flexor Stretches

Muscles Stretched
Muscles in front of the hips and thighs

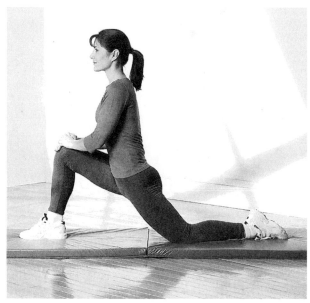

Begin by kneeling on the floor. Bring your right knee in front of you and place your foot flat on the floor. Your left knee should be resting on the floor. Slowly lean forward to extend your left leg back, keeping your shin and knee on the floor, as shown. You should feel a stretch in the front of your right hip and thigh. Make sure your right knee isn't extending farther than your toes. (If it is, move your right leg farther back.) Hold this stretch for 20 to 30 seconds, then switch sides. Repeat four times.

Hip/Quad Stretches

Muscle Stretched
Iliotibial band (outside of legs from hips to knees) and quadriceps

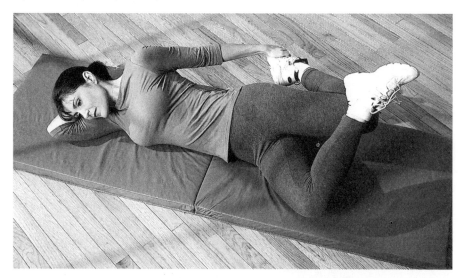

Lie on your right side with your right arm extended under your head. Bend your left knee and use your left hand to pull your heel up toward your buttock. Take your right foot and place it on top of your left knee, as shown. Apply a downward pressure with your right foot, pushing your left knee toward the floor. Hold for 20 to 30 seconds and then repeat on the opposite side. Repeat the stretch four times on each side.

Inner Thigh and Groin Stretches

Muscles Worked
Inner thighs and groin

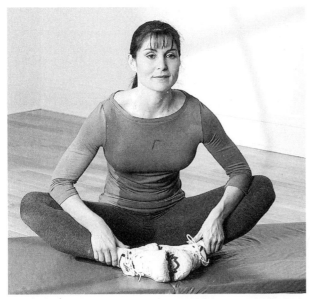

Sit on the floor with your back straight. Place the heels of your feet together and drop your knees out to your sides. Clasp your hands around your ankles. Using your forearms, slowly press your knees toward the floor until you feel a stretch. Do not force your knees to the floor. Hold for 20 to 30 seconds. Repeat four times.

Hamstring Stretches

Muscles Stretched
Backs of thighs

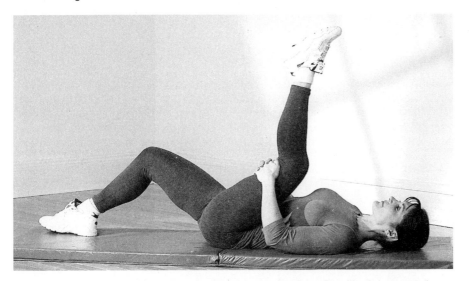

Lie on your back, keeping your lower back pressed to the floor. Bend both knees and keep your feet flat on the floor. Bring your hands to the back of your left thigh and slowly straighten and raise your left leg. Gently pull your leg in toward your torso until you feel a stretch in the back of your leg. Hold for 20 to 30 seconds, then repeat with the other leg. Repeat four times with each leg. As this stretch becomes easier, keep the resting leg straight out in front of you instead of bent, for more of a stretch.

Calf Stretches

Muscles Stretched

Gastrocnemius and soleus (backs and sides of calves) and Achilles tendon

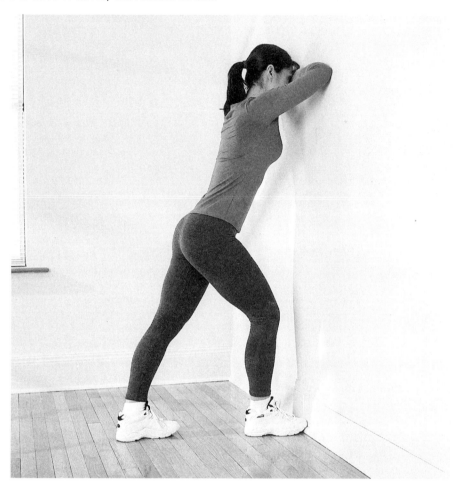

Stand with your forearms against a wall and your right leg out in front of you with the knee bent. Your knees shouldn't extend past your toes. Keep your left leg straight and your foot flat on the floor. Slowly lean forward on your right leg until you feel a stretch in the back of your calf. Hold for 20 to 30 seconds. This will stretch the upper part of the calf. Then slightly bend your left knee and repeat to stretch the lower part of the calf. Hold each stretch for 20 to 30 seconds, then switch sides. Repeat four times with each leg.

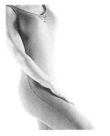

Workout-Friendly Clothes

Remember when "play clothes" consisted of a pair of shorts, an old T-shirt, and sneakers? That combination will still work if you rely on housework or casual strolls for exercise. But if you're jogging, cycling, or playing any kind of sport, you'll need a few sports-specific items—an exercise bra, shoes geared for your activity of choice, and a few other comfort or safety items.

Finding workout clothes is easier than ever, thanks to forward-thinking women like Anne Kelly, owner of Junonia, a women's fitness catalog company catering specifically to women who look for support as well as style when they exercise, but who find shopping for exercise clothes a challenge. As a size 16 petite who herself exercises, Kelly could wear a unisex size XL, but even at that size, "all I would see was one pair of black bike shorts on the rack.

"Larger women are built differently and need clothing designed for them," Kelly says. "Because of their size, larger women generate more heat. If you're wearing a big, floppy sweat suit, you're not getting any support and you're hot," she says. High-tech fabrics offer support, "bounce control," smooth lines, and water- and heat-dispersion systems that wick away perspiration and keep women cool.

Junonia is just one of a growing number of suppliers who offer a colorful array of exercise gear for larger women, from basics like bras to sports-specific gear. Woman's View, a division of Sears for women size 14 and up, now offers cotton/spandex leggings in sizes up to 4X (50 to 52 inches) in 11 colors, for example. The Lane Bryant catalog company offers cross-training shoes up to size 13 D and 11 EE. Lane Bryant stores (which aren't affili-

ated with the catalog) offer leggings, unitards, exercise bras, and short- and long-sleeved workout tops made in a variety of high-performance fabrics in sizes 14 to 28 (3X). At the upscale end, a new manufacturing company, A Big Attitude, of Los Angeles, has created a sporty line of fitness wear available at Nordstrom department stores and specialty women's clothing boutiques.

Manufacturers say the clothing sells well.

"Plus-size women have been conditioned into wearing shapeless clothing to exercise," says Cynthia Tivers, founder of A Big Attitude and author of several exercise books and creator of a workout video for plus-size women. "Many plus-size women worked out in private because they couldn't wear what others wore, and they felt stigmatized," says Tivers, who believes all women deserve choices that are attractive, supportive, and practical. Her designs give larger women features they told her they appreciate, such as sleeves and longer tops, but they also allow women to move freely and check out their form, just like everyone else who exercises.

Finding the right workout gear starts with what's probably one of the most appreciated—and most cursed—items in an active woman's wardrobe: the exercise bra.

Finding the Perfect Exercise Bra

Women who exercise need support for their breasts, but they often have to put up with chafing, uncomfortable moisture, and the annoyance of having to be a contortionist to get the thing off after a sweaty workout.

If you've yearned for an exercise bra that's as comfortable and attractive as your regular bra, take heart. There are now more styles than ever before. The key to good fit is to find the style that works best for you.

"Women need to make some decisions about what they need in a bra and what kind of bra wearers they are," says Missy Park, founder of Title 9 Sports, a women's athletic apparel supply company based in Emeryville, California. "If you're primarily concerned about the look of your silhouette, for example, you'll want to get an isolation, or encapsulation, bra. Don't even bother looking at pullover compression bras."

Here's a rundown of the different styles to help you decide what's right for you.

Encapsulation/Isolation Bra

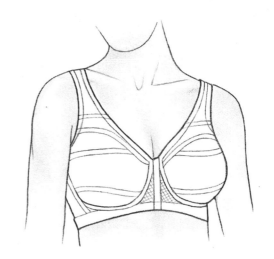

You want: Support for larger breasts (D cup or larger), to avoid flattened breasts, or to have a curvier silhouette (all breast sizes).

Look for: A bra that holds each breast separately, known as an encapsulation or isolation bra. Some isolation bras have preshaped cups that provide even more curve.

Compression Bra

You want: Support for small to medium breasts (A, B, or C cup), or to avoid looking too busty.

Look for: A bra that hugs your breasts up against your chest wall, known as a compression bra. For maximum compression, some of these bras are made with more material and fit like a snug, cropped tank top. The extra material, particularly in the back, holds your breasts tightly and supports their weight better than the regular compression style.

X/Y-Back Bras

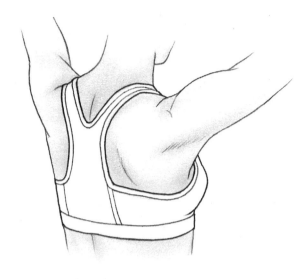

You want: To control bouncing.

Look for: A bra with straps that run down the middle of your back. These X- or Y-shaped straps, made of the same material as the bra, pull your breasts up and help control bouncing better than straps that fit straight over your shoulders. The thicker the straps, the more support and control the bra provides.

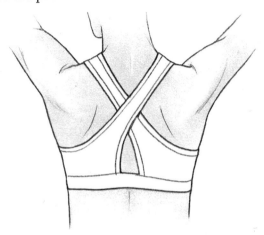

Bra Top

You want: To cover your midriff if you prefer to work out in just an exercise bra.

Look for: A bra that looks like a tank top, with the bra built in. Known as a bra top, this style stretches to just below your belly button, so it doesn't expose your midriff. This style isn't as supportive as a cropped exercise bra, however, so it's best used by women who are smaller-breasted (although larger-breasted women can use it for low-impact activities).

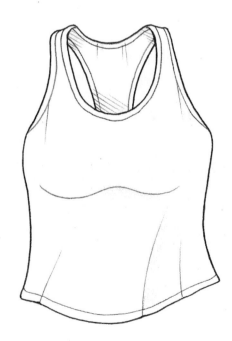

Closure Bra

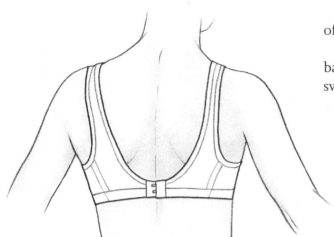

You want: A bra that's easy to put on and take off.

Look for: A style with closures in the front or back so you don't have to wrestle your tight, sweaty bra up over your head after a workout.

Once you've determined your style, it's time to consider fabric. "Unless you're wedded to cotton (which gets soaked easily), you will want a bra that's lined with moisture-wicking fabric, such as CoolMax, that dries quickly and pulls the sweat away from your body," says Park. There are other materials to consider as well. If you want maximum bounce control, get a bra made with nonstretch shoulder straps; for breathability and moisture management, get one made with mesh materials; and for reduced chafing, look for soft materials such as Supplex nylon.

Once you've narrowed down the style and fabric that fit your needs, it's time to try out a few brands. "Finding the perfect exercise bra is like finding the perfect pair of sneakers," says Park. "The only way to tell if a bra is right for you is to take it for a trial run, walk, tennis match, golf game, or whatever exercise you normally do." Remember, for sports such as soccer and running, you'll need to choose a style and fabric that have more motion control than you'd need for activities such as inline skating and walking.

It's important that the bra you choose is comfortable and that you don't experience any chafing, wetness, or unwanted exposure, bouncing, or flat-

tening. For the best fit, start by trying on an exercise bra in the same size as your regular bra, says Park. Full-figured women will be glad to find exercise bras that accommodate women who wear DD cups or sizes of 38, 40, and higher.

Once you find a bra you like, buy two or three so that you can wash and wear one to test it out. If it meets your needs, you don't have to go back to buy more, and if it doesn't, you can return the unused ones and try something different.

Other Must-Have Gear

Aside from the right bra, your apparel is dictated more by the kind of exercise you do and the weather than anything else. Whatever activity captures your fancy, one rule applies: Choose clothing that feels good, urges Mike May, spokesman for the Sporting Goods Manufacturing Association in North Palm Beach, Florida. "You don't want your clothing to hinder the natural movement of your body in any way," he says.

Besides, the right fitness wear can enhance your attitude as well as your performance, points out Ellen Glickman-Weiss, Ph.D., associate professor of exercise physiology in the department of exercise, leisure, and sports at Kent State University in Ohio. Workout-friendly clothing helps you stick with exercise, rather than dropping out because you're cold, wet, sore, or uncomfortable.

Walking, jogging, cycling, and hiking. High-tech outerwear is drawing the praises of winter walkers, joggers, cyclists, and hikers alike. If you're ambulating by foot when the snow falls, wear running tights and multiple thin layers of clothing. Select fabrics made from CoolMax, Capilene, or other specialized fibers designed to wick away your body's moisture, yet protect you from the elements.

Windproof pants and jackets, a hat, and gloves will keep you jogging through winter's chilliest days. Some joggers like balaclavas that cover the head, neck, and most of the face; you'll find them in sporting goods stores and fitness-wear catalogs.

In summer, clothes that help sweat to evaporate as you work out help your body to dissipate heat and cool itself more efficiently, says Dr. Glickman-Weiss. Choose lightweight, light-colored, loose-fitting fitness wear that covers as little body surface area as possible. Apply a sunscreen lotion with a sun protection factor (SPF) of 15 or higher at least 30 minutes before you head outdoors to exercise.

Also, think visibility. Like many busy women, Ruth Barnes, past president of the California Association of Bicycling Organizations of Los Angeles, finds that she often cannot work out until evening, when peace comes to streets clogged with commuters earlier in the day.

"If you exercise at night, whether it's cycling, walking, or jogging, be aware that you can become a part of the dark. Sporting goods stores offer jackets that have strips of glow-in-the-dark material incorporated into the design. Even at dusk, it's a good idea to avoid gray, navy, green, and other colors that blend into the background and camouflage you. Wear bright colors, such as yellow, red, and purple, so you can be seen," Barnes says.

Bright clothing is in demand for active women of every size, so manufacturers have responded by creating fashionable, functional styles that weren't available when attitudes pushed heavier women toward dark, bulky designs. Larger women have more choices than ever. "Try something new and look in

the mirror," urges Catherine Lippincott, director of public relations for Lane Bryant Stores in Columbus, Ohio. "You might be surprised."

Cycling. Walking and jogging gear can double as cycling gear. In addition, women-specific cycling items are a real blessing for two-wheelers of every stripe—stationary cyclists, road cyclists, and mountain bikers, says Barnes.

Padded cycling pants and shorts. Women's cycling shorts cost about $30 a pair and will make for a much more comfortable ride. Bicycling pants designed for men contain padding in the seams that chafe most women "in the wrong places," Barnes says delicately. "I just plain don't recommend unisex shorts." Champion and Danskin make bike shorts for large women.

One common-sense tip: Like leotards and swimsuits, cycling shorts should be washed out every time they're worn to prevent fungal and yeast infections.

For extra protection, you may want to pony up for a bicycle saddle made specifically for women. There are many different kinds and many innovative shapes. One design is a saddle with slits in the middle to avoid rubbing your genitals as you ride. If you can't find one at any of the cycling shops in your area, try the Bike Nashbar catalog.

Even with padded shorts and a woman-friendly saddle, you can expect a little discomfort in the early days and weeks of riding. "It will go away," Barnes counsels. It will take about a dozen rides to form your buns to the saddle.

Gel-filled gloves. These reduce the pressure on your fingertips and hands during long rides. The main feature to hunt for is fit, says Barnes.

"Women's hands tend to be smaller than men's, so some companies now offer select sizes just for women. I prefer gloves that are washable," she says.

Swimming and water aerobics. For honest-to-goodness water exercise, wear suits that favor freedom of movement over fashion, says Marti Boutin, a training specialist for the Aquatic Exercise Association headquartered in Nokomis, Florida.

"When you're exercising, there's the comfort factor and the modesty factor," says Boutin. In water aerobics, for example, "you don't want your suit to

(continued on page 194)

Workout-Wise Shoe Choices

Buying athletic shoes can be tough even for experienced sports enthusiasts, so it's no wonder that beginning exercisers often feel confused. It's easy to be swayed, not to mention perplexed, by the ergonomic wonders added to sports shoes these days. And the variety is daunting. The key is to find the right shoe for your chosen activity (or activities). The chart below will help. It was created by James McGuire, D.P.M., a physical therapist and director of the department of physical medicine and the Foot and Ankle Institute of the Temple University School of Podiatric Medicine in Philadelphia. If you have special foot problems, he suggests that you consult a podiatrist for individualized advice.

Keep in mind, though, that these are only guidelines. You'll go home with the right shoes if you buy them from a knowledgeable salesperson who can answer your questions about the way they're constructed. And always try before you buy;

many sporting goods stores have indoor areas where you can jump, jog, or kick some balls to test the shoes. If the salesperson doesn't offer you the opportunity to test the shoes, ask. If the answer is no, ask if you can return the shoes after you've worn them. If the answer is still no, buy your shoes elsewhere.

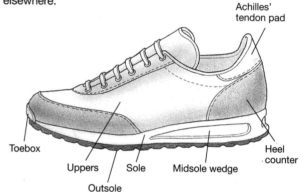

Activity	What to Look For
Aerobics classes, badminton, jumping rope, rowing, stairclimbing, stepping, and table tennis	Thickly cushioned flexible forefoot with a metatarsal break for flexibility (this means that the shoe bends easily); reinforced midfoot (reinforced shank or wedge construction); firm heel counter; unflared outsole; shock-absorbing heel; removable insole to allow for replacement when worn or for orthotics when prescribed by a podiatrist. Tennis, aerobics, and cross-training shoes are very similar and can usually be interchanged.
Belly dancing	Usually done barefoot, but if that's painful, try a soft, flexible dance shoe.
Bicycling	Cycling shoes are specifically designed to fit the toe-pieces on the pedals, but they don't work for mountain biking, where you need to pull your feet off the pedals for balance. You can use a low-cut, light hiker that easily slips off the pedals if necessary (see *Hiking*). Cross-trainers are also a good choice. Road cycling shoes should have a flexible toe, rigid shank, and low-cut, firm heel counter.
Bowling	A typical bowling shoe is an oxford-style lace-up with a flexible slider or smooth sole, a reinforced shank to support the midsole, and a reinforced heel counter to resist pronation.
Cross-country skiing	Cross-country ski boots should have a waterproof exterior, custom toe design to fit your specific binding mechanism, a flexible forefoot to allow for a smooth glide, and a reinforced midfoot and heel counter to prevent pronation and support the rear of the foot. Almost any supportive footgear, such as cross-training, running, or walking shoes can be used on ski machines (see *Aerobics Classes* or *Housework* for construction details).
Dancing	Can be done barefoot or with toe shoes or dance flats. Shoes must give minimal resistance to motion and allow the dancer to create a beautiful "line" or appearance to the foot and ankle during movements. Shoes for tap dancing and other specialty dances are usually chosen more for their appearance during performance than for the structure of the shoe. Try to maximize support for the rear-foot and midfoot and choose a lace-up design over a slip-on when possible.

Activity	What to Look For
Downhill skiing	Rigid molded shell with a mechanism to allow for forward flex during turns; ankle and Achilles tendon padding; removable insole to allow for custom foot-beds or orthotics if needed; auto-molding of the liner or heat or injection molding to improve fit and comfort is advisable, when available.
Elliptical training, Spinning, stationary cycling	Running, walking, or cycling shoes are appropriate as long as they are comfortable (see *Jogging*, *Housework*, and *Bicycling*).
Fencing	Flexible upper to allow for quick movements of the foot; flexible sole to allow the fencer to rise on her toes; reinforced heel counter to allow for rear-foot support; lace closure for increased midfoot support.
Gardening	Waterproof or water-resistant outer material; flexible toe to allow for kneeling; firm midsole and reinforced heel counter to provide rear-foot support. Many people prefer gardening clogs, which have a rigid sole and a very specific last or shape that makes them very comfortable for some foot types and very uncomfortable for others.
Hiking	*Light hikers:* Similar to walking shoes but with a more rigid shank and stiffer forefoot for climbing; padded, reinforced heel counter; removable insole (and extras to use if the originals get wet); ¾ or low construction.
Housework, power walking, and walking	Flexible forefoot; roomy toebox; slight rocker-sole (a design that facilitates rolling off the toes and reduces ankle motion); rigid shank; reinforced heel counter; padded collar and Achilles tendon area; roller heel (a beveled rounded-off heel); removable insoles; slight heel elevation is fine.
Ice skating	Skates with removable insoles, if possible, to allow for a more customized fit.
Inline skating	Skates with removable insoles, if possible, to allow for a more customized fit.
Jogging and treadmill training	Running shoes with a wide, flexible toebox; metatarsal break for flexibility; straight or in-lasted sole, depending on your foot type; firm, reinforced midfoot with no cutouts to decrease support; firm, reinforced heel counter with a padded collar and Achilles tendon padding; padded tongue; shock-absorbing outer sole, particularly in the heel; a flared heel is fine as long as the flare is not excessive.
Racquetball and squash	Tennis shoes or cross-trainers with a thickly cushioned forefoot and a metatarsal break for flexibility; reinforced shank or wedge construction; firm heel counter; unflared outsole; shock-absorbing heel; removable insole.
Snorkeling	Can be done barefoot or with water shoes or swim fins. Wearing water shoes anytime you are walking where you are unsure of the bottom is recommended (see *Swimming*).
Swimming and water aerobics	Water shoes that drain easily, dry quickly, and provide a cushioned, protective layer between your feet and the ground; these shoes protect your feet from injury or an infection that could be picked up while walking barefoot at the lake, beach, or around pools.
Tennis	Tennis shoes have a thickly cushioned forefoot and a metatarsal break for flexibility; reinforced shank or wedge construction; firm heel counter; unflared outsole; shock-absorbing heel; removable insole.
Yardwork	Flexible forefoot; extra toe room; rigid or reinforced shank; reinforced heel counter; padded collar and Achilles tendon area; waterproof outsole; water-resistant upper; removable insole. Light hiking shoes or construction-type boots are best.

ride up." For more information on swimsuits for women with figure problems, see page 320.

Downhill and cross-country skiing. Winter sports clothing has come a long way since the soggy jeans and clumpy down jackets you may have worn when you went skiing with your friends in high school. Whether making tracks on windswept downhill slopes or traversing open plains, layering with lightweight, moisture-wicking fabrics is the key to staying warm, dry, and unencumbered, says Mike Lloyd, manager of Christy Sports in Colorado Springs, Colorado. Add or remove layers as the temperature falls or rises, or as you step up your activity or wind down.

Layer 1: Begin with thermal underwear, top and bottom. A variety of newer polyester fabrics have been created to wick moisture away from the skin, according to Lloyd. Some are woven and others have hollow fibers to pull moisture away—something cotton cannot do. All of these fabrics "keep you drier, and in turn, that keeps you warmer," he says.

You may be thinking, "Polyester next to my skin? Won't it feel rough or make me feel clammy?" Well, think again, says Lloyd. The new polyesters are soft and comfortable, and they wick moisture and wear well. They don't pill, and they can be tossed in the washing machine and dryer.

Layer 2: If it's very cold—10°F or below—add an insulating layer of wool, fleece, or a combination of the two for warmth. This layer should be moisture-wicking, too.

If it's breezy or windy, add an uninsulated shell of nylon, polyester, or one of the newer silky microfiber materials.

Layer 3: If it's snowing or drizzling, take advantage of outerware made from one of the waterproof, breathable fabrics that allow moisture out, but won't let it in. This lets your perspiration evaporate while keeping you dry, enabling you to stick to your exercise program even in wet weather. Choose among various well-known brands, including Durepel, Gore-Tex, and Mem-Brain.

For more information on workout shoes and exercise apparel, visit our Web site at www.banishbbt.com.

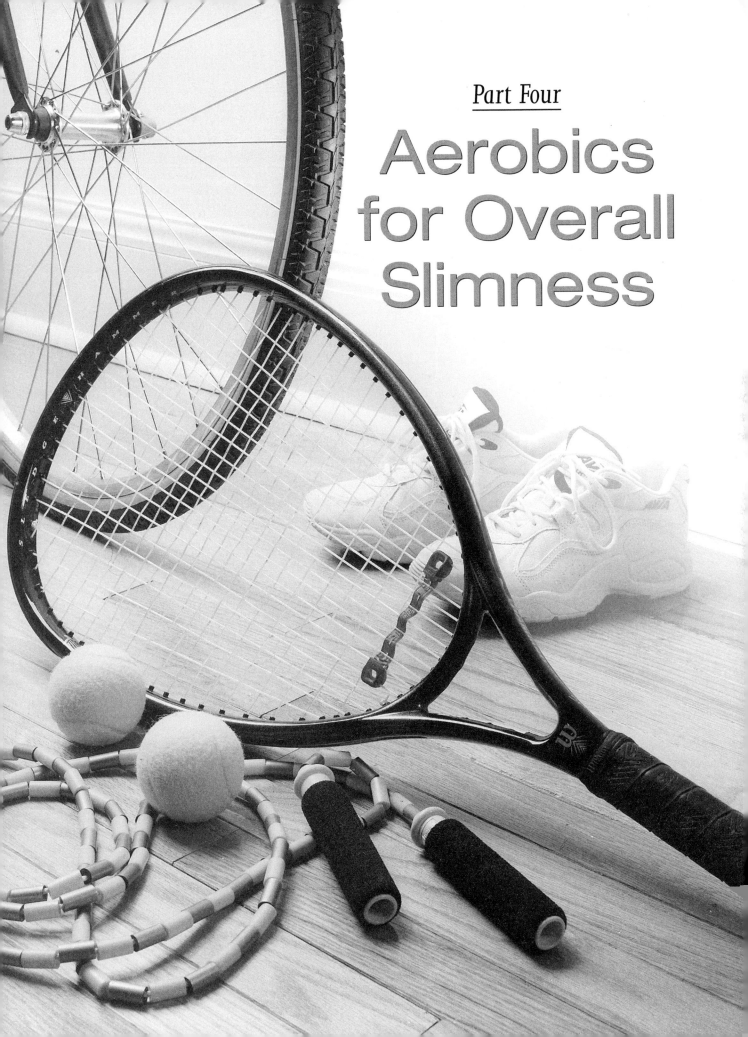

Part Four

Aerobics for Overall Slimness

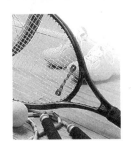

25 Ways to Work Off Fat and Calories

Thanks to a daily aerobic workout that consisted only of walking (coupled with weight training), Barbara Evanson lost 23 inches, mostly from her waist, abdomen, and hips.

"I am quite overweight and have a long way to go," says Barbara, 51, a certified nursing assistant who lives in Cadott, Wisconsin. "But I can't believe I started to see changes in just one month! Sometimes I just can't find time to walk. But on those days, I spend one to two hours at a time weeding my garden."

You'll be happy to learn that working out aerobically doesn't mean you have to run or join an aerobics class to lose weight and shape up—unless you want to. Everyday activities like walking and gardening count. They can and do burn fat and calories just like more strenuous workouts and can help women just like you flatten their abs, trim their thighs, and tuck their butts.

How It Works

Aerobic exercise works this way: Your exertion demands an increased flow of oxygen to supply energy. When you breathe in, the oxygen pours from your lungs into your bloodstream. Your heart then pumps it to your muscles. There, the oxygen is used to break down carbohydrate, fat, and protein into the energy that your muscles need to function.

Aerobic activities are big calorie burners, and—along with a diet that controls fat and calories—they go a long way toward melting away fat. That's because causing your heart to pump at a faster, sustained rate will increase your metabolism during the exercise, burning more calories, and it may eventually increase your metabolic rate, the rate at which you burn calories as you go about your daily business. Metabolic changes, in turn, improve your body's ability to burn fat and make your muscles better able to use oxygen for this purpose. As your level of aerobic fitness increases, your heart, lungs, and muscles become more efficient, so you can do more without getting tired.

Once you become more physically active, people may start noticing that you look leaner and more muscular. Most aerobic activity doesn't build muscle, but your muscles will look more toned, and you'll lose fat, so you'll look leaner. For that reason, you'll probably notice that your clothes fit better before you actually see your weight change on the scale.

Looking good isn't the only benefit to shaking a tail feather. You'll feel good, too. Evidence shows that participating in aerobic exercise can help reduce symptoms of depression and anxiety and make you feel generally better emotionally. A study conducted by the department of human performance and health promotion at the University of New Orleans, for example, found that 36 women and six men who enrolled in step aerobics classes of varying intensity felt less tense, depressed, fatigued, and angry after the more intense workouts than they did after the less intense workouts.

Some experts say that exercise elevates your mood simply by freeing your mind from everyday concerns. "It may be just that you're having fun," suggests Charles Corbin, Ph.D., professor in the department of exercise science and physical education at Arizona State University in Tempe. "You're doing something you like." Given that many women blame unwanted weight gain, in part, on a tendency to overeat when they're tired, bored, tense, or angry, the psychological benefits of aerobic exercise can play a part in your success.

No one is exactly sure why exercise elevates mood. Other experts say that during and after exercise, your brain releases endorphins, chemical substances associated with pleasure. You've probably heard athletes or others refer to this as an endorphin high. But everyday exercisers like you can enjoy the same uplifting effect.

How Hard Do You Have to Work?

Experts say that to reap the health benefits of aerobic exercise, you need to work at moderate intensity to raise your heart rate for at least 30 minutes a day three to five times a week.

If you're aiming to lose weight, you need to exercise aerobically at a moderate intensity for 30 to 60 minutes most days of the week. "Thirty minutes is the point at which fat is being used as the primary energy source," says Laurie L. Tis, Ph.D., associate professor in the department of kinesiology and health at Georgia State University in Atlanta.

How do you know what's moderate intensity? One way is to calculate your target heart rate. To do this, subtract your age from 220. This tells you your approximate maximum heart rate. You don't want to work at your maximum (nor should you). Instead, you need to calculate your target heart rate zone—a range, depending on your fitness level, that's 60 to 90 percent of your maximum. To do that, multiply your maximum rate by 0.6 if you want to exercise at 60 percent of your maximum (low intensity), which is good for beginners, 0.7 for 70 percent of your maximum (moderate intensity), or 0.8 for 80 percent (high intensity).

This isn't as hard as it sounds. To calculate her target heart rate zone, for example, Sarah, the 52-year-old described in earlier chapters, would subtract 52 from 220 for her maximum heart rate of 168. To work out at 70 percent of this maximum rate, she would multiply 168 by 0.7 for a target heart rate of 118.

You can make sure your heart rate falls within your target range while you exercise by placing two or three fingers—but not your thumb, which has its own pulse—lightly in the inside of your opposite wrist below the base of your thumb. Count the beats for one minute to get the pulse rate, which is the beat of the heart as felt through the walls of the arteries, or count for 15 seconds and multiply by four.

Experts say that if you're new to aerobic exercise, you can aim for a target heart rate of 60 percent. Once you're in pretty good shape, you can work up to 90 percent.

If you have no patience with numbers, there are a few other, simpler ways to tell if you're exercising hard enough, says Michael Youssouf, a certified trainer and manager of trainer education and advancement at The Sports Center at Chelsea Piers in New York City. You're doing fine if you're breathing hard, but not so hard that you can't carry on a conversation. Or if you've broken a sweat. Or you simply *feel* like you're working.

Want another way to rate intensity? Ask yourself how much longer you can carry on the activity. The activity should take enough out of you that you wouldn't be able to continue for hours, but you shouldn't be working so hard that you need to stop right away, says Youssouf.

As you continue to get in shape, what used to be strenuous becomes easier, so you must add to the duration, intensity, or frequency of the exercise, or start doing a different, more challenging activity, says Youssouf. For each of the aerobic activities described in the pages that follow, experts have prescribed beginner, intermediate, and experienced levels to help you get started and progress. These levels are not just for safety; they have a built-in success ratio, explains Youssouf. Assign yourself 20 to 30 minutes a day, and make your workout part of your daily routine. Find a level you can do, and if you enjoy it, you'll keep at it. When you're ready to move on to the next stage, you will.

Work Hard (but Not Too Hard)

Just as one-size-fits-all clothing tends not to fit any woman well, a strict and uncompromising exercise routine is uncomfortable for most individuals. All a woman needs to do is find some activities that allow her to work within a range that gets her heart pumping. Throughout this section, you'll hear from dozens of women, each of whom tamed their trouble spots by doing something different. Some walked off the unwanted bulges. Some took up inline skating. Others found weight-loss nirvana on "new" equipment like elliptical trainers. Others turned to old standbys like stationary bicycles and cross-country ski machines.

For them, like many women, the key to sticking with an aerobic exercise program was to make it fun or interesting. "A lot of times, it's just a matter of finding an activity that you like," says Dr. Tis. "If you don't like walking, then try biking, mountain biking, or inline skating." Better still, try a mix of activities. Maybe on Mondays you play tennis, Wednesdays you attend an aerobics class, and Fridays you go bicycling with your family.

Only you can decide what works best for you. For some women, sticking with one form of exercise rather than doing a mix is best because they like to excel at one thing, says Martin Hoffman, M.D., professor in the department of physical medicine and rehabilitation at the Medical College of Wisconsin and director of the sports performance and technology laboratory, both in Milwaukee. So, for example, if you enjoy running, you may be motivated to do just this exercise by constantly trying to improve the time or distance of your runs. As you shop for an aerobic activity that suits your purposes, you'll also learn how to maximize the body-shaping benefits by maximizing your effort or frequency.

Another time-honored approach for women just beginning an exercise program—and one that works—is to find an exercise buddy, says Dr.

Hoffman. "If you know that your friend is going to be there at 6:00 in the morning to go for a walk with you, you won't decide you're too tired today and sleep in."

By simply walking 30 minutes a day at a moderate pace, you will lose 5 to 15 pounds after one year, depending on your size, says Dr. Corbin. "The best form of exercise for weight control is the kind of exercise you will actually do," he adds.

Exercise or other physical activity can also become a time to maintain or strengthen family ties or friendships, says Dr. Tis. Go cycling with your kids and use the time not only to burn calories but also to talk with them. Or take your husband along on your evening walks, and make the most of this time to yourselves.

Dr. Tis exercises regularly with one of her colleagues "and it's our talk time. We work out and have 30 minutes away from the phones and the office and are able to just talk."

Getting Started

Before you start an aerobic exercise program, ask your doctor for advice if you answer yes to two or more of the following.

- You are over the age of 45.
- You are less than 55 and past menopause and not taking estrogen-replacement therapy (which protects your heart).
- You smoke cigarettes.
- You have or have ever had high blood pressure or high cholesterol.
- You're sedentary—that is, you work at a desk, have no physically active hobbies or pastimes, or don't currently exercise regularly.
- You have a family history of heart disease, high blood pressure, or high cholesterol.

If your foray into fitness takes you to a health club or other group setting, don't be intimidated by how other women look, or whether they are more proficient on treadmills, stairclimbers, or various other exercise machines, advises Dr. Tis.

"It's been my experience that if you can get

through some of those initial insecurities, you'll be surprised at how much exercise boosts your self-esteem," Dr. Tis says. "Just remember, you are there to improve your health and well-being. You want to feel good now, and 25 years from now. So this is a commitment to yourself. You will feel more comfortable, and everything will start to fall into place."

Start by gently warming up: Walk at an easy pace for five minutes to get your blood circulating. Then do some gentle stretches (no bouncing) before you start your aerobic activity. When you've ended your activity, allow your body to cool down. Walk for about three to five minutes. Then do some gentle stretches, which will help increase or maintain flexibility, says Dr. Tis.

When starting out, don't be discouraged if you can only do, say, 10 minutes on a particular exercise machine, cautions Dr. Tis. The next time, lighten the tension and ease the pace and try for 15 minutes. Then try to build upon that gradually.

"This isn't a competition or a race," points out Dr. Tis. "You have to stay within your abilities so it's comfortable."

How much should you increase your performance by before leveling off? "The rule of thumb is 10 percent per week," says Dr. Tis. "That's probably a little low. The thing to remember is that you can either increase your pace or your time, but you shouldn't increase both at the same time."

For example, say that you're walking at 3 miles per hour on a treadmill for 20 minutes at a time. You're cruisin'—hardly huffing, scarcely sweating. Here are your options: You can increase your time on the machine to 22 to 23 minutes. Or you can stay at 20 minutes, but increase your speed to 3½ to 4 miles per hour. Or you can do neither, but make the degree of incline a little steeper.

"You can either increase the intensity, increase the time, or increase the resistance on some of the machines, but do only one increase a week," advises Dr. Tis. If you are really enjoying working out, you could keep the intensity and duration the same, but add an extra day. And remember, take one day off a week, no matter how fit you are.

No matter which method you choose, you'll be on your way toward the body you desire.

To banish your belly, butt, and thighs, you can choose from more than two dozen types of activities, from walking or gardening to vacuuming and yard work, described in the pages that follow. (Leg lifts and other forms of resistance workouts can play a role in banishing your belly, butt, and thighs, but for different reasons.)

For more information on these and other aerobic forms of exercise, visit our Web site at www.banishbbt.com.

Aerobics Classes and Videotapes

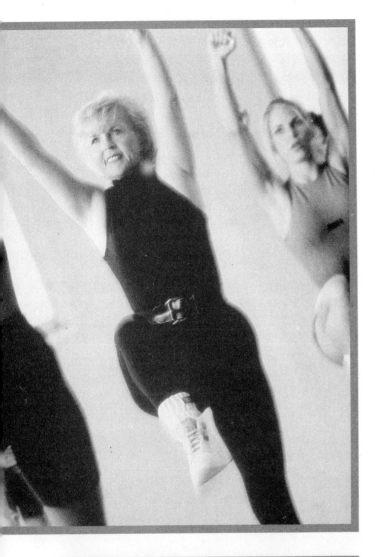

The fat-blasting, muscle-toning, heart-strengthening moves of aerobics workouts have come a long way since their disco-inspired beginnings as choreographed calisthenics. Today's aerobics classes and videotapes challenge you to kickbox, jump rope, do tennis swings, and more, with background tunes ranging from reggae to golden oldies.

For weight loss, an aerobics workout can hardly be beat, says Laurie L. Tis, Ph.D., associate professor in the department of kinesiology and health at Georgia State University in Atlanta. For muscle toning, aerobics also incorporates resistance exercises that add up to a sleek physique.

Body-Shaping Benefits

Doing aerobics on a regular basis contributes to weight loss and body-toning in several ways.

- You'll burn fat more efficiently.
- You'll tone muscles from head to toe, improving your appearance, strength, and stamina.
- You'll improve your flexibility, which extends your range of motion and improves muscle performance, balance, and coordination.

Psychological Benefits

Research shows that aerobic exercise imparts increased feelings of well-being and self-confidence while relieving stress, depression, symptoms of premenstrual syndrome, and sleep problems. A group of women surveyed by the Melpomene Institute, a research organization devoted to studying the link between women's health and physical activity, described an after-exercise "glow," the feeling of more energy, well-being, and exhilaration.

"A good aerobics workout gives you immediate gratification for having done something good for yourself," says Jennifer Sherman Bolger, program manager with FitLinxx, a fitness center in

Aerobics Stats

Calories Burned*	Body-Shaping Potential
228 per half-hour	Tones abdominals, hips, thighs, buttocks, and depending on type of aerobics performed, also other major muscles

*Based on a 150-pound woman. If you weigh more, you'll burn more calories; if you weigh less, you'll burn fewer.

San Diego. "Women develop a lot more confidence in their abilities to do anything that they want to do."

The Right Footwear

Shop for cross-trainer shoes, which provide good cushioning, support, flexibility, and traction for performing the variety of exercises that aerobics workouts entail, advise experts at the American Council on Exercise (ACE). If you have high-arched feet, look for a shoe with added shock absorption and more ankle support. If your feet tend to be more flat, look for less cushioning and greater support and heel control.

For a proper fit, allow a half-inch between the end of your longest toe and the end of the shoe.

Your shoe should also be as wide as possible across the forefoot without allowing your heel to slip. A well-fitted shoe does require a breaking-in period. If your feet are blistering after a few days, take the shoes back. Finally, replace your shoes regularly. They lose their cushioning after three to six months of regular use, making you more susceptible to knee and ankle injuries.

What Else You'll Need

Aside from a good pair of shoes, you'll need clothing suited to working up a sweat. And if you'll be exercising on your own, you'll need aerobics videotapes.

Clothes. Look for "breathable" fabrics in a blend of cotton and synthetic fibers that whisk

She Did It!

Jana Lost 40 Pounds—And Has Kept It Off

When Jana Trabert's family moved to the United States from Korea when she was 12, her introduction to this new world included junk food, TV, and weight gain.

"The American lifestyle is so sedentary," says the 33-year-old interior designer. "Even though I'd been thin in Korea, by my freshman year in high school here, I weighed 150 pounds, and I'm only five feet two inches tall. I felt fat, yucky, and totally self-conscious."

Jana decided to diet the weight away. "I tried every diet in the book, including starvation," she says. "My girlfriends and I would even read about bulimia and try to get ourselves to throw up after we ate. Nothing worked, of course, and I was ruining my body and my health."

It was in college that a friend suggested Jana take an aerobics dance class with her at a local YMCA. She was hooked immediately.

"It was fun," Jana says. "And I started noticing a difference in my body, both on the scale and in the way I looked and felt, after just a couple of months." Working out three times a week, she shed 40 pounds and has kept it off. "I realized that I have to make this my lifetime regimen, along with healthy eating. But I like it. I'm thrilled to have discovered something that really works."

While Jana has kept up with her aerobics regimen for about 15 years, these days she does her workouts at home, having traded crowded gyms for her family room, where she plugs in her favorite aerobics exercise videotapes.

"I try to set a certain day and time to do it," Jana says, "but sometimes I get busy—especially since becoming a mother—and I have to just fit it in. And I do. It's not always easy, but it makes me feel great."

Take It to the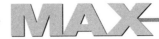

Kick It up a Notch

Droves of women experienced at aerobics who want to power their workouts have found the answer: Martial arts–inspired aerobic workouts like Tae Bo with Billy Blanks, and Karate Integrated (KI) Aerobics, among others. Held at many fitness centers but also available as video workouts, these fast-paced aerobic workouts set to music incorporate kicks, punches, and other moves often found in other high-intensity aerobics classes. "In short, they're an Americanized version of martial arts," says Ginny Whitelaw, Ph.D., a chief instructor of aikido at the Aikido Association Atlanta in Georgia, and the author of *Body Learning*.

Tae Bo is probably the best-known form of martial arts–inspired aerobics. But similar versions abound, and classes go by names like "cardio kickboxing" and "aerobo-tae." The number of calories you can burn per session varies with the type of routine offered. Nevertheless, experts say that you can figure on burning roughly 280 calories per half-hour—about the same as any intense aerobics class.

To find a martial arts–type aerobics class in your area, call your local gym or fitness center. And by the way, experts emphasize that kickboxing-type aerobic routines are geared to intermediate or experienced exercisers, not beginners.

---

sweat away from your body, allowing you to keep cool. For more details, see Workout-Friendly Clothes on page 187.

If the temperature in your workout area varies, wear clothes in a couple of layers that you can take off or put back on as needed.

Videotapes. Aerobics videotapes are a great way to exercise at home—you get to enjoy lively music as you follow the moves of other in-shape exercisers bounding across your TV screen. Tapes are available in a wide range of aerobics styles, from traditional choreographed floor aerobics to workouts that help tone specific muscle groups.

Consider the following when choosing a videotape, advises Jill Ross, director of product acquisitions at Collage Video in Minneapolis, which specializes in exercise videos.

- Type. Look for a workout and music that sparks your personal interest.
- Time. Figure out realistically how long your workout will be. If your time is limited, use 30-minute videos and put a couple of them together at those times when you can do a longer workout. If you're a beginner, decrease the time or the intensity of your routine if it feels too difficult.

- Intensity. Don't overestimate what you can do, or you risk getting discouraged right off the bat, says Dr. Tis. You're probably a beginner if you haven't even taken a walk in at least six months or you're very overweight. If you walk or do some other form of exercise at least two or three times per week, start at an intermediate level.

Getting Started

Here's what you need to get started and keep going with an aerobics exercise program.

Learn the basics. Many aerobics exercises require a degree of motor skill and coordination, which could take time to develop. Start with an introductory class or videotape workout described as low-impact or no-impact, which means less stress to your joints, advises Lauri Reimer, director of aerobic instructor training for the Aerobics and Fitness Association of America. As you get comfortable with the exercise program, gradually move into a more advanced workout.

Warm up. Prepare your body and mind for exercise with a 5- to 10-minute warmup of the muscles you will use during your workout, advise experts at ACE. For example, walk in place to warm up your legs. Follow with "static" (gentle with no bouncing) stretching of those same muscles. Warming up helps your body burn calories more efficiently by increasing your core body temperature. It also helps your muscles work faster and more forcefully, improves muscle elasticity and muscle control, and prevents the buildup of pain-provoking lactic acid in the blood.

Monitor your intensity level. The talk test is a good, commonsense way to judge whether you're working out at a safe pace, says Richard Cotton, chief exercise physiologist for the American Council on Exercise in San Diego. You should be able to carry on a conversation at the same time you're exercising. If you can't, slow down.

An aerobics workout will burn fat, strengthen your muscles, and help your heart grow stronger as long as you're exercising at a higher than usual heart rate—your "target heart rate" (generally between 60 and 90 percent of your estimated maximum heart rate), say experts. If you're just starting out, you want your heart rate during the aerobics portion of your workout to be at the lower end of your target heart rate range. Be sure to monitor your pulse rate during your exercise routine. You should not exceed your maximum heart rate.

Aim for 30 to 60 minutes. Make it your goal to exercise for at least 30 minutes—either at a single stretch or accumulated throughout the day, say experts. If you're an absolute beginner, start out doing only 10 to 15 minutes during the aerobics portion at a low- to moderate-intensity level. As you grow stronger, gradually add workout time without increasing intensity.

Add toning exercises. Most aerobics classes are followed by a few minutes of exercises specific to muscle strengthening. Look for a class that focuses on your "problem areas." Or add toning exercises with light weights to your home workout.

Cool down. As few as three minutes of moderate movement like walking after a workout enables your heart and muscles to slowly return to their normal state, says Dr. Tis. Gentle movements and stretches may also help increase or maintain your flexibility and minimize muscle soreness.

Work out several days a week. In order to lose weight, experts recommend that you exercise at least four or five days a week.

Aerobics Workouts

Beginner

10 to 20 minutes, 3 days a week; target heart rate 60 to 65 percent of maximum

Intermediate

20 to 30 minutes, 3 to 5 days a week; target heart rate 65 to 75 percent of maximum

Experienced

Minimum 20 to 30 minutes, 3 to 5 days a week; target heart rate 75 to 90 percent of maximum

The best approach to exercise intensity is to work at your own pace, says Lauri Reimer, director of aerobic instructor training for the Aerobics and Fitness Association of America. "In a class, don't worry about keeping up with the people in the front row."

Do 5 leg kicks instead of 10 if that's all you can handle right now. Jump, but skip the arm-reaching part of jumping jacks. Just keep moving. "The point is to do as much as you can and aim for improvement over time," Reimer says.

Monitoring your heart rate can help you ascertain whether you're working out at a safe and effective intensity. For maximum weight loss, work out for 30 to 60 minutes at moderate intensity most days of the week, says Laurie L. Tis, Ph.D., associate professor in the department of kinesiology and health at Georgia State University in Atlanta.

Bicycling

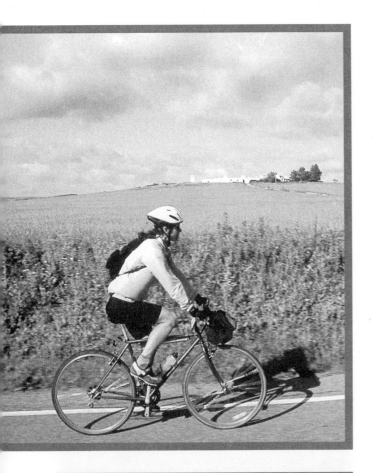

You say the last time you rode a bike, it was a pink two-wheeler with a banana seat and streamers hanging off the handlebars? Well, you've grown up, and so has the bicycling industry. According to the National Sporting Goods Association, 45 percent of all adult bike riders are women. And more and more bikes are designed for women. No, women's bikes don't have pink paint and streamers. But they do have seats and frames designed for the female anatomy. And they're sturdy and easy to ride—even if you've never been on a bike in your life.

"If your knees, ankles, or hips bother you when you walk, then cycling might be a great, pain-free way to exercise and lose weight," says Edmund Burke, Ph.D., professor of exercise science at the University of Colorado in Colorado Springs and coauthor of *Fitness Cycling*. "Unlike walking or running, cycling isn't a weight-bearing exercise—the bicycle, not your bones and joints, supports your weight."

Bicycling Stats

Calories Burned*	Body-Shaping Potential
130–345 per half-hour, depending on your speed and terrain	Strengthens and tones all the muscles of your lower body, including your butt, thighs, and calves

*Based on a 150-pound woman. If you weigh more, you'll burn more calories; if you weigh less, you'll burn fewer.

Body-Shaping Benefits

"The body-shaping benefits of cycling are primarily from the hips down," says Dr. Burke. "Bicycling works the muscles in your buttocks, front and back thighs, and lower legs." These are the largest muscles in your body, and when you use them to perform high-intensity work, such as cycling, you burn a lot of calories. (Remember, calories are a form of energy, and it takes energy to do physical work.) So if you bicycle regularly:

- You'll strengthen and tone the muscles of your lower body during your workout.
- You'll burn off a fair amount of stored calories—or fat.

Psychological Benefits

If you're like a lot of women, you probably have wonderful memories of exploring your neighborhood by bike as a kid, riding with your friends for hours. Yet somewhere along the way toward adulthood—probably once you got your driver's license—your bike started to gather dust in the garage, becoming a forgotten relic of the past. And that's a shame.

"You'll enjoy riding a bike as an adult just as much as you did as a kid," says Dr. Burke. "Bicycling gets you outside just like walking does, but it expands your terrain. When you get on a bike, you can see more of the world."

She Did It!

Saturday Bike Rides Helped Lynn Lose 26 Pounds

Like many women, Lynn Hoerle, 43, of Inverness, California, found that some of life's rites of passage, such as turning 30, starting a new relationship, and moving to the suburbs, brought something else into her life—weight gain.

"At five-foot-seven, I had always weighed about 125 pounds," says Lynn. "But in my thirties, I found myself weighing 156. I struggled with the extra weight, but I was too busy with work to do anything about it."

Lynn, an office manager, did buy a mountain bike at one point, but it sat in her garage for three years, unused. "Then my mother and brother died within a few months of each other," Lynn says. "I realized then that there was more to life than just going to work, so I promised myself I would get out more."

One thing Lynn did was sign up for a six-week mountain-biking class being held on Saturdays at the local community college. "I learned a lot about biking, but I also learned a lot about Mount Tamalpais, a recreation area where a lot of Northern Californians go to bike and hike," she says. "I made friends with someone in the class, and together we decided to continue meeting on Saturdays to ride together. We'd get out our maps and our guidebooks and just figure out where we wanted to go."

Lynn so enjoyed biking with her friend on the weekends that together they took biking vacations to Washington, Idaho, Montana, and even Alaska. "Within the next couple of years, I joined WOMBATS

(Women's Mountain Bike and Tea Society, a national biking organization) and met more women with whom I could bike every few days," says Lynn. "My whole network of friends expanded immediately. I loved it."

With regular bicycling, Lynn noticed a change in her body shape. "My legs were definitely leaner and stronger," she says. But she was still pushing 156 pounds up and down those hills. "Being heavy really affected my riding. At one point, I almost hung it all up because I couldn't keep up with everyone else."

Lynn didn't want to give up the riding and the friendships that had come to mean so much to her. "So I decided I would just have to lose the weight," she says. She followed a structured weight-loss program that included healthier meals. "I basically cut out the junk. No more double chocolate chunk ice cream, no more hunks of cheese after dinner, no more bags of chips."

Lynn now weighs 130 pounds and combines road racing trips with her mountain biking outings. "Sometimes, I'm one of the oldest women on the group rides," she says. "Riding motivates me to become fitter, so I can keep up with my friends." She's so motivated, in fact, that for the first time, she recently put on a bathing suit and joined her friends in the hot tub after a long ride.

"They'd never seen me in a bathing suit before," Lynn says. "And I felt great, because I didn't feel like an outsider anymore."

If you typically walk an hour a day for exercise and cover 3 to 4 miles, you can cycle for the same amount of time and cover 10 miles.

The Right Footwear

Unless you're competing in the world-famous, multi-day Tour de France bike race, you can cycle in comfortable, lightweight sneakers, as long as the soles have enough grip to stay put on the bike pedals, says Dr. Burke.

"Be sure to tuck the laces under the tongue of your shoe, though, so the laces don't get tangled in the pedals, chain, or chain guard," he adds.

Also, don't tie your laces too tightly, or your feet will fall asleep while you ride. To keep your feet comfortable, choose socks made of blends of cotton and synthetic fibers like polypropylene, which wick moisture away and let your skin breathe.

What Else You'll Need

Aside from the right footwear, you'll need a bike and a helmet—both of which you should purchase at a bike shop, where they sell and service bikes. Even if you have an old Schwinn you want to resurrect, you need to take it over to a bike shop for a tune-up before you head out down the driveway. It's almost sure to need new tires and some oil to lubricate the chains and gears.

"Bike shop owners know which bikes are good for beginners," says Dr. Burke. Bike shops usually work in tandem with their customers to keep their bikes working well, which means you'll be safer and your bike will last longer.

If you need a bike, you can choose from three types.

- Road bike. This bike looks like a 10-speed, which you may have ridden as a teenager. It has drop handlebars (they curve under) and smooth, narrow tires. These bikes are designed for speed, not comfort.

- Mountain bike. These bikes have flat handlebars (they don't curve) and fatter tires than road bikes. It's easier to balance on them. The tires are knobby for better traction. They're designed for riding on unpaved trails, over rocks and roots and such—but they function well on paved paths, too.

- Hybrid bike. These bikes have gears, handlebars, and frames similar to mountain bikes, but with narrower tires for the smooth ride of a road bike. Experts tend to recommend hybrid bikes for adult women interested in bicycling.

"Hybrids generally have sturdier frames than road bikes, so they provide lots of stability," says Tim Blumenthal, executive director of the International Mountain Bicycling Association in Boulder, Colorado. "They're easy to ride on pavement. And if you want to ride in parks, hybrids can handle dirt trails and unpaved roads."

The right fit. Experts at bike shops are better equipped to measure you and your new equipment properly than salespeople at a department store. Ask for a bike designed especially for women. These have a steeper seat tube (the vertical tube) to position you correctly, and a shorter top tube (running from the seat tube to the head tube and handlebars) to accommodate women's shorter torsos and arms. Or they may steer you toward a man's bike that the specialists reconfigure to fit you (moving handlebars or changing the seat, for instance, so you don't have to reach as far for the handlebars).

Proper fit is essential. "If your bike doesn't fit you properly, it will be too uncomfortable for you to ride regularly," says Dr. Burke. If you're not experienced at riding a bike with multiple gears, you may want to consider a bike with gears that are clearly numbered, to help you learn how to shift.

A comfortable seat. If you're serious about getting in shape, you'll be spending a fair amount of time in the saddle. So whichever style of bike you choose, you also need to feel comfortable in the saddle.

"You have to find a good bike with a comfortable seat, or else you'll be putting pressure on parts of your body that don't respond well to intense friction and excess weight," says Dr. Burke. So by all means, ask about special seats made for women. Some feature a wider back and narrower, cut-out nose that takes the weight off delicate tissues for a more comfortable ride. Others use a soft material on the underside with less bracing (used for stiffness) than seats for men's bikes, so that the saddle flexes to absorb impact.

A helmet. When you cycle outdoors, you must always wear a helmet to protect your head from impact if you collide with the pavement (or anything else). Many helmets are specially designed for women—a big help if, for example, you want to pull your hair back in a ponytail when you ride. Helmets sold in bike shops are almost always of equal quality because all are made to the same safety specifications. Further, the Consumer Product Safety Commission requires all helmets made or sold in the United States to meet federal safety standards. Consider a helmet with a vent to help keep you cool, and those with reflective stripes and removable visors for riding at night and in the sun. Plan to wear a cap under your helmet only if the helmet is designed to accommodate a hat—otherwise, you compromise fit and safety.

Getting Started

Once you have a well-oiled bicycle that suits you to a "T," it's time to head out into the wide world of road cycling.

Get to know your bike. Before taking off on a 10-mile trek, ride around your neighborhood or an empty parking lot to get to know the gears and brakes on your new equipment.

Practice shifting gears. "Most people who are new to biking keep their bikes in one gear because they aren't sure how to shift and haven't taken the time to get to know which gears will help them on which terrain," notes Dr. Burke.

Bicycling Workouts

Beginner

Cycle nonstop for 20 minutes on flat terrain, 2 or 3 times a week for 3 to 4 weeks.

Intermediate

Beginning on flat terrain, cycle fast for 20 to 30 minutes, then include a couple of hills or shift to a harder gear for 5 minutes at a time, without necessarily going fast. Do this 3 times a week until you work your way up to riding comfortably 60 minutes each time.

Experienced

Extend one of your regularly scheduled rides, probably on the weekend, to at least 1½ to double the time or distance of a weekday ride. Vary the speed and intensity as you ride: Climb hills, ride quickly for a few minutes, and use more intensity at other times.

When you first start to cycle, don't try to conquer hills or ride for a set amount of time, says Edmund Burke, Ph.D., professor of exercise science at the University of Colorado in Colorado Springs and coauthor of *Fitness Cycling*. Instead, choose flat terrain. "You want to feel successful each time you ride, so you look forward to getting on the bike again the next time. For the first few weeks, just think of your rides as being a nice, easy way to spend your leisure time."

Your next goal will be to change the intensity of your workout and make it just a little bit longer, perhaps an hour total. "Change one thing in the beginning, such as adding hills or using a higher gear," says Dr. Burke. "And always give yourself some time to recover from the change in intensity before you make another change during the ride."

As you progress, take longer, more challenging rides at least once a week, says Dr. Burke. "You can ride solo," he says. "But I think it's helpful to join a biking club and ride with a group. Everyone will be doing the same ride, in terms of intensity and distance, which inspires most people to the next level of fitness."

Technically, the best way to figure out whether you're using the right gear for a specific terrain is to count your pedal strokes. To do this, count your pedal revolutions (on one leg) for 15 seconds, then multiply that number by four. Efficient riders do 80 to 100 revolutions per minute on flat roads, and about 60 to 85 revolutions on hills. But for beginners, pedaling and counting while looking at your watch and trying to see where you're going is a bit tricky. An easier rule of thumb: Use the lower (smaller) gears on steeper terrain, and the higher (larger) gears on flatter terrain. Then practice until you get a feel for the combination that enables you to pedal the most efficiently. If you're struggling, downshift. If the wheels are spinning with little or no resistance, upshift.

"Don't be afraid to play with your bike in the beginning," urges Dr. Burke.

Experiment with hand positions. Some hand positions feel better than others. You might feel comfortable riding with your hands close together, while another bicyclist may prefer grasping the very edges of the handlebars.

Follow through when you pedal. Good pedaling involves technique. You have to use your leg muscles on the back end of the pedaling stroke—that is, when you're bringing the pedal back up and bending your leg to pedal efficiently. To do this, just imagine that you're scraping mud from the bottom of your shoe. In other words, press your leg down, apply force when your foot is at the bottom of the stroke, then use your leg muscles to pull the bottom of your leg back up toward your butt, says Dr. Burke.

Lean forward—or stand—on the hills. As you progress and begin to feel more comfortable on your bike, you'll spend more time out of the saddle. For instance, when you go into a turn, you'll lean forward, out of the seat. When you go up hills, you'll stand in order to get more power to your legs.

Watch out for cars, both moving and parked. If you ride on roads and streets, you probably know enough to pay attention to moving vehicles. But you also need to be aware of parked cars. Many street accidents take place when someone who has just parked her car opens the door straight into the path of a bike rider. "It takes practice to learn how to ride on crowded roads," cautions Blumenthal. "You should ride with traffic, not against it. Keep your eyes and ears open; both are important." That means no Walkman.

Take a lesson. Many bike shops offer clinics and classes for novice riders. You'll learn, for example, that as with driving a car, it's usually best to brake before a turn, rather than during one.

Cross-Country Skiing

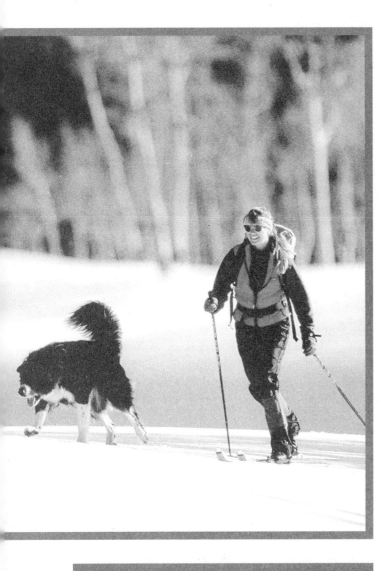

Some 5,000 years ago, the enterprising natives of what is now Scandinavia began strapping large animal bones to their feet to better traverse their homeland's snow-covered terrain. Over time, bones gave way to boards, and cross-country skiing was born.

In the United States, cross-country skiing has become a popular wintertime activity—though more for recreation than transportation. Part of its allure is its simplicity. You can step into a pair of skinny skis and go just about anyplace that is snow-covered—across a meadow, a woodland trail, even a golf course.

Body-Shaping Benefits

Cross-country skiers get a tremendous all-over workout. Here's what you can expect if you decide to glide, according to Christopher Proctor, M.D., a physician for the U.S. Ski Team and an orthopedic surgeon in Santa Barbara, California.

- You'll tone your entire body as you strengthen the major muscles in your feet, legs, buttocks, abdomen, back, arms, and shoulders.
- You'll improve your chances of permanent weight loss, because cross-country skiing is one of the best ways to burn calories and fat.
- You'll get a fabulous aerobic workout and improve your cardiovascular fitness.

The Right Footwear

In cross-country skiing, choosing the right footwear is just as important as choosing the right skis. A knowledgeable salesperson at a reputable ski shop can get you properly outfitted. Here's what you'll need, says Carole Lowe, ski instructor and co-owner with her husband of Rendezvous Ski Tours in the Grand Teton Mountains near Jackson Hole, Wyoming.

Boots. Expert cross-country skiers usually invest in ultralight boots that resemble tennis shoes,

Cross-Country Skiing Stats

Calories Burned*	Body-Shaping Potential
486 to 1,116 per hour, depending on the speed and terrain	Tones the abdomen, buttocks, hips, thighs, calves, arms, shoulders, and upper and lower back

*Based on a 150-pound woman. If you weigh more, you'll burn more calories; if you weigh less, you'll burn fewer.

Lowe says. But beginners should stick with classic boots, which look more like hiking boots and provide light ankle support.

Bindings. As their name suggests, the bindings hold the toes of your boots against your skis. They leave your heels free to rise with each step in a normal walking motion. Bindings are standardized to fit certain types of boots; have the salesperson verify that your bindings and boots are compatible as well as check that your boots and skis are compatible.

Socks. Socks should be warm but not too thick. You can find wool-silk blends of ski socks at ski shops, but the best ski socks are made of high-tech polyester, such as Thorlo brand wick socks,

according to Lisa Feinberg Densmore, a former member of the Women's Pro Ski Tour, producer and host of numerous ski fitness videos, and instruction editor for *Mountain Sports and Living* magazine in Hanover, New Hampshire. "The poly variety not only wicks moisture but also inhibits odor. They help keep your feet dry and toasty as you ski," she says.

What Else You'll Need

If you're new to cross-country skiing, consider renting the necessary equipment to start. A complete package including skis, poles, boots with bindings, gaiters (described a bit later), and even

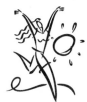

She Did It!

Skiing Helped Kim Avoid Midlife Weight Gain

Five years and 25 pounds ago, Kim Neifert turned to cross-country skiing as a way to keep exercising through the winter. "I started out just wanting to avoid midlife weight gain," recalls the 39-year-old teacher of emotionally disturbed teenagers. But she came to relish her peaceful excursions into the snowy countryside near Lehighton, Pennsylvania.

"I almost always go alone or with my dog, Honey," Kim says. "I have a very stressful job. Skiing gives me a chance to get back to nature and clear my head."

She first got interested in cross-country skiing while watching it on TV during the Olympics. She figured that it didn't look too difficult. And she was right.

"I'm not extremely coordinated, but the technique was easy once I got going," she explains. "It's a very rhythmic motion that seems to come naturally."

Even before she started losing weight, Kim no-

ticed her abdomen, hips, inner thighs, and upper arms—especially her triceps—becoming firmer and better toned. Once she made dietary changes to complement her exercise routine (she also walks year-round and kayaks when weather permits), the pounds began to disappear.

Kim appreciates the fact that cross-country skiing—unlike running—is gentle to her knees, ankles, and feet. She also loves the convenience and cost-effectiveness. Once you have the equipment—Kim got hers for Christmas after one wildly successful trial run on rental skis—"you can go whenever you want for nothing," she says.

Kim prefers to do her skiing in state parks and on open-space trails—mostly on weekends, in the gathering dusk after school, or on nights made silvery white by a full moon. "I even mark my calendar," she says of her moonlit outings. "I can't begin to describe how beautiful those evenings are."

the trail fee costs $20 to $30 a day—about what you'd pay to rent downhill ski equipment. So for a relatively modest fee, you can go on a few trial runs before deciding if cross-country skiing is for you.

Whether you rent or buy, follow these guidelines when selecting equipment and preparing to hit the cross-country trail.

Skis. Cross-country skis are sometimes called skinny skis—presumably for how they look but arguably for what they can do for your figure. They are lighter and thinner than downhill skis, and they range in length from 180 to 200 centimeters. The pair you choose should be roughly 10 centimeters longer than your height. To check

Take It to the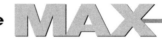

Push Yourself to Ski Harder, Longer

You have mastered the basic leg and arm movements, and you have glided all around town. Now you want to add some variety to your cross-country skiing routine to maximize the fun. These tips will help you do just that.

Do things differently. Incorporate bird watching into your outings. Or invite family members or friends to ski with you. "Cross-country skiing is a lifetime activity with lots of variations," says Carole Lowe, ski instructor and co-owner with her husband of Rendezvous Ski Tours in the Grand Teton Mountains near Jackson Hole, Wyoming.

Add some fancy footwork. Skating is a technique in which you push your skis out to the sides rather than sliding them forward. The foot movements resemble ice skating. This type of cross-country skiing gives you an outstanding aerobic workout. But it is best done on snow where ski tracks haven't been set yet or on ground courses, says Christopher Proctor, M.D., a physician for the U.S. Ski Team and an orthopedic surgeon in Santa Barbara, California.

Center yourself. Cross-country ski centers are popping up throughout snow country. These facilities offer marked trails, lessons, races, and a fireplace-cozy lodge in which to wind down afterward. Most charge a trail fee of about $10 a day. Lessons cost another $6 (for a quick orientation) to $15 (for longer instruction).

Go wild. Wilderness lovers may want to blaze their own trails through the backcountry. The U.S. National Park Service, the U.S. Forest Service, and some state parks provide maps for this purpose. When you request park maps, also look into policies on permits, regulations, and services. To ensure your safety, many national parks require you to register for a backcountry pass, and state parks may require special-use permits. Also inquire at the park office about the possibility of avalanches and dangerous animal sightings. Pack a compass and emergency supplies. And above all else, says Lowe, take along a buddy.

Travel hut to hut. Backcountry hut systems, such as the one maintained by Rendezvous Ski Tours, offer a way to combine cross-country skiing and winter camping. First, you ski on a trail for two to five hours until you reach a hut stocked with food, a stove, and sleeping bags. Then you stay in the hut for several nights, skiing into the surrounding wilderness during the day. The cost of such an adventure is about $150 a day.

Get ready, get set, ski. Skiers with a competitive edge can participate in 5-K, 7.5-K, 10-K, 15-K, 30-K, and even 50-K races, says Steven E. Gaskill, Ph.D., an exercise physiologist at the University of Minnesota in Burnsville, former head coach of the U.S. Nordic Combined and Cross-Country Ski Teams, and author of *Fitness Cross-Country Skiing*.

length, stand one ski at your side, then raise your adjacent arm overhead. You should be able to comfortably cup your hand over the end of the ski, says Lowe.

Also, look for skis that are textured on the underside, says Lowe. The grooves provide traction on the snow, eliminating the need for waxing (which serves the same purpose).

Poles. Cross-country poles are designed to propel the skier forward. This is why they are longer than downhill poles. Beginning cross-country skiers should choose traditional-style poles that reach shoulder-height, Lowe says.

Gaiters. If you are going to ski in snow that is higher than your ankles, Lowe suggests wearing gaiters, waterproof sheaths snapped on over your boots and pants legs. They'll keep the snow from getting in the tops of your boots.

Under- and outerwear. Dressing in layers allows you to adapt to changes in body temperature and weather conditions while you are skiing. Lowe says that she wears four layers for ski outings on cold, snowy days. Her first layer consists of tights and a long-sleeved undershirt, both made from moisture-wicking material (such as Capilene or Thermax). Then she adds a shirt, a wool sweater, and a jacket or fleece pullover on top. On the coldest days, she also wears insulated ski pants rather than basic ski pants. The jacket-and-pants outer layer, she says, should be made of material that is labeled waterproof or moisture resistant and breathable, such as Gore-Tex.

Cross-Country Skiing Workouts

Beginner

25 to 45 minutes on a level or gently rolling trail, using the classic skiing technique

Intermediate

45 to 75 minutes on a prepared trail with rolling hills, using the classic technique or the skating technique

Experienced

65 to 100 minutes on a packed, hilly trail, using the classic technique or the skating technique; alternate 3 to 5 minutes of high-speed skiing (at the fastest pace you can sustain) with 10 to 15 minutes of recovery skiing (in which your heart rate slows to about 65 percent of maximum)

All cross-country skiers—outdoors and indoors, regardless of skill level—need to warm up before working out, says Steven E. Gaskill, Ph.D., an exercise physiologist at the University of Minnesota in Burnsville, former head coach of the U.S. Nordic Combined and Cross-Country Ski Teams, and author of *Fitness Cross-Country Skiing*. Gently stretch your hamstrings by propping each leg, in turn, on a low table or stool and bending forward until you feel tightness, not pain, in the back of the leg. Add a few toe touches and shoulder rolls, and you're ready to go.

During workouts, beginning skiers should be able to talk easily. If you can't, you're pushing yourself too hard. If you're an advanced skier, you may want to train in intervals, periodically picking up the pace or pushing up hills but always recovering to the point where you can speak in full sentences, with equal amounts of time pushing and recovering, says Dr. Gaskill.

Keep in mind that how hard and how long you work ultimately determines the degree of physical benefit that you get from cross-country skiing. "Long and slow movement, for example, can teach your body to burn fats more efficiently, while high-intensity skiing will especially affect your aerobic fitness as well as calorie loss," says Dr. Gaskill. "Most people start out by basically walking on their skis. But even that gives a little more of an upper-body workout than regular walking. Once you learn to glide on the skis and push with the poles, cross-country skiing uses about as much muscle as any activity you could devise."

A hat. A warm hat is a must. Without one, you lose 25 to 40 percent of your body heat through your head. For cross-country skiing, you can wear the same kind of cap you'd wear for other outdoor winter sports—knit, fleece, and so forth.

A backpack. A backpack comes in handy for carrying any clothes that you shed as you warm up. Stock it with plenty of water and high-energy snacks. Snack on fruits, nuts, and sports bars, suggests Dr. Proctor. "Don't worry about the calories. You'll burn them off pretty darn fast," he adds.

Sunscreen and sunglasses. Due in part to snow glare, the sun's rays are no less harmful in winter than in summer. Protect yourself by slathering exposed skin with sunscreen that has a sun protection factor (SPF) of 15 or higher. Also, wear sunglasses or goggles that screen out 100 percent of the sun's ultraviolet rays (the label should say so). Even on sunless days, eyewear safeguards your eyes against wind and snow, says Dr. Proctor.

Getting Started

You may have heard the expression "If you can walk, you can cross-country ski." True, both activities use the same basic one-foot-in-front-of-the-other movement. But cross-country skiing has a bit more to it than that.

"I probably skied for five years before I even knew there was a technique," Lowe says. "When I wanted to stop, I just fell down."

Most expert cross-country skiers recommend taking a few lessons to learn the mechanics of striding efficiently, getting up hills, and, yes, stopping. Cross-country ski centers offer individual and group lessons as well as guides.

That said, the following pointers can help ensure a safe and enjoyable cross-country experience.

Get into the rhythm. Cross-country skiing is about rhythm. Breathe in as you slide one ski forward; breathe out as you slide the other ski forward. With each stride, move the opposite arm forward, just as you do when walking, says Lowe.

Give yourself a head start. Cross-country skiing takes stamina and strength. You can have fun at any level. But the better shape you are in, the longer and more challenging ski journeys you can take, says Dr. Proctor. If you're planning a weekend-long cross-country outing, he recommends that you do a bit of running, bicycling, in-line skating, or hiking three times a week for 12 weeks in advance of your trip. Your body will be better prepared, so you will feel better and have more fun.

Take time to acclimate. If you plan to head into the mountains for your ski outings, you need to adjust to any altitude higher than 5,000 feet or so. If you are a flatlander, take it easy on your first day and be sure to drink three to four quarts of water and avoid alcohol.

Classic altitude illness has been described as feeling like a hangover. It is marked by headache, fatigue, loss of appetite, nausea, and vomiting. If you experience these abnormalities, Dr. Proctor strongly recommends that you stop skiing until your symptoms disappear. Take altitude illness seriously—one extreme form known as high-altitude pulmonary edema (HAPE) is a potentially deadly accumulation of fluid in the lungs. If you have shortness of breath and a cough and you feel weak and tired, seek medical attention immediately.

Know where you're going. Beginners should stay in an area familiar to them or on the marked trails of a cross-country course. Never venture into the wilderness unless you are accompanied by an experienced backcountry skier, says Lowe.

Cross-Country Ski Machines

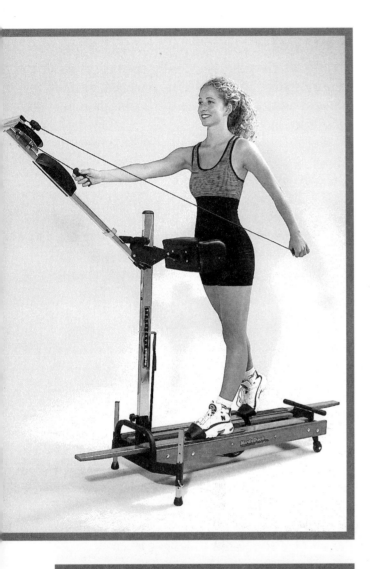

Even if you live in sultry Miami, you can cross-country ski—on a ski simulator machine. These gizmos approximate the sliding-and-gliding motion of traversing snowy trails.

And what a workout!

"I just feel it's the best workout out of any," says Jodi Paul, racquetball program director at the Allentown Racquetball and Fitness Club in Allentown, Pennsylvania. "You use your upper and lower body at the same time, whereas most equipment uses one or the other." Paul has owned a cross-country ski simulator for eight years, swears by it, and teaches members of her club how to use the machine.

Body-Shaping Benefits

Here's what experts say you can expect if you use a cross-country ski machine as part of your body-shaping program.

- You'll get an all-around workout that works both your upper and lower body, raising your heart rate more and burning more calories than if you used exercise equipment that works just one or the other.

- You will work all your main muscles—quadriceps, hamstrings, hips, and glutes—as well as your back, arms, and shoulders.

Psychological Benefits

As with other forms of exercise, women using cross-country ski machines can benefit emotionally, says Martin Hoffman, M.D., professor in the department of physical medicine and rehabilitation at the Medical College of Wisconsin and director of the sports performance and technology laboratory, both in Milwaukee. The rhythmic motion and the solitary nature of the exercise can be peaceful. Cross-country ski simulators take practice, though, so be patient. The

Cross-Country Ski Machine Stats

Calories Burned*	Body-Shaping Potential
Burns 254 to 339 calories per half-hour, depending on intensity	Tones the quadriceps, hamstrings, hips, buttocks, back, arms, shoulders, hips, and thighs

*Based on a 150-pound woman. If you weigh more, you'll burn more calories; if you weigh less, you'll burn fewer.

psychological benefits don't kick in until you master the machine. First, concentrate on proper technique.

The Right Footwear

Unlike outdoor skiing, you needn't concern yourself with boots and bindings. Your feet will be inside toe cups on the machine, so you need only wear a pair of comfortable cross-trainers or running shoes. Paul prefers running shoes, because their pointier toes fit more snugly in the footholds.

What Else You'll Need

If you're buying a cross-country ski machine for your home, you need to have a roomy area in which to use it. On most models, the skis extend beyond the simulator—figure on an overall length of about eight feet and a width of about three feet.

Other machines are shuffle-type skiers that don't extend beyond the machine's body. But some users say they don't really simulate cross-country skiing, says Paul. "Still, they give a good workout and may be worth a look if space is a consideration."

Since fewer and fewer manufacturers are selling cross-country ski machines, most likely, you'll be using a machine at a gym or fitness center. Either way, here's what to look for when choosing one.

Consider the design. Ski machines come in two basic types. One, called a dependent system, links the skis with poles that you move back and

She Did It!

Becky Skimmed Off Pounds on a Ski Machine

Becky Warner bought a cross-country ski machine for her home because she wanted an alternative to her exercise video workouts. Then her marriage unraveled, and she hit the ski simulator with a renewed zeal.

"I'd take out all my frustrations on that poor machine," says Becky, age 46, a homemaker from Bethlehem, Pennsylvania. A year later, Becky, who is five feet five inches tall, had gone from 154 to 127 pounds, dropping three dress sizes—from a 12 to a 6. Her hips are trimmer, plus her arms, back, and calves are shapelier. "I feel like I have more energy," she adds.

The marital crisis is over, but Becky continues using her ski simulator because it just wouldn't feel right if she didn't. "I'd feel guilty if I wasn't doing it," she says. "It's so much a part of my routine that if I don't do it, I miss it."

Like many women, Becky found that using a cross-country ski machine took some getting used to. "I felt kind of clumsy, but I tried to start out slow and just keep after it. Once you get the rhythm down, it's very comfortable."

Eventually, Becky worked up to doing five miles on the machine, regardless of how long it took. Today she does six miles three or four times a week. It takes her anywhere from 65 to 80 minutes. She sets both the arm and leg movements at a moderate tension or resistance.

In addition to the body-shaping benefits, Becky says she also feels better mentally after a session on her ski machine. "I know I've done something good for my body," she says. "I feel like I've accomplished something. And it's cheaper than a shopping spree at the mall."

Take It to the 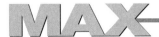 MAX

A Hard Machine Made Easier

A cross-country ski simulator gives a great full-body workout, but it's a tough piece of exercise equipment to master. To make working out easier while maximizing the benefits, follow these suggestions from experts.

Create tension. When you begin on the machine, make sure that there is some leg tension, even if it's only on the lowest setting. Otherwise, your feet may slide back too easily.

Set the rhythm. The hardest thing to learn on this machine is how to develop a rhythm in which your arms and legs are moving in conjunction, not at odds with each other. Try perfecting just your leg movements at first, resting your hands on the handlebars or bumper pad in front of you until you do.

Then gradually begin coordinating arm motion with that of your legs.

Position your legs. As you begin the lower-body movement, keep one foot forward and one back as though you're walking, rather than side-by-side.

Bend your knees, please. You should have "soft" knees—slightly bent—when you're using this machine.

Go all the way. Practice a full range of motion with your arms and legs when skiing in your home or gym.

Perfect your posture. Don't lean forward on the ski simulator. You should stand upright when using it. If you rest your stomach on the bumper pad in front of you, you may be propelled off the back of the simulator.

---

forth or up and down with your hands. One foot moves forward, and the other automatically moves back. These machines are easy and safe to use, but they aren't as challenging as independent systems and may become boring.

An independent system works each foot separately and uses a cable, rather than poles, that you pull with your hands. This type of machine takes longer to learn, but the independent foot action is smoother and more enjoyable to use. Also, an independent machine forces you to use your upper body, so it gives you a more balanced workout.

Check the machine's features. Your ski simulator should be sturdy and have separate resistance settings for the legs and arms, so that you can increase the tension on either one or both as you become more proficient in the use of the machine. It also should have a mechanism to adjust for arm length. This will enable you to use the machine comfortably regardless of your height. Some machines have electronic monitors that tell you how fast you're moving,

how many calories you're burning, how long you've been on the machine, and how far you've traveled.

Get more, pay more. If you find a store that sells cross-country ski simulators, be aware that they go for about $450 or more. Don't buy the bargain-basement machines. "Those aren't even worth considering," says Dr. Hoffman.

Getting Started

Ski simulators are hard to get the hang of, but enthusiasts say they are worth the effort. Establishing a rhythm while moving your arms and legs is difficult.

"There's a big learning curve," says Laurie L. Tis, Ph.D., associate professor in the department of kinesiology and health at Georgia State University in Atlanta. "It takes practice."

Master the leg action first. To speed up the learning process, work on the leg motion alone, then practice the arm action by itself, before trying the two movements together.

Warm up your legs. Warm up for 5 to 10 minutes before a workout on a ski simulator recommends, Dr. Tis. Start out at a leisurely walking pace for a few minutes, then gradually increase the speed or resistance for a few minutes and let this serve as your warmup. This will help you avoid strain and injury.

Give it time. Don't be discouraged if the machine initially feels as strange as dancing on a water bed. "For most people, their first time on is not the time to judge whether they are going to like it or not," says Dr. Hoffman. If you're considering buying a machine, he recommends trying one out at your local Y or fitness center several times before making a purchase.

Cross-Country Ski Machine Workouts

Beginner

For the first 1 to 3 months, do only the lower-body movement of the machine. Aim for 30 strides per minute for 15 to 20 minutes, 3 times a week.

Intermediate

Add movement of your arms as well as your legs. Increase your pace by about 10 percent to 33 to 35 strides per minute. For the first month at this new rate, stick to the 15 to 20 minutes, 3 times a week, then gradually increase your time.

Experienced

Increase the resistance a couple of notches for your arm and leg movements. Aim for 40 strides a minute for 30 minutes, 5 times a week.

On some cross-country ski machines, you can elevate the front of the machine to simulate a hill. You might assume this would give you a more taxing workout, but it doesn't, says Martin Hoffman, M.D., professor in the department of physical medicine and rehabilitation at the Medical College of Wisconsin and director of the sports performance and technology laboratory, both in Milwaukee. While the incline does create more tension on the forward movement of your leg, simple laws of gravity make it too easy when your leg comes back down.

Instead of toying with the machine's incline, manipulate the appropriate dials to increase resistance or tension on your arms, your legs, or both.

Another option: Speed up the rate of movement from, say, 40 to 60 cycles per minute. Some of the better models have a speed-monitoring system that enables you to gauge this.

Dancing

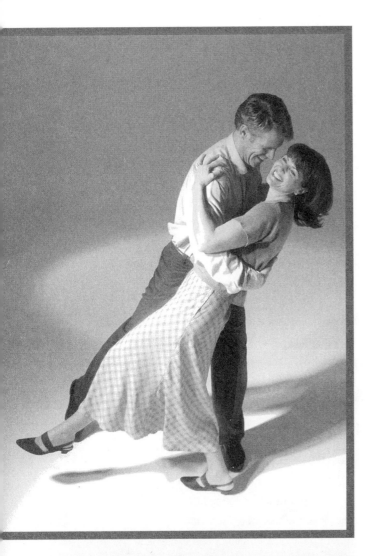

Shall we dance?

The answer is a resounding yes.

Comprised of movement, energy, rhythm, and design, dance has ancient roots as a form of celebration, entertainment, and courtship. Although it can be vigorous exercise, only recently has it begun to be appreciated for its fitness benefits.

"People see it as just having fun, but social dance can be just as good a workout as playing basketball or running," says Phil Martin, a dance instructor and lecturer in the department of kinesiology and physical education at California State University in Long Beach.

Martin completed a study with Betty Rose Griffith, Ph.D., to observe the aerobic-conditioning effects of dancing. They found that dancers' heart rates were within their "exercise benefit zone" (60 to 85 percent of estimated maximum heart rate) after doing the samba, the polka, swing dances, or the Viennese waltz.

Many folk dances are also highly aerobic. "You can reach 85 percent or higher of your maximum heart rate," Martin notes.

Body-Shaping Benefits

If you dance regularly, you can expect to see these results.

- Your entire lower body will be toned, especially your calves, thighs, buttocks, abdomen, and hips.

- You will strengthen the major muscles of your lower body, including your hamstrings, quadriceps, and gluteals. Some dance moves, such as pulling your partner forward in swing dancing, work the triceps, biceps, deltoids, and pectoral muscles.

- You'll lose weight and improve your cardiovascular fitness. Country line, folk, jazz, swing, samba, salsa, polka, and tap dancing may provide an aerobic workout. Other forms of dance, such

Dancing Stats

Calories Burned*	Body-Shaping Potential
Per half-hour: ballroom, 105; aerobic, 201–276; modern, 147; country line, 150	Tones the muscles of the calves, thighs, abdomen, buttocks, shoulders, arms, and upper back

*Based on a 150-pound woman. If you weigh more, you'll burn more calories; if you weigh less, you'll burn fewer.

as modern dancing or ballet, may be aerobic or not, depending on the moves and tempo.

Psychological Benefits

According to a study at Reed College in Portland, Oregon, dancers are happier and more secure, confident, creative, coordinated, exhilarated, intelligent, and energetic than their nondancing counterparts. Perhaps this is because dancing requires concentration, creativity, and in most cases, social interaction, which provide health benefits that go beyond the physical ones, says Martin, who met his wife on the dance floor.

"Dancing can bring on euphoria," Martin says, recalling people reluctantly dragged along to

She Did It!

Lisa Dances the Night—And the Pounds—Away

Lisa Deslauriers wasn't looking for a way to lose weight or get in shape. Recently divorced and feeling introverted, she wasn't even particularly interested in dating.

All that and a lot more began to change one afternoon when a co-worker confided that he'd lost his dance partner, who had recently gotten engaged. "Do you want to try it?" he asked.

It took a few months of classes for Lisa to learn the Lindy Hop, a variation of swing dancing. Then, to the rhythm of the big band sounds of the 1930s and 1940s, Lisa found a new life.

"I basically started going out every single night. There were a lot of supportive people in the community willing to dance with a beginner, and it was fun. All of a sudden, I said, 'Wait a minute, I'm good at this!'" she recalls.

Over the next few years, the 33-year-old technical support whiz for a Boston-area computer company found herself buying a new wardrobe for swing dancing. While she was purchasing new clothes for swing dancing, she realized that she also had to buy new clothes for work because she'd dropped a size or two from dancing.

"I had always worn clothes that were probably too big for me. But my body image changed, and I started wearing things that fit me more appropriately," she says.

Lisa was stunned to realize she had lost 20 pounds despite an occasional ice cream cone after a night of spinning on the dance floor. But the weight-loss goals she realized were always secondary to the pure entertainment of swing.

"It became important to me to be able to dance the whole night and still be able to breathe easily enough to talk," she said. That was to happen soon enough.

The most remarkable change of all, Lisa says, is the change she saw in herself. "I used to be very shy. I was the type of person who would much rather do things by myself," she explains.

Caught up in the burgeoning swing dance movement, she suddenly found herself developing a reputation as someone who "got things done." She could stand up in front of a crowd and announce club activities or the next dance. And she came to look forward to meeting a new partner and engaging in conversation for the three minutes it took to complete a dance.

Swing dance, by keeping people at a socially acceptable distance as they get to know each other, helped her to grow more confident.

"I'm a totally different person," she says.

classes by partners or friends who wound up becoming enthusiasts of samba or swing.

Dance enhances mood, relieves stress, and lends variety to life. It can be a way for newcomers to town or singles to meet new people, and a way for married couples to get off their couches and reinvigorate their relationships.

Besides, Martin adds, "It's really fun. Many people take one dance class and make a lifetime hobby of it."

The Right Footwear

Okay, so it's time to put on your dancing shoes, which range from cross-trainer tennis shoes to ballet slippers to tap shoes, depending on the type of dance you do. When purchasing dance shoes (excluding tennis shoes), go to a specialty store where you can be fitted by an expert. Modern dance is often done barefoot. Here are some things to look for when you choose.

Tennis shoes. For social dancing, you'll need a pair of shoes that turn easily on the floor without being too slippery, says Martin. Generally, a tennis shoe with some padding is a good idea if you plan to dance all evening, since your feet may burn the next day from the constant impact. If you find that the studio or stage where you dance is sticky, you may need a leather or suede-soled shoe. Ballroom dance shoes are available, but they range from $70 to $150—a purchase you may want to put on hold until you've danced enough to know if it's right for you. Ballroom shoes are ideal for dancing, because they have suede soles that allow you to glide and turn but aren't too slippery. The rest of the shoe is usually made out of leather, which is lightweight and flexible. Keep the shoes clean with a shoe polish brush. Wax buildup on the soles of ballroom shoes can cause them to harden and lose friction.

Cowboy boots. For country line dancing, Martin says you can wear tennis shoes like the ones mentioned above or cowboy boots. "Look for cowboy boots with low heels, so you can dance more easily and comfortably," he suggests. Also, buying boots with leather material will keep your feet cool.

Socks. Socks should keep your shoes on without your feet slipping, but definitely shouldn't make your shoes too snug, since your feet may swell a bit over the course of a night out on the dance floor. "Sometimes, a really thick sock can throw you off balance because it's too mushy," Martin warns. Socks that have cotton blend material help reduce slipping because they reduce sweat.

Ballet shoes. These run about $20 to $30 and should be somewhat snugger than street shoes since they are leather and will stretch, says Lori Binkly, owner of Karabel Dancewear in Burbank, California. Your toe should touch the end when you're standing flat, but it should not be scrunched to fit in the shoe. If the shoes are too roomy, the leather will crinkle when you stand on your toes, she notes. Make sure the store has shoes that accommodate the width, not just the length, of your foot.

Tap shoes. Jazz tap shoes are available in an oxford and Mary Jane style, among others. Mary Janes are low-heeled strap shoes. Both the oxford and Mary Jane styles are best for beginners, since it is harder to learn in a high-heeled shoe, Binkly says. For about $60 to $70, you can get such a shoe with the taps and rubber already in place, rather than having to take them to a shoemaker for customizing.

What Else You'll Need

Modern and ballet dancers generally wear comfortable leotards, tights, and perhaps leg warmers. Square dancers and folk dancers may wear costumes, while country line dancers wear jeans and Western shirts. Aerobic and jazzercise dancers wear fitness clothing, from exercise bras to leggings or shorts.

Social dancing is generally done in casual street clothing, not exercise wear. Women shouldn't wear slippery fabric that may slide out of their partners' grasp or belts that could catch on an outstretched hand, cautions Martin.

Since dance is so varied, it's a good idea to call before the first class to be sure your footwear is permitted on the dance floor and your apparel is appropriate for the crowd.

Getting Started

To find beginning dance classes in your neighborhood, check your local newspaper, telephone book, or city parks and recreation activities bulletin.

Start simple. Some dances are easy to learn. You may want to begin with a class that features cha cha, salsa or mambo, and rumba. "If you're a real couch potato, start with the fox-trot," advises Martin.

Take it slow. Until you learn the steps, you may not feel like you're getting a workout. Don't worry—your concentration now will pay off in major fitness benefits within a few weeks.

Spice your workout with variety. "A variety of dances and intensities can be an excellent sub-stitute for walking or running," says Steven F. Loy, Ph.D., professor of kinesiology and director of the exercise physiology laboratory at California State University at Northridge. Remember: One dance will not tone every muscle, increase your strength and flexibility, and provide a fat-burning aerobic workout.

Play, stop, rewind. If you love the notion of dancing but can't overcome your shyness at learning with others, brush up on the important steps at home by watching dance videos. Martin's Sodanceabit tapes include West Coast and East Coast swing, waltz, polka, cha cha, two-step, country line, and social and folk dance aerobics. For a free catalog, write to Sodanceabit, 15550 Carfax Avenue, Bellflower, CA 90706. Dance Lovers USA video collection also provides a wide variety of dances. You can receive a brochure by writing to Dance Lovers USA, P. O. Box 7071, Asheville, NC 28802.

Dancing Workouts

Beginner

Try a class that offers a slow waltz, fox-trot, or rumba. Dance at a level that allows easy conversation.

Intermediate

Dance the Viennese waltz, samba, or salsa.

Experienced

Do the polka or the East Coast swing, also called the jitterbug. You can also country line dance.

"Because you can easily reach your maximum heart rate when you dance, it's a good idea to consult your physician before you start out," says Steven F. Loy, Ph.D., professor of kinesiology and director of the exercise physiology laboratory at California State University at Northridge. "Also, if you're just starting out, begin with a beginner dance. When you feel you can do this with ease, you can try an intermediate-level dance and so on." Dr. Loy also says that he doesn't recommend doing any one dance for more than half an hour.

Variety not only adds to the fun of social dancing but also enables you to work different muscles and change your aerobic pace. No one form of dance will tone every muscle, increase your strength and flexibility, or by itself get rid of a lot of weight, says Dr. Loy. To shape up and lose weight, you should combine different forms of dance and change what you eat.

"Keep in mind that the speed of the music and your own energy level make a lot of difference," Dr. Loy says. "You can be doing swing and not putting much effort into it, while the person next to you might be bouncing off the ceiling."

Elliptical Training

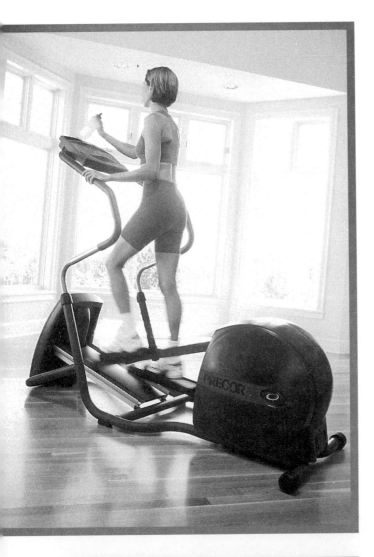

An elliptical trainer is about as close as anything comes to a perfect exercise machine. It looks like a combination treadmill, cross-country ski machine, and a stepping machine, and it combines the movements (and benefits) of hiking, cross-country skiing, and biking. Working out on the trainer feels like standing on a cross-country ski machine, but instead of your feet moving back and forth, the machine forces them to move around in an oval (or elliptical) pattern.

Using the elliptical trainer doesn't create any impact, so it's easy on your joints. And it's versatile: You can use it to climb or glide. For your effort, you'll get a calorie-burning workout that pumps your heart like an all-out run without the same stress and strain on the joints in your body—the ideal workout routine for overweight women who don't have the wherewithal to jog. Even though most women burn hundreds of calories on the elliptical machine, they feel as if they're just strolling along. As a result, you can get rid of unwanted accumulations of fat on your belly, butt, or thighs without having to push yourself as hard as you do on other machines.

"We compared 16 men and women who each used an elliptical trainer, a treadmill, an exercise bike, and a stair stepper," says John Porcari, Ph.D., professor of exercise and sports science at the University of Wisconsin-La Crosse. "Even if you use the elliptical trainer at the same intensity as running on the treadmill, the impact is the same as walking, so it puts less stress on your feet and legs. You get the same workout as running with only half the potential for injuries. It's an outstanding piece of equipment."

Elliptical Training Stats

Calories Burned*	Body-Shaping Potential
500–600 per hour	Tones muscles of the entire lower body and burns fat

*Based on a 150-pound woman. If you weigh more, you'll burn more calories; if you weigh less, you'll burn fewer.

Body-Shaping Benefits

Here's what you can expect when you use an elliptical trainer regularly.

- When you move forward on the machine, you'll work your quadriceps (the big muscles on the

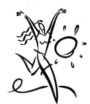

She Did It!

Lisa Is 45 Pounds Thinner—With a New Rear View

At the age of 35, Lisa Andruscavage found herself weighing 221 pounds and wearing a size 24. "At five feet four inches, my weight was really starting to affect my health," says Lisa, a mother of two from Allentown, Pennsylvania. "In fact, I took three weeks off from work because I felt like my heart was actually tired, as if my body were going to shut down."

At that point, Lisa figured she'd never lose weight, so she went out and bought all new clothes in larger sizes. But she also prayed that the answer would come.

And it did. When she returned to work, Lisa found out that her employer had begun offering a Weight Watchers program on-site. "I felt that it was a sign from God," Lisa says. "I decided to give it one more chance."

Lisa joined Weight Watchers, and because they advise their clients to exercise through their time on the program, she decided to start going to her company's gym again.

She hadn't tried exercise for years. "I'd had a number of miscarriages, and I'd stopped exercising when I was pregnant with my second child because I didn't want to overdo it," she says.

Lisa's first stop back at the gym was the stationary bicycles, but she didn't like them. "Boring," she thought.

Right next to the bicycles, however, was a piece of equipment Lisa had never seen before—an elliptical trainer. "I asked someone to show me how to use it," Lisa says. "I was able to do only five minutes, at level one with zero resistance. I thought, 'I'll never be able to do this.'"

Fortunately, Lisa stuck with it. "For me, the elliptical trainer is more interesting to use than the bike," Lisa says. "It didn't hurt my butt or my knees. Also, I have carpal tunnel syndrome, and the elliptical machine is easier on my hands than the other machines."

Within four months, Lisa was able to train for 30 to 35 minutes at a time, four times a week. "I keep the resistance low, but I move really quickly on a high ramp level," Lisa says. "That really works for me." The machine indicates that Lisa burns more than 300 calories per workout.

The results? In one year, Lisa has lost 45 pounds, and her percentage of body fat has gone down 14 percent. She's also down to a dress size of 16. "I've lost most of the extra weight in my legs and butt," she says. "In fact, many people notice my weight loss from behind. They'll come up and say, 'I was behind you and I didn't recognize you.'"

The way she looks isn't the only thing that keeps Lisa motivated. "I like the way I feel," says Lisa. "Sometimes people get on the machine next to me and they have to stop after 10 minutes. It makes me feel so fit—especially if they are really thin. I understand now that you do not have to be really skinny to be fit and healthy."

Lisa loves the elliptical trainer so much that she and her husband have decided to invest in one for their home. "I can't walk on a treadmill or for long distances because I get lower-back pain, so the elliptical trainer is a perfect purchase for us," Lisa says. "I'm going to put it center stage in my living room."

front of your thighs) and gluteus muscles (that shape your backside).

- You'll tone and slim your entire lower body.
- You'll notice that your legs are shapelier than ever, since elliptical training uses all the muscles of the legs, large and small.
- You'll burn approximately 10 calories per minute while you work, and as a bonus, you'll continue to burn calories at a higher rate for a few hours afterward.

Psychological Benefits

If you have tried treadmill running and found it boring, or if you're ready for a change, an elliptical trainer offers varied programs to keep you moving for a long time to come. Most converts find they love elliptical trainers simply because they're so easy to use, says Dr. Porcari.

The Right Footwear

Because your feet don't leave the elliptical trainer's surface, any lightweight athletic shoe will suffice, says Gregory Florez, owner of Fitness First, a personal training company in Chicago and Salt Lake City. Just be sure not to tie the laces too tightly, or your feet will start to feel numb.

To keep your feet dry and blister-free, pair those shoes up with athletic-wear socks of synthetic or cotton/synthetic fiber blends that "breathe," advises Florez.

What Else You'll Need

An elliptical trainer has various settings: resistance, speed, and, usually, ramp. You can program just one setting at a time, or all three together.

As with a stationary cycle, resistance on an elliptical trainer determines how much effort it will take for you to keep your feet moving. Ramp levels describe how high or low you've set the angle of the ellipse. For instance, a high ramp mimics hiking, while a low ramp mimics cross-country skiing. As you move, you determine the speed at

which you move on the trainer. The resistance will, of course, affect the speed at which you *can* move, but how you respond to the resistance is under your control. You could, for example, choose a low resistance and move quickly, or you could put the resistance up high and not be able to move smoothly. Ideally, says Florez, you want to be able to move at a comfortable, moderate speed, interspersed with occasional bursts of high intensity as well as high speeds.

Quality elliptical trainers are expensive and may cost up to six times as much as a treadmill or stationary bike, putting them out of range for many home exercisers. So most likely, you'll use a trainer at a gym or fitness center, at least at first. If you fall in love with elliptical training and want to buy a machine for your home, here are some buying tips from experts.

Go for range. Look for a variety of ramp settings and intensity levels in an elliptical machine. If the ellipse itself isn't expansive and doesn't offer ramp and intensity changes, then the workout isn't nearly as effective.

The Precor EFX models, for example, use an oval-shaped collection of gears, pedals, and flywheels that allows the legs to move in their full range of motion, giving you a good workout. At retail, they sell for approximately $2,000 to $2,700. If you try less expensive machines, with less of an elliptical shape, you may find that you don't get the same range of motion, says Florez.

If you can afford it, consider a model with a control panel that offers various preprogrammed courses and records how many calories you've burned.

Skip the handles. Some machines come with handles that allow you to move your arms back and forth—with resistance—while you're on the elliptical machine. "That doesn't increase calorie burning very much," says Florez. "To burn more calories, it's much more effective to buy a machine without handles and work your legs at a higher intensity without leaning on your arms."

Try various settings. As with a treadmill or stationary bike, you'll want to get a sense of how the machine feels at different settings. Try different combinations of ramp and speed settings. Also, vary the resistance, which enables you to work at different levels of intensity. The higher the resistance, the more power you'll need to exert to get your feet moving.

Measure twice, buy once. Elliptical trainers are long—up to five feet long and over four feet tall at their highest point. Measure the machine you're going to buy and the space in which you plan to use it.

Don comfortable clothes. Elliptical trainers don't require a special outfit. As with most workouts, your best bet is a layer or two of loose-fitting, comfortable clothing made of fabrics that wick sweat away. That way, you can peel off a layer as you work up a sweat. After a few workouts, you'll find what works best for you, says Florez.

Getting Started

When you first step onto an elliptical trainer, you'll probably start going backward. "This just tends to be the natural movement," says Florez. That's fine for a minute or two, but studies (and personal trainers) have found that going backward doesn't work the legs as effectively as forward motion. You will burn slightly more calories by going in reverse, says J. Zack Barksdale, an exercise physiologist at the Cooper Aerobics Center in Dallas, but not enough to make up for the potential strain you're putting on your knees.

Instead, simply place your feet on the foot pads and push forward slightly. The trainer will begin to move your legs in the elliptical shape; all you have to do is follow along. The higher the level of resistance, the harder you'll have to push.

Go slowly. While you may be tempted to power your way through the virtual hills and val-

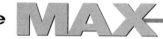

Take It to the MAX

A Workout with Options Galore

One sure way to increase your aerobic output on an elliptical trainer is to pump your arms as you work out. But to give your lower body a total workout, mix and match the settings to mimic a number of sports. Each leg motion works different muscles in different ways, says J. Zack Barksdale, an exercise physiologist at the Cooper Aerobics Center in Dallas.

Cross-country skiing motion. To simulate cross-country skiing, set the ramp level on low. This exercise emphasizes the butt and hamstring muscles. Unless you're practicing for a skiing race, try to keep the pace and resistance level at a moderate level, so that you can move smoothly.

Hiking motion. If you want to stay in shape for weekend hiking excursions, or if you just want to reap the benefits that hiking brings to your quadri-

ceps and butt, keep the elliptical trainer's ramp setting on high and increase the intensity on the machine, which will simulate climbing.

Jogging motion. Love running, but it hurts your knees? Head over to the elliptical machine. If you keep the ramp setting at middle height, you'll be moving in a motion that is close to running. Although the movement will be similar, you won't have the strain of impact to contend with.

Put it all together. With so many options, the elliptical trainer serves as a cross-trainer. You can mix and match the different ramp and intensity levels to create all types of workouts. For instance, you could move from sport to sport within one workout, or you could simply do a different "sport" each time you get on the equipment. Either way, your lower body reaps an amazing array of workout benefits.

leys over which the elliptical machine can take you, stay in the midrange of the ellipse at first, advises Barksdale, who has put numerous people on elliptical training programs. "The wide range of motion the ellipse machine can take you through is great, but you need to work up to it."

Furthermore, people with lower-back problems may find this kind of exercise jarring, so consult your physician before working out on an elliptical trainer, Barksdale notes.

Keep your hands free. Getting your balance on an elliptical machine can be a little tricky at first. But bear in mind that you'll burn far more calories if you let go of the handles than if you hang on, says Barksdale. Allow your arms to swing freely, or try a little of a pumping action, he advises.

Keep your head straight. It may be easy to get distracted and look around or talk to someone while you're on the trainer, but twisting your torso is a no-no. To keep your knees in line with your feet and avoid injury, always point your head straight ahead, warns Barksdale.

Elliptical Training Workouts

Beginner

2 or 3 times a week for 10 to 20 minutes at a time in a slow rhythm

Intermediate

2 or 3 times a week for at least 20 minutes, using a pre-programmed workout that doesn't include intervals

Experienced

2 or 3 times a week, for 20 to 60 minutes of interval training, either pre-programmed or self-directed

"At first, start off with 10 minutes of elliptical training at a low intensity," says J. Zack Barksdale, an exercise physiologist at the Cooper Aerobics Center in Dallas. "Do this twice a week for one week, then begin to change the workouts. To do this, increase something every week, but don't increase two things at once. For example, in the second week, you could increase the number of times you exercise from two times to three times. Then, in the third week, you might increase your intensity. In the fourth week, you could increase from 10 to 20 minutes. Keep making changes in your workout every week in order to see the most results. And make sure you include other kinds of aerobic activity in your weekly exercise routine, in addition to the elliptical trainer."

Gardening

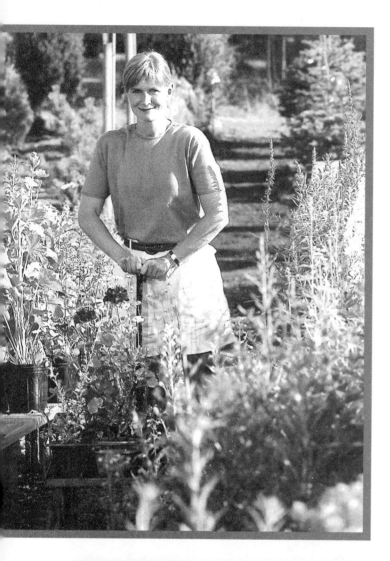

Mary, Mary, quite contrary, how does your garden grow? With silver bells and cockleshells and lots of terrific, body-shaping exercise.

"Gardening involves stretching, repetition, and even resistance principles similar to those of weight training, while also expending calories," says Barbara Ainsworth, Ph.D., associate professor of exercise science and director of the Prevention Research Center at the University of South Carolina in Columbia.

"It's a challenging workout without being as stressful as jogging or a similar exercise would be to the body," notes Richard Cotton, chief exercise physiologist for the American Council on Exercise in San Diego.

Besides making it easier to lose weight and keep it off, helping your garden grow can reduce your risk of heart disease, diabetes, colon cancer, and high blood pressure as well as build stronger and healthier bones, muscles, and joints.

Body-Shaping Benefits

Gardening provides excellent whole-body exercise, says Cotton. Here's how.

- Walking and other large-muscle movements provide an aerobic workout. Gardening activities like raking, sweeping, hoeing, and shoveling are the most aerobic because they are sustained activities.

- You'll exercise your back, chest, abdomen, buttocks, legs, arms, and shoulders with the pushing and pulling movements of digging and tilling. Your arms and shoulders will get exercise as you plant, weed, and do sit-down digging. Finally, you'll exercise your legs and buttocks with the repetitive up-and-down of moving along a flower or vegetable bed.

- Gardening offers the kind of sustained, moderate, fat-burning workout that, when performed three to five times a week, can help you lose weight and keep it off.

Gardening Stats

Calories Burned*	Body-Shaping Potential
Planting seedlings: 48 per 10 minutes Hoeing: 62 per 10 minutes Digging: 86 per 10 minutes	This head-to-toe workout tones arms, shoulders, chest, back, buttocks, abdomen, and legs.

*Based on a 150-pound woman. If you weigh more, you'll burn more calories; if you weigh less, you'll burn fewer.

The Right Footwear

Because of the many positions your feet will be in as you garden, you'll want to find shoes that have flexible toes and rear-foot support. Also keep in mind that you'll want shoes that will protect you from bug bites. You might want to check out a pair of gardening clogs, which can be very comfortable for certain foot types.

What Else You'll Need

The gardening tools and supplies you need will depend on the size and character of your garden.

Tools. One day you may very well need an industrial-strength soil tiller to dig up the acre behind your house, but for starters, stick to a few hand tools such as a shovel, cultivator, and hoe, says Cotton. As your ambitions and competence

She Did It!

Gardening Keeps Kate Slim and Young

Kate Flynn lost 25 pounds, wears a size 6 or 8, and looks more like 39 than 49—thanks to gardening, her favorite form of "exercise."

"During my childhood and young adult years, I'd always been self-conscious about my weight," says Kate, who is a clinical therapist and single mom in Pittsburgh. "All my female relatives were chubby, and I saw myself gaining weight and starting to look just like them."

Kate tried running, aerobics, and even walking, but without much success. "I found I couldn't run every day," she says. "And it was hard on my knees—I felt like I was killing my body. I enjoyed aerobics classes, but raising two young sons on my own made it hard to get to class. And raising two growing boys, I couldn't afford it.

"As for walking, I have a wheaten terrier that needs to be walked, but the dog stops to sniff so often that it really isn't much of a workout," says Kate.

When Kate bought a little ranch home for herself and her boys, she plunged into gardening in a big way—with big results.

"I was determined to make the most of the space—I ripped out parts of the lawn and planted beds of medicinal herbs, shrubs, and ornamental grasses, plus a few vegetables. There are three of us, but you know how kids feel about vegetables and gardening," she adds.

Because she hates the heat and humidity, Kate gets up early to garden in the mornings. "I start out with easy stuff, like pulling weeds, then do some planting, and quit before it gets hot," she says. "Some nights I do more work after sundown, working under floodlights. So I end up getting some exercise every single day during the growing season."

Make no mistake about it, says Kate: Gardening is a real workout. "I'm moving constantly—pulling weeds, carrying buckets of mulch and clippings, raking the soil flat."

For Kate, exercise, not dieting, is the key to staying in shape. "I have the metabolism of a snail, so being active is the only answer for me. Plus, when you get some exercise, you feel you 'earn' what you eat and don't feel guilty about every single bite of food."

Kate says working out has really helped keep her firm. "My legs were always heavy, but now they're much slimmer."

Plus, she looks much younger than other women her age. "When I go out, people who meet me for the first time always think I'm 37, 38, or 39. They never think I'm the age I am."

grow, work up to long-handled, stand-up tools, which give you more of a full-body workout.

Other stuff. Find yourself a cushiony mat you can kneel or sit on while weeding, gardening gloves to protect against abrasions and keep dirt at bay, and clothing that breathes when you sweat in the heat and that keeps you cozy in cooler weather. Don't forget to wear at least some sunscreen and a hat to ward off damaging ultraviolet rays. Kathi Colen, urban agriculture coordinator for SLUG, the San Francisco League of Urban Gardeners, goes even further. She never gardens without sunglasses, a wide-brimmed hat, long sleeves, and long pants, for all-over protection from both sun exposure and wayward twigs and branches.

Getting Started

You dream of sweeping hillsides, abundant with fruits and flowers. Great, but start small, advises Maria Gabaldo, horticultural therapist at the Chicago Botanic Gardens in Glencoe, Illinois, and former president of the American Horticulture Therapy Association of Denver. Cultivating your green thumb in a "container garden" on your porch will do just fine, she says.

If you have a large plot of land to work with, before you even start, warm up by taking a brisk walk around your property. Breathe in the fresh air and take in the wonders of nature all around you. Then you'll be ready to get down to work, says Suzanne DeJohn, horticulture staff coordinator at the National Gardening Association in Burlington, Vermont.

Either way, here's how to get started.

Set reasonable goals. Don't expect to dig and plant your garden all at once, says DeJohn. "Do one thing at a time, a little at a time."

Choose the right time. During hot weather, avoid working in stressful midday heat by gardening before 10:00 A.M. and after 2:00 P.M. Also, try working when you're usually most energetic. If you're a morning person, hit the dirt when the sun comes up. If you don't get revved up until later in the day, save gardening for the late afternoon or evening.

Warm up. A 5- to 10-minute warmup helps prepare you for the effort of gardening and makes you less prone to injuries, says Cotton. He suggests a warmup specific to the task. For details on how to stretch, see Stretch into Shape on page 180.

Drink plenty of water. To avoid dehydration, which can lead to fatigue and muscle cramps, have

Gardening Workouts

Beginner

Weeding or planting seeds or seedlings for 10 minutes at a time

Intermediate

Tilling with a long-handled tiller, or hoeing or other chores for 30 minutes at a time

Experienced

Digging or spreading fertilizer or mulch or other chores for 45 minutes at a time, 5 days a week

If you're new to gardening, it's best to start with 10-minute sessions and low-level activities, such as weeding or tilling with a hand tiller. These work only a few muscles compared to full-body movements such as digging a garden plot from scratch, explains Richard Cotton, chief exercise physiologist for the American Council on Exercise in San Diego. "That's not always possible, however, if you have to dig your gardening bed from scratch, which is a very high intensity activity. At the very least, alternate easier and harder activities." For example, dig for a few minutes, then spend a few minutes gently raking dead vegetation.

As you grow stronger, work into longer or more intense gardening sessions. To lose weight, garden for 35 to 45 minutes at least five times a week, Cotton recommends.

a glass of water before you begin gardening, and sip frequently from a jug or water bottle while you're out there, advises Dr. Ainsworth.

Aim for variety. Engaging in a variety of movements every time you garden trains a variety of muscles, making you stronger and more toned overall, says Cotton. It also reduces the risk of overstressing specific muscles and joints. For example, dig for 10 minutes, then switch to planting or weeding, then to watering, and then to tossing weeds and twigs into a basket.

Bend and lift smartly. Gardening can put a real strain on your lower back, says Dr. Ainsworth. Instead of bending at the waist to weed or plant, squatting down on one knee, with the other knee bent, is a safer, healthier posture. When lifting, use your legs instead of your back.

Hold tools up close. Even the lightest tools can strain your muscles when they're used for the repetitive motions of gardening. To reduce the strain, hold tools closer to your body, suggests Dr. Ainsworth. Rather than stretching for weeds and placing your back in an unsupported position, dig up the ones that are nearby with a hand shovel held close to your side. Then either switch sides after you've pulled all the weeds that are close to you or do one side of a row and then come back down the other side. To include more stretching while gardening, reach with your whole torso, making sure your back is supported under your feet and legs, she adds.

Hiking

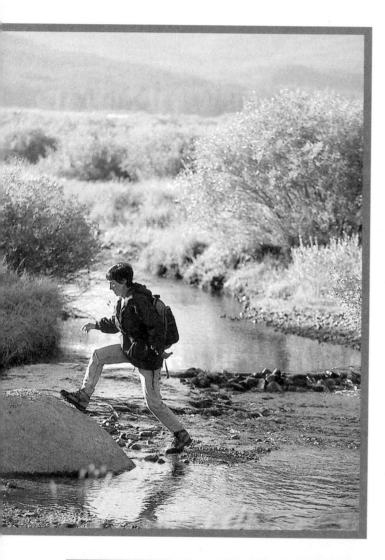

Breathe deeply. Smell the clean air, the flowers, the pine trees. Look around. See the blue sky, the green leaves, the white daisies, the yellow buttercups. Listen. It's quiet. Even the birds and crickets sound peaceful and serene. Stop. Take a drink from your water bottle and feel how cool the water is against your throat. Walk and feel the crunch of leaves underneath your feet, the craggy bark of the maples and oaks against your fingers, the crisp air drifting over your face. Oh, look! A doe and her fawn.

"Hiking is like walking with one major difference: It takes you to new and exciting terrain," says Dan Heil, Ph.D., assistant professor of exercise physiology at Montana State University in Bozeman. So if you have been walking or running and hanker for variety, take to the trails.

Body-Shaping Benefits

Physiologically, hiking is walking turned up a notch or two. Here's how you can benefit.

- You'll burn more calories by hiking than by walking, since climbing hills or walking on uneven terrain takes more energy.

- When you carry a pack of some kind (which most people do), the extra pounds further pump up your calorie burning.

- You'll give your quadriceps, hamstrings, gluteus maximus, and gluteus minimus (the major muscles in your hips, thighs, and buttocks) a good workout, since hill walking forces your leg and thigh muscles to work even harder and more intensely than walking on flat terrain.

- If you use hiking poles, you'll tone your arm and back muscles, too.

The Right Footwear

You don't have to hoist a heavy overnight pack and sleep in a tent to hike. But you do need more than ordinary sneakers. You can get by with run-

Hiking Stats

Calories Burned*	Body-Shaping Potential
250 per half-hour	Tones the legs and buttocks; will also increase aerobic endurance

*Based on a 150-pound woman. If you weigh more, you'll burn more calories; if you weigh less, you'll burn fewer.

ning or walking shoes, especially for short hikes on relatively flat terrain. But your feet will be a lot happier in hiking boots, especially if you have problems with weak ankles or balance.

Look for boots or trail shoes with lugged rubber soles. "You need a shoe with traction over rocks, dirt, leaves, and tree roots—all of which are slippery, especially when wet," says Dr. Heil. "And you need ankle support for stability." Whatever you do, don't wear loafers.

What Else You'll Need

Like fitness walking, hiking calls for a few other essentials.

Proper clothing. Thinking blue jeans? Think again. "Jeans are 100 percent cotton, which holds moisture against the skin if it gets wet from inside or outside the body," says Dr Heil. "Instead, wear nylon shorts or hiking pants and pullovers made from fabrics such as polypropylene or CoolMax, which keep moisture away from your body and dry quickly. In extremely cold weather, wear three layers. Use fabrics such as CoolMax, polypropylene, or ThermaStat blends as an inner layer to wick moisture away from the skin. As a middle layer, insulate by trapping a layer of warm air next to your body with fleece, wool, or BiPolar fabric. The outer layer should shield you from weather extremes. Wind jackets and pants of either Gore-Tex or Gore-Tex and fleece are all good outer protectors." If the weather is clear and only mildly cold, an inner and middle layer will suffice, adds Dr. Heil. You can find these clothes in sporting goods stores.

"If it's cool enough to wear a jacket, then you also need gloves and a hat, since the largest source of heat loss is through the head and extremities," says Dr. Heil.

An extra pair of socks. If you're going on a long hike—more than half a day or so—wear two pairs of socks. The first (closest to your feet) should be made of a lightweight material that wicks away moisture, such as CoolMax. The outer layer should be made of a thicker material that protects your feet from rubbing against your shoe, like wool. "Switch to a new pair of both layers of socks about midway through the trip," says Dr. Heil. "It really feels better and is good for your skin."

Food. Okay, if you're just going for a 15-minute loop through the park, you will probably survive without something to eat. But if you're heading out for a couple of hours or longer, count on getting hungry. "You want snacks that are high in complex carbohydrates, such as granola bars, bananas, or a sandwich," says Dr. Heil.

Water. Anytime you exercise for an hour or more, you need to drink water to avoid even mild dehydration. So always carry bottled water or a water purifier. "Never drink water from a stream or creek, because you don't know what might be upstream," says Dr. Heil. "Waste from livestock or wildlife may be just a few hundred yards away, or decomposing animals could be nearby, and you don't want to drink water that's passing over those areas before it makes its way down to you."

A walking stick. You can buy one, or you can simply use a sturdy stick you find on your trail (unless you're hiking in the desert). "Walking sticks are great if you have a back problem, bad knees, or trouble with balance," says Dr. Heil. "It's a third point on the ground. In fact, experienced hikers prefer two poles, which turn them into four-legged creatures." And they come in handy when crossing small streams.

One avid pole-user is Diane Benedict, manager and trip leader for Mountain Fit, an organization in Bozeman that plans hiking adventures. "When descending, I find poles helpful to lessen the impact on my knees," she says. "And using one or two poles turns hiking into a great upper- and lower-body workout."

A map. Unless you can actually see the entire area that you're walking while you're walking, you need a map. "Call hiking clubs, walking clubs, a visitors bureau, or a park headquarters where you plan to hike," suggests Dr. Heil.

Getting Started

You'll enjoy hiking more—and you'll be less likely to feel sore the next day—if you prepare ahead of time, says Benedict. Her suggestions are as follows.

Practice on stairs. The one type of walk you can't practice for in a gym is going downhill. "Coming down is what usually bothers people the first time they're out on a long hike, so climb down stadium stairs or just use the stairs in your office to get your quadriceps and knees ready for the descents," says Benedict.

Practice with your pack. Sure, your pocketbook weighs a ton, but how often do you sling it behind you and carry it up hills for seven or eight hours? If you're preparing for a long hike, load up your pack when you're going short distances. This way, you'll find out just how much weight you're comfortable with, and you'll also get to know the ins and outs of your pack.

Practice with your poles, too—it takes time to get used to using them before you can build up speed.

Adjust your stride. When you walk on flat terrain, you tend to take long strides. "But hiking requires small steps to remain steady on uneven ground," says Benedict.

Hiking Workouts

Beginner

20 to 30 minutes of hiking on a trail or on a beach 3 times a week

Intermediate

40 minutes of hiking 5 or 6 days a week, plus a long hike (60 minutes) up and over a mountain on Saturday

Experienced

Longer hikes on rockier terrain, which take 2 to 4 hours; for highly experienced hikers, adventures that last for more than 4 hours

"Distance, terrain, and weather conditions can make a hike challenging," says Dan Heil, Ph.D., assistant professor of exercise physiology at Montana State University in Bozeman. So few hikers worry about speed. "Hiking isn't a race," he says. "If anything, it's leisurely, because even when the terrain is challenging, you're taking time to notice just how beautiful nature is."

Hiking a mile on a trail isn't the same as walking the same distance on the flat. Distances can be deceiving. So pay attention to guidebook estimates of how long a trail is, the elevation gained, and how much time it takes to hike. "Time, distance, and ascent will help you determine what hike you want to do on any given day," says Diane Benedict, manager and trip leader for Mountain Fit, an organization in Bozeman that plans hiking adventures. A conservative rule: Allow an hour for every 1½ miles of trail, plus ½ hour for each 1,000 feet ascended.

Housework

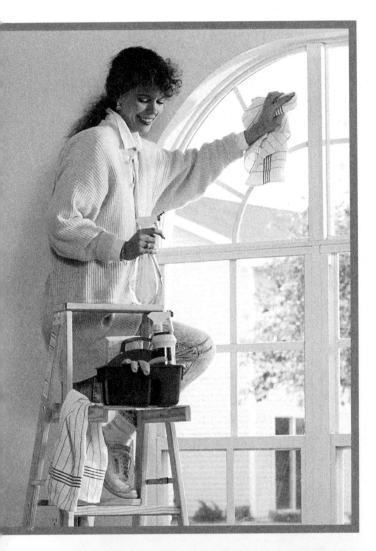

They're the words you've been waiting to hear: Cleaning your house counts as exercise!

Health and fitness experts, researchers at the Centers for Disease Control and Prevention, and the U.S. Surgeon General all agree that the "everyday exercise" of picking up dirty socks, scrubbing floors, and slaving over a hot stove qualifies as just the moderately intense sort of physical activity you need to stay healthy and fit.

"It may seem that spending 15 to 20 minutes vacuuming a couple of rooms doesn't come to much, but in the long term, people who do quite a lot of housework will reap significant benefits in terms of calorie expenditure, fitness, and health," says Russell Pate, Ph.D., an exercise physiologist at the University of South Carolina in Columbia.

Body-Shaping Benefits

Because it engages all of your major muscle groups, housework builds strength, endurance, and flexibility, says Thomas P. Martin, Ph.D., professor in the health, fitness, and sport department at Wittenberg University in Springfield, Ohio. Here's how.

- Picking up clutter and carrying it from one room to another and—an even greater challenge—carrying it up and down stairs works the muscles of your arms, shoulders, legs, and buttocks, Dr. Martin says, while your back and abdominal muscles stabilize your body.

- You'll primarily work your upper body by pushing a vacuum, but walking with your vacuum from one end of your home to the other works your legs and midsection.

- Scrubbing a floor or washing windows helps maintain strength in your arms and back, while the stretching motion maintains flexibility, says Dr. Pate.

The effort you expend cleaning your house also efficiently burns calories, especially when it comes to more strenuous tasks such as scrubbing

Housework Stats

Calories Burned*	Body-Shaping Potential
30 to 50 per 10-minute period	Tones arms, shoulders, chest, back, buttocks, abdomen, and legs

*Based on a 150-pound woman. If you weigh more, you'll burn more calories; if you weigh less, you'll burn fewer.

floors or lugging heavy objects up and down stairs, Dr. Martin notes.

Getting Started

Anyone who has spent a weekend spring-cleaning only to wake up stiff and sore on Monday morning knows that even informal types of exercise call for certain precautions. Here's what you need to know.

Take it slow. Work yourself up slowly to doing housework for extensive periods, especially strenuous tasks. "Don't be a spring-cleaning athlete," Dr. Martin advises. "People make this mistake all the time. They give their whole house a big cleaning once a year, but if they haven't done so since last spring, they're going to end up aching all over."

Start your day with stretches. Honestly, now, are any of us likely to stop and stretch out our hamstrings before laying hands on a broom? "I don't know how many people are going to stretch before they sweep the carpet," says Dr. Martin. "That would be nice, but what's probably most practical is to do a simple stretching routine every day when you get out of bed in the morning."

Alternate activities. To avoid overworking particular muscles, switch from one task to another, suggests Dr. Pate. "It's a good idea to move

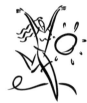

She Did It!

She Dismissed Her Housekeeper—And Shaped Up

While in her late forties, Julie Cooney of Riverside, Illinois, became determined to start exercising regularly. She had put on extra pounds during menopause, she says, and while she didn't feel terribly overweight, she did feel awfully out of shape.

Cooney dragged herself to a health club to which her daughter had given her a one-year membership.

"I went once, and I hated it," she recalls. "You have to dress, get organized, drive to the place, find a parking spot, get undressed, put on your workout clothes, get into step with everybody else in class, then undress again, shower . . . all that!

"I asked myself, 'What am I doing here? I can do more exercise at home.'"

At just about the same time, Cooney's cleaning lady announced her retirement, so Cooney decided not to replace her. Instead, she reclaimed her mop, vacuum, and dirty laundry, and she turned cleaning her house into an exercise regimen.

"I try to do everything very deliberately," says Cooney, now 61. "I have three floors to vacuum, plus hardwood floors everywhere to mop. I'm constantly picking things up and climbing up and down stairs to put them away. I have lots of windows to wash, and when I do, I stretch as much as I can and alternate arms. When I'm doing laundry, I throw everything on the floor. Then I sort it all out with a kind of ballet movement, bending down for each piece and throwing it in a sweeping motion, whites to the right and darks to the left.

"There's always housework to be done, so I figure I may as well get the most out of it," Cooney says. She does occasional cleaning all week long, then a once-a-week cleaning, a schedule that has kept her fit and trim.

"It really is a wonderful way to stay in shape," Cooney says. "I'm five foot seven, about 125 pounds, with good muscle tone and flexibility. I feel great, better than I felt in my forties."

the work around to various muscle groups and move the stress around from joint to joint and tissue to tissue." For example, do a little bit of vacuuming, then put in a load of laundry, and then scrub the bathroom sink.

Perceive your exertion. If you've been pretty sedentary and you're now determined to tackle your housework with fervor, be sure to pay attention to how you feel every step of the way, cautions Dr. Martin. Exercise experts call this "rating your perceived exertion." "Ask yourself how you feel about the intensity at which you're working," he says. "If you feel like you're starting to push the envelope, if you're feeling tired or getting short of breath, slow down and go to a different, less strenuous activity."

Position yourself properly. The bending, lifting, twisting, reaching, and other often demanding movements of housework can play havoc with muscles and joints, says Dr. Pate. "My general advice would be not to force yourself into positions you're not accustomed to or that feel abnormal. In particular, don't do so over and over again or over a long period of time."

For instance, don't get down on your hands and knees to scrub the floor for a half-hour if you're not used to being in that position. Instead, ease into it for a few minutes, then switch to another task and come back to the floor later—if you feel okay. And avoid stretching yourself into postures befitting a contortionist to reach beneath the couch or behind the refrigerator.

Bend and lift smartly. Housework can put a real strain on your vulnerable lower back. Use proper technique to protect yourself: Bend and lift with your legs, not your back.

Think, "30 minutes a day." Weight-loss experts recommend 30 minutes or more of moderately intense physical activity on a daily basis, says Dr. Martin. "We're generally talking about a brisk walk or its equivalent. Carpet sweeping could be the equivalent. Pushing a vacuum, washing windows, scrubbing floors—all of these qualify."

As with any other form of exercise, if you've been pretty sedentary up to now, start out with 10 to 15 minutes of housework two or three days per week and build from there.

Housework Workouts

Low Intensity

Doing laundry, making beds, ironing, washing dishes, putting away groceries, cooking, vacuuming

Moderate Intensity

Sweeping the garage, sidewalk, or outside of the house, washing windows, mopping vigorously

High Intensity

Moving household furniture, carrying heavy boxes, climbing or carrying items up stairs

You can make almost any everyday chore aerobic by aiming to reach your target heart rate zone, says Thomas P. Martin, Ph.D., professor in the health, fitness, and sport department at Wittenberg University in Springfield, Ohio. Just monitor your heart rate while you work. "For starters, go for about 50 percent of your estimated maximum heart rate."

Use this formula for estimating your maximum: 220 minus your age. For example, if you're 40 years old, your estimated maximum heart rate is 180, making for a 90-beats-per-minute rate at 50 percent.

"As you build endurance, gradually push yourself to higher levels: Work faster or more continuously, without stopping and starting. Don't exceed 85 to 90 percent of your maximum heart rate, however," Dr. Martin says.

Inline Skating

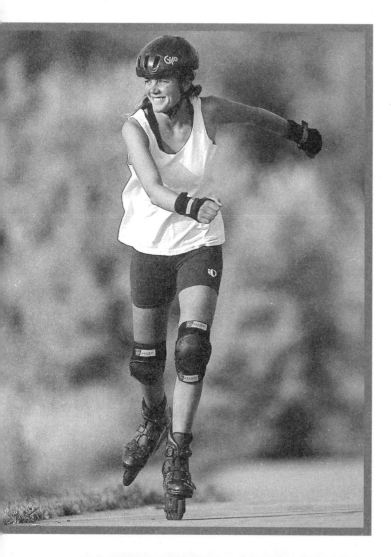

Want to exercise without feeling like it's exercise? Try inline skating. Far from the rickety ride you may remember from your childhood roller skates, inline skating is so smooth you almost feel like you're flying, says Kalinda Mathis, executive director of the International Inline Skating Association (IISA) in Wilmington, North Carolina, and an enthusiastic skater herself.

Further, if you're looking for a way to burn major calories while trimming your thighs, inline skating is made-to-order.

"Inline skating will give you legs to die for," says Carolyn Bradley of Wayne, Pennsylvania, who is an examiner for the International Inline Skating Association instructor certification program. "It's one of the best workouts you can get."

Body-Shaping Benefits

If you're game, here's what you can expect from regular inline skating.

- You'll tone and strengthen your lower body and torso, including your calves, thighs, buttocks, and to a lesser degree, your tummy.

- You'll get a cardiovascular workout roughly comparable to running, without stressing your joints as much.

- You'll burn about as much fat and calories as treadmill running, stepping, or rowing, but have a lot more fun along the way.

Psychological Benefits

Simply put, inline skating feels a lot more like playing than working. And that's no small perk in a world where grown-ups have few opportunities to let loose and have wind-in-your-face, fast and giggly fun.

"You're outside, not in the gym. You're moving fast. The word a lot of people use to describe the feeling is freedom," says Mathis.

Inline Skating Stats

Calories Burned*	Body-Shaping Potential
340–476 an hour, depending on how vigorously you skate	Tones the legs, especially the calves and inner and outer thighs, and the buttocks and abdomen

*Based on a 150-pound woman. If you weigh more, you'll burn more calories; if you weigh less, you'll burn fewer.

You can skate by yourself, focusing on your thoughts, or with a crowd. You can even do it with your kids, solving the problem of when to exercise for busy mothers.

Whether you prefer to go solo or social, inline skating is a stress-relieving activity, according to Mathis.

The Right Footwear

Inline skates are nothing like the metal contraptions you clamped to your play shoes with a skate key when you were in grade school. Basically, an inline skate is more like a sturdy ice skate with a series of wheels, bearings, and a brake built into a double-shelled boot with a buckle and lacing.

She Did It!

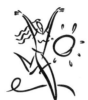

Nicole Skated Off Her "Stress Weight"

Nicole G. Lambros, 34, knew it before her doctor broke the news. At five feet two inches and 140 pounds, the makeup artist and hairdresser from Sunrise, Florida, realized she was carrying too much "stress weight," put on after her divorce as she adjusted to a cross-country move and life as a single mom.

"My doctor told me I had to lose 20 pounds, and he sent me to a nutritionist," says Nicole. "The nutritionist told me I could lose the weight in a month by taking pills and going on her diet plan. But it would cost $600, and I didn't have $600."

The next morning, Nicole put on her tennis shoes and started walking. Walking became jogging. Pretty soon, she was doing two miles a day, but she was bored. So she slipped into her son's inline skates.

"My son had a pair of Rollerblades, and when he went to his dad's for the summer, I put them on and off I went," she says with a giggle.

Nicole had an edge: She had figure skated as a child, so inline skating came easily. In fact, she wowed a group of single, divorced men, who were stunned by how quickly she learned to balance, turn, and stop. "You've bladed before!" they accused her.

"I loved it from the very first minute," she admits. The only adjustment she had to make from figure skating was braking, which is done with the back of inline skates and from the front in figure skates.

Her newly found athleticism came as a surprise to Nicole, who admits to being so intimidated by the hard-bodied women at her gym that she can't work out. She had quit figure skating at 16; her last foray into sports was in junior high school. Inline skating was the first activity that ever captured her interest as an adult.

Within six months, Nicole began to notice major changes in her body, especially in her buttocks, but also in her legs, abdominals, lower back, arms, and chest. She wasn't dieting, but her weight was dropping—10 pounds, 15, then 20 within the year.

"Clients of mine who are personal trainers were saying, 'What are you doing? You look great!'" says the beautician. Her doctor was amazed—and very pleased.

Nicole now skates every morning, and she loves the way she looks and feels. But she says the changes in her life have gone beyond the physical.

"Skating opened up my mind. It's my natural Prozac," she says.

The number one criterion in choosing a skate is comfort, says Mathis. Since skate prices start at about $100 and a quality pair of skates will cost between $150 and $300, it makes sense to rent several styles and brands before you commit. Some local sports equipment shops will rent them by the day.

Women's skates for women's feet. Most women prefer skates designed for women's feet, notes Mathis. They're built on a narrower last (the mold used for making footwear) than men's skates.

Start with a recreational skate. Compared to recreational skates, fitness skates are lighter, have a lower-cut boot, and larger wheels (76 to 80 versus 72 to 76 millimeters). As a beginner, you'll probably want to start on a recreational skate; later, you may want to switch to a more high-performance fitness skate should you commit to power workouts on wide, smooth surfaces.

What Else You'll Need

When you walk or run, you're generally traveling at a speed of 3 to 8 miles per hour—a pretty leisurely clip. Inline skaters travel on hard surfaces at much faster speeds—anywhere from 10 to 25 miles per hour. Pebbles, deep sidewalk cracks, or other objects can trip up your wheels. Sooner or later, you'll fall. Unless you wear protective gear, you can fracture your wrist, arm, or collarbone, cautions Richard A. Schieber, M.D., of the National Center for Injury Prevention and Control in Atlanta. Here's what you'll need.

Wrist guards. When you fall, you tend to fall forward, putting your hand out to break your fall. Padded, plastic wrist guards dissipate the impact—you slide along the ground on impact, saving your wrist from a sprain or fracture from the impact. "Wrist guards are absolutely necessary," says Dr. Schieber.

Knee and elbow pads. Injuries to the knees and elbows are less common than injuries to the wrists, but you still want to protect them from scrapes and other injuries. Protective pads help cushion your fall so you don't leave part of your skin behind.

Helmets. Since a collision with the pavement or a vehicle can be catastrophic, you want to protect your brain. A biking helmet might be better than an inline skating helmet, because it must meet certain standards. All bicycle helmets made or sold in the United States have to meet federal safety standards set by the Consumer Product Safety Commission (CPSC). Dr. Schieber recommends a CPSC-certified bicycle helmet, but he says any helmet is better than none.

Clothing. What you wear to skate should accommodate your pads (jeans may not be comfortable with knee pads) and otherwise be comfortable and nonrestrictive. Most skaters choose exercise shorts on warm days or leggings on chilly days, plus comfortable tops that allow them to freely pump their arms.

Getting Started

Inline skating may look easy, but don't let that fool you into thinking you can just strap on a pair of skates and hit the sidewalk. Watching the neighborhood kids whiz by, it certainly doesn't seem like a dangerous sport. But if you don't know what you're doing—and don't know how to stop or brace yourself for a fall—you could get hurt.

"Learning some basic moves and wearing the right equipment can greatly minimize your chances of hurting yourself," says Craig Young, M.D., medical director of sports medicine at the Medical College of Wisconsin in Milwaukee.

First, learn how to brake. In a study of more than 300 recreational inline skaters by doctors at the department of orthopaedic surgery at the Medical College of Wisconsin in Milwaukee, nearly 15 percent stopped by skating off into the grass. Another 3 percent stopped by voluntarily falling. Neither method is much fun.

Proper braking on inline skates isn't difficult, says Mathis, but it doesn't come as second nature to newcomers. Save yourself time—and potential bruises: Call a sporting goods store that sells inline skates or your local parks and recreation department, and sign up for an individual or group lesson, so an instructor can show you how to glide, stride, and most important, stop.

Dr. Schieber agrees. He strongly urges taking lessons from an instructor (as opposed to a friend). "When inline skating, you go fast from the first stroke," he notes. "You might not have the needed balance and agility from the start, and you need to learn how to fall. Remember, the skate is attached to your foot. You can't just 'jump off' at the first sign of trouble." Contact IISA at 201 North Front Street, Suite 306, Wilmington, NC 28401, for a list of instructors if you can't find one on your own.

Find a smooth, safe place to get started. Bradley, a former figure skater, recommends an empty parking lot, maybe early on a weekend morning, or an uncrowded bike path. "Definitely don't start skating on the street," she says.

The ideal place for any inline skating is a roller rink, adds Dr. Schieber.

Relax. Bend your knees and keep your hands in front of you as you glide your feet slowly and smoothly in front of each other, says Mathis. The rhythm will soon come easily to you.

Skate often. Inline skating may feel a little awkward at first, acknowledges Mathis. Commit to skating in short but regular sessions. "Practice really does make perfect in inline skating. The body starts to memorize where it should be over your skates to be comfortable," she says.

Inline Skating Workouts

Beginner

Skate for 15 to 25 minutes, alternating between 10 slow strides and 10 fast strides.

Intermediate

Skate for 40 minutes, starting with 10 fast, then 10 slow strides. Then do 20 fast strides and 10 slow strides.

Experienced

Skate for 60 minutes using shorter, faster strokes. Abbreviate the glide between strokes.

As you become comfortable on skates, you can intensify your workout by bending more deeply at the waist, says Craig Young, M.D., medical director of sports medicine at the Medical College of Wisconsin in Milwaukee. "This works the large muscle groups of the legs harder," he explains.

Some experienced skaters assume a stance that looks like a speed skater taking a turn, with hands clasped behind their backs as they bend low into their strides. Using this technique, your buttocks get the workout, says Dr. Young.

You can intensify your aerobic workout and burn more calories by skating into the wind and skating up hills, Dr. Young notes. And of course, you can give ice skating a whirl and get a similar workout.

Jogging and Treadmill Running

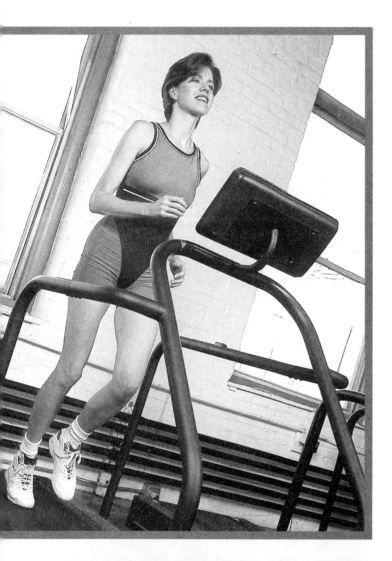

Jogging gives you more bang for your buck than walking, since it uses the same muscle groups but burns calories faster, says Ellen Glickman-Weiss, Ph.D., associate professor of exercise physiology in the department of exercise, leisure, and sports at Kent State University in Ohio.

"You can generally figure on burning 100 calories a mile," says Dr. Glickman-Weiss. "Walking one mile may take you 15 to 20 minutes; jogging will take you half as long. Both are tremendous for overall fitness benefits," she explains. Simply defined as running slowed down, jogging offers less risk of injury than full-out running, while providing top-notch aerobic benefits.

Body-Shaping Benefits

Whether you jog on a treadmill or through a dew-sprinkled park, slow running provides a wealth of physical payoffs.

- You work both the large and the small muscle groups of your calves, thighs, buttocks, and hips, and in a less pronounced way, your waist and abdominal muscles.

- You burn calories and use up fat stores, big time.

- You'll raise your metabolic rate even after your running shoes are back in the closet. According to researchers at the University of Colorado, the resting metabolic rates of middle-aged women runners stayed steady as they grew older, while sedentary women gained weight and body fat as their resting metabolisms slowed. In the long run, older runners burn up to 600 additional calories a week (equal to nine pounds a year!) even when they're at rest. "That doesn't even count the calories burned when they run," notes Pamela P. Jones, research assistant professor of kinesiology and applied physiology at the University of Colorado at Boulder.

Jogging Stats

Calories Burned*	Body-Shaping Potential
102 per mile	Firms the calves, thighs, buttocks, and to a lesser extent, the abdomen

*Based on a 150-pound woman. If you weigh more, you'll burn more calories; if you weigh less, you'll burn fewer.

The Right Footwear

Fortunately for joggers, manufacturers have come a long way in designing shoes to accommodate the sizes and running styles of virtually any woman, at prices that generally range from $50 to $100. Here's what to look for, according to Dr. Glickman-Weiss.

Shoes for *your* feet. Reading running shoe reviews can help you decide which of the dozens of shoe makes and models might best meet your needs, says Dr. Glickman-Weiss. Also consult knowledgeable salesclerks at sporting goods stores or athletic shoe stores. Take your old shoes along. Worn spots show whether you run more on the outside or the inside of your foot and which areas need the most support.

Enough wiggle room. A wide toebox is vital to give the front of your foot enough room when

She Did It!

Cynthia's Second Attempt at Jogging Did the Trick

Cynthia Smith didn't set out to lose weight. "I really just wanted to do something to improve my overall health," says the a 45-year-old sales executive from Venice, California.

Nevertheless, Cynthia knew she could stand to lose a few pounds. "I had some extra weight around my hips and abdomen, and I felt heavy," she recalls. "I just didn't feel attractive." Cynthia had tried "scattershot approaches" to dieting coupled with a roller skating routine for aerobic fitness back before the invention of inline skating. But she had a lackadaisical attitude toward the diets, and roller skating did not work off the pounds. So she began to search for an exercise routine that would fit into her busy traveling schedule and be enjoyable.

"I did some running in my twenties and really loved it," says Cynthia. So she decided to try it again.

"The first day, I ran entirely too fast," she admits. "I went home after only about a quarter-mile, winded and discouraged." But a fellow runner and friend coaxed Cynthia to slow down her pace and just trot, and within two weeks, she was able to complete a two-mile loop around her house without stopping. She eventually graduated to 30- to 40-minute jogs at dusk, on the beach or the street.

Cynthia's renewed efforts at jogging paid off, physically and mentally. "After only a few months of jogging, I started feeling trimmer and more toned," she remembers. "I went from 134 pounds to 124 pounds, I dropped a dress size, and my clothes fit me better." At five feet six inches, Cynthia says the 10 pounds she lost wasn't the only benefit. "I just feel so much more toned and healthy," she says. Jogging also took away her cravings for heavy, fattening foods. "Instead, I always want to eat something light for dinner, such as a salad with turkey, or fish and fresh vegetables."

When she started to see positive changes in her body, Cynthia began to lift weights at the gym to which she had previously belonged, but seldom attended. Sure enough, weight lifting further toned her hips, legs, and abdomen.

"Plus, my runs are therapeutic," adds Cynthia. "They clear my head, and I get ideas." She doesn't always feel like lacing up her running shoes and heading out. "But I always feel better physically and emotionally after I'm done," she says. "Jogging after a hard day at work is a tremendous tension reliever. Everything that builds up during the day just sort of vaporizes."

Take It to the MAX

Run Longer, Not Faster

If jogging is your sport of choice, but you have trouble getting out there as often as you'd like—or you're starting to get bored—make it more fun, says Ellen Glickman-Weiss, Ph.D., associate professor of exercise physiology in the department of exercise, leisure, and sports at Kent State University in Ohio. She offers these tips.

Vary your route. If you run outdoors, alter your route, run with friends, or make it a family activity. While Dr. Glickman-Weiss generally enjoys the solitude of solo runs, she sometimes invites her husband to jog along. And from time to time, her eight-year-old son accompanies her on his inline skates.

Say okay to a 5-K. The next time you see a charity run announced in the newspaper, sign up, encourages Dr. Glickman-Weiss. The competition, free T-shirt, and opportunity to help raise money for causes like breast cancer, arthritis, or Alzheimer's research will motivate you to stick with your program.

If you've been jogging faithfully at a leisurely pace—about six miles per hour—and you're not seeing the results you're looking for, your best bet is to increase your distance, not your speed, says Dr. Glickman-Weiss. In one study of 1,837 women who ran recreationally (not to compete), the women who ran the most miles per week had the narrowest waists and hips, regardless of how fast they ran.

You don't need to run every day. Running too fast—or too often—can increase the risk of knee, hip, or tendon problems, or other common injuries. Three to five days a week is fine. And if you're just starting out, you shouldn't run more than 15 miles a week, cautions Dr. Glickman-Weiss. At that point, the stresses on your muscles, joints, tendons, and ligaments outweigh the body-shaping benefits. There are other, better ways to maximize your efforts than going all-out, all the time. Here's how.

Increase your weekly distance by no more than 10 percent a week. If you're jogging three days a week for 30 minutes a day, for example, and covering three miles, increase by no more than one mile total the first week, and so forth, says Dr. Glickman-Weiss.

Stick to flat, smooth surfaces. If you run outdoors, you can run longer while minimizing impact if you stick to a soft, smooth, unbanked cinder track or an artificial surface. The same goes for soft, smooth dirt trails, says Dr. Glickman-Weiss. Avoid asphalt and concrete.

Alternate jogging with other activities. Swimming, water aerobics, cycling, stairclimbing, rowing, or cross-country skiing gives your feet and legs a welcome respite from the constant pounding of running, while working other muscle groups than running would alone, says Dr. Glickman-Weiss.

the force of your foot is pushed forward. Women with wide feet may want to check out running shoes designed specifically for women, from companies like Ryka, which makes shoes exclusively for women, to New Balance and Saucony, among others.

All-weather, all-surface tread and materials. If you're going to be running in rain and snow, look for a shoe made from weather-tight fabric, with a hard-core outer tread. If you're a treadmill runner, this isn't important.

Replacements, as needed. Buy a new pair of shoes every six months or 600 miles. At that point, the shoes start to fall apart, even if they still look good. You can prolong the life of your running shoes by wearing them only to run.

Treadmill Tips

If you find that rain, sleet, and snow keep you from jogging, try treadmill running at a gym. If you find yourself sticking to it (and you can afford it), consider a treadmill for your home. To save money, shop at a secondhand sports equipment store.

Choose a body-friendly model. Some treadmills have a built-in suspension, like shock absorbers on a car, to minimize the impact on weak hips or knees, says Edmund Burke, Ph.D., professor of exercise science at the University of Colorado in Colorado Springs and author of the *Complete Home Fitness Handbook*.

These machines approximate the impact of running on a soft surface, says Dr. Glickman-Weiss. They're also sturdier and better able to accommodate heavier walkers and runners than lightweight units that you can stow under a bed, she adds.

Go for a test jog. If you decide to buy, go to a reputable fitness showroom dressed for action. Run on many treadmills, looking for a shock-absorbing platform, plus a belt wide and long enough for your comfort, and handrails you like.

Know you can stop. So you can stop without risking an injury, make sure the treadmill has a device that will immediately stop the belt in case you run into trouble, advises Dr. Burke.

Getting Started

Unless you're already in shape, work up to jogging gradually. Start out walking, then increase the distance and then the intensity of your walks.

Jog at a slow pace for 10, then 15, then 20 minutes, making sure you're not so out of breath that you can't talk to a partner while running, says Dr. Glickman-Weiss. When you're ready for more, run longer, not faster.

Jogging Workouts

Beginner

Alternate jogging and walking for 20 minutes a day, 3 to 5 days a week.

Intermediate

Jog 40 minutes at least 4 or 5 days a week.

Experienced

Jog for an hour, up to 5 times a week, not to exceed 30 miles a week. Beyond 30 miles, there is really no extra benefit, and your risk of injury increases.

To be sure you're working hard enough (but not too hard), keep track of your heart rate as you jog, says Ellen Glickman-Weiss, Ph.D., associate professor of exercise physiology in the department of exercise, leisure, and sports at Kent State University in Ohio.

To determine your ideal maximum heart rate range—an intensity that's neither too easy nor too hard—subtract your age from 220. Multiply that number by 0.6—that's your lower-limit heart rate for exercise. Next, multiply the same number by 0.9—that's your upper limit.

Make sure your heart rate falls within this range while you exercise. First, take your pulse while walking or marching in place. Place your first two fingers (never your thumb, which has its own pulse) on the inside of your wrist below your thumb, or below your jaw, next to your windpipe. Count the beats for 15 seconds. To get your heart rate, multiply the count by four. If you find it difficult to take your pulse while exercising, get a sports watch that monitors your heart rate, suggests Dr. Glickman-Weiss.

Jumping Rope

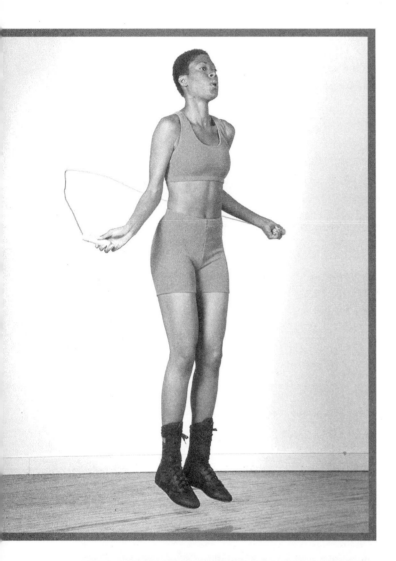

For the busy woman on a budget, jumping rope is the ultimate calorie-burning exercise. It doesn't take a lot of time, it's inexpensive, and it's high-intensity.

Body-Shaping Benefits

Women who want to lose weight are ideal candidates for jumping rope, says Ken Solis, M.D., an emergency room physician at Beaver Dam Community Hospital in Greenfield, Wisconsin, and the author of *Ropics*, a book of exercises he developed for the jump rope. Among the rewards:

- You'll burn calories—lots of them. Jumping rope is on a par with running when it comes to calorie burn.
- You'll improve endurance, coordination, balance, and timing.
- You'll strengthen your bones as well as your muscles; this is a great bonus, because it helps prevent osteoporosis.

The Right Footwear

Since you're going to be doing a lot of bouncing on the balls of your feet, wearing the right shoes is important. Otherwise, you could sprain an ankle or tear a tendon. You'll need a quality pair of aerobic or cross-training shoes to give you cushioning and support in all the right places, says exercise phsiologist Carla Sottovia, assistant fitness director at the Fitness Cooper Center in Dallas. When you're in the store, cast your inhibitions to the wind and jump up and down to make sure the shoes fit right. As for those old tennis shoes, running shoes, or sneakers in your closet—use them for other sports, she says.

What Else You'll Need

Once upon a time, an old clothesline may have served as a jump rope. Now you have many more

Jumping Rope Stats

Calories Burned*	Body-Shaping Potential
110–130 per 10-minute session	A high-level calorie burner. Firms up the buttock and thigh muscles. Also develops calf muscles.

*Based on a 150-pound woman. If you weigh more, you'll burn more calories; if you weigh less, you'll burn fewer.

choices—and it's also important to choose the right bra and mat. Here are the possibilities.

Spring for the swivel. The rope should swivel within the handles or at the handles, so that the rope doesn't twist on itself while you're jumping, says Dr. Solis.

Choose right. Jump ropes are made of many materials. Starting out, you might choose a segmented rope (otherwise known as a beaded rope) or a rope made of woven cotton or synthetic material. The segmented or beaded ropes have a nylon cord at the center that is strung with cylin-

drical plastic beads that look like hollow noodles. A woven rope, made of nylon, cotton, or polypropylene, resembles the old-fashioned kind of jump rope, and it won't sting as much if you happen to swat your back, Dr. Solis notes from personal experience.

After you've advanced a bit, you might choose a speed rope or licorice rope. They're made from vinyl plastic, and they're light and fast. Leather ropes are just as fast as speed ropes, but they wear out sooner. Some advanced jump ropers who are in very good physical condition choose weighted

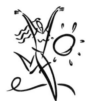

She Did It!

How Heidi Skipped Four Inches off Her Hips

Heidi Zarder was a certified group exercise instructor in Germantown, Wisconsin. Now, being an exercise instructor is not exactly a sedentary job. But even so, after Heidi had her third child, she began to wonder whether she would ever get rid of the extra pounds she'd put on during pregnancy. Her normal workout routine just wasn't getting results.

Then, eight months after her daughter was born, she started jumping rope. "It made all the difference," says Heidi. "In one month, I lost four inches off my hips."

The new exercise was actually the result of Heidi's profession. "The local YMCA wanted me to lead classes that mixed different forms of exercise," says Heidi. "One week called for rope jumping. In order to teach, I had to practice myself."

Heidi had a wood deck behind her house, and that became her happy jumping ground. "I made sure I didn't jump or bounce too hard," says Heidi. "I would work on it for 10 to 15 minutes, watching myself in the reflection of the patio door. Then I'd

get tired, go inside, and come back out to practice again when I felt ready."

Heidi knew she had reached a plateau in her efforts to lose weight, and skipping rope was the boost she needed to lose the last few pounds. "Many people who go to step and aerobic classes never lose any weight," notes Heidi. "That's because they reach a plateau and need something to kick in a higher amount of calorie-burning. Rope skipping can blast you through the plateau."

One unforeseen problem, however, was bladder control. "After three kids, bouncing up and down could trigger leakage," says Heidi. "To handle this, I just avoided drinking anything with caffeine. I limited how much water I drank before I worked out. Instead, I drank plenty of water *while* I was exercising."

Now, when she teaches aerobics classes, Heidi includes rope skipping. It has been a popular addition to her classes at a local college. "It's great for coordination," says Heidi. "But most everyone uses it as a tool for weight loss. It simply burns a lot of calories."

Take It to the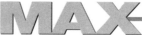

Jump . . . for Joy!

Rope skipping can be intense—but with music in the background, and maybe some kids or friends to keep you company, it's fun, too. Plus, it travels well. Just pack your jump rope and shoes, and you can skip rope wherever you go. It's a great way to be sure you'll get a workout in during your hotel stay, notes exercise physiologist Carla Sottovia, assistant fitness director at the Fitness Cooper Center in Dallas.

Here are some guidelines to keep in mind as jumping becomes a regular part of your life, according to Ken Solis, M.D., an emergency room physician at Beaver Dam Community Hospital in Greenfield, Wisconsin, and author of *Ropics*, a book of exercises he developed for the jump rope.

Warm to the task. Start out with an easy, two-footed jump. Wait a few minutes, until your muscles get warmed up, before you try jumping faster. After you feel comfortable and warm jumping with both feet, you can try a light jog step, says Dr. Solis.

Alternate between high- and low-impact jumping. "You can't expect to do high-impact jumping for a half-hour," says Dr. Solis. "So you have to combine it with low-impact moves." When you stop to take a breather, try marching in place for a while.

Mix and match. For a high-intensity interval workout, you can combine jumping rope with circuit training. For instance, after a warmup, you might alternate jumping with pushups, triceps dips, and squats.

Be very varied. There are many variations on jumping rope, and if you observe some advanced rope-skippers, you'll get some ideas. One variation is the heel dig jump: With each jump, you bring one leg in front of your body as if you were digging in your heel. It looks like a variation on a Cossack dance without the deep squat or the funny hat.

If you're feeling more ambitious, you might try criss-crossing your arms when you jump—though don't be surprised if you get tangled up at first. Or try jump-rope jacks, where you land with your feet apart on the first jump, then bring your feet together on the second jump: It's like jumping-jacks, with the rope going all the time. If you want to observe some challenging variations on rope jumping—including moves like the Samurai Whirl or the 360-Degree Rotation—don't miss the world championships of rope jumping, which airs every year on ESPN.

Join others. Skipping rope with others helps you beat boredom and stick with your routine. Many classes are held in conjunction with kick boxing or martial arts classes, and they're offered at aerobics studios. Local gyms, YWCAs, kick boxing schools, and martial arts schools are likely to have information. Just call and ask.

ropes that can weigh up to six pounds. Needless to say, you don't want a weighted rope until you're very confident about your swinging and timing, says Dr. Solis.

Measure for leisure. When a rope is the right length, you can hold it at waist-level and hardly move your hands, and it will clear your head and feet with no problem. (If you have to circle your arms around, the rope's too short; if it bounces and hits your ankles, it's too long.) To get a comfortable length, stand with one or two feet in the middle of the rope, then lift the handles as high as they'll go. If they reach your armpits, you have what you want, says Dr. Solis. Some ropes are adjustable, and others can be shortened just by putting in a couple of overhand knots near the handles.

Cradle your top. You probably know by now whether you're more comfortable in an exercise bra—but this is a sport where you might even want two. Women who take a bra size 36 or larger usually do best by layering two running bras on top of each other, and then wearing a close-fitting T-shirt or tank on top of that, says Sottovia.

Find the space. "Even though it's convenient to skip rope at home, it's sometimes hard to find enough room above you and around you," says Dr. Solis. If you're average height, you'll need at least a nine-foot ceiling, with plenty of space around you. The lawn won't work, because the rope gets tangled in the grass, and carpet slows you down. So you might head for the basement, garage, or patio. That's fine, as long as you're on a surface that has a little give to it, like wood or hard rubber, says Dr. Solis. You don't want to jump on hard concrete or

Jumping Rope Workouts

Beginner

5 to 20 minutes of easy, 2-footed jumping, paying attention to form. Start out with 5, 1-minute sessions between other interval activities. Work up to doing 1-minute jumping intervals for half the time. Do this combination 3 or 4 times a week.

Intermediate

20 to 40 minutes of 2-footed jumping—or alternating between 1-footed and 2-footed jumping—3 or 4 times a week. Jump for 2-minute intervals, broken up by 3 minutes of another activity, so you are jumping two-thirds of the time.

Experienced

Alternate 3 minutes of rope skipping with 3 minutes of other activities for a total of 40 to 60 minutes.

When it comes to choosing an aerobic exercise, think of jumping rope as the polar opposite of walking. It takes about 50 minutes to burn 100 calories when you walk, whereas you'll easily burn over 100 calories in just 10 minutes of jumping rope. Likewise, most of us can keep up a nice walking pace for at least an hour or two—which would be the equivalent of a marathon in rope jumping.

Once you get the general rhythm of jumping, try to ex-

tend your workout until you can jump for two to three minutes before taking a break. At that point, rope skipping can become the aerobic segment of an interval workout. "Jump for up to three minutes, then do three minutes of weight training or resistance work," suggests exercise physiologist Carla Sottovia, assistant fitness director at the Fitness Cooper Center in Dallas. "You'll notice a big change in the shape of your lower body if you alternate lower-body routines with high-intensity rope skipping a couple of times a week."

Since it is nearly impossible to jump straight through your workout, combine rope work with intervals of other cardiovascular activities. Some moves you can vary your workout with are squats, walking briskly around the gym, and riding a stationary bike, says Ken Solis, M.D., an emergency room physician at Beaver Dam Community Hospital in Greenfield, Wisconsin, and the author of *Ropics*, a book of exercises he developed for the jump rope.

You can also use rope skipping as the high-intensity portion of a less-intense, regular workout. For example, if you like to walk, you can take your usual route, then return home for a minute or two of jumping rope, says Sottovia. This will raise your heart rate and increase the intensity of your routine.

Just remember that it takes more than a few tries to catch on to the rhythm of the whirling rope and coordinate it with your bouncing feet. Even if you jumped rope frequently when you were younger, the body doesn't have instant memory of its former moves—and besides, there's the age factor. Your leg muscles may complain in ways they never did before. Be patient with yourself.

tile, he warns. Those surfaces don't give you any bounce, and they're murder on your joints.

Go to the mat. You can convert a thick carpet to a jump-friendly surface by using a plastic mat that is usually sold to be placed under an office desk or chair, says Dr. Solis. These are available at larger office supply stores.

To convert the floor in a garage or spare room into a jump-friendly surface, invest in plastic interlocking tiles, says Budd Pickett, executive director of the United States Amateur Jump Rope Federation (USAJRF). These are not soft mats, but flooring used in indoor courts for sports such as volleyball, gymnastics, and jump roping, he explains. To locate a store near you that sells interlocking tiles, write to Sport Court at 939 South 700 West, Salt Lake City, UT 84104.

A hard rubber mat or flooring is good, too, according to Dr. Solis. Avoid squishy aerobics mats because they have too much give, he adds.

Getting Started

"If you're just starting out and haven't skipped rope in years, don't set out to jump for a certain amount of time," says Dr. Solis. Instead, ease into it.

Skip the skip. Begin jumping with both feet, but try to do it without that little skip between jumps. Jump just high enough to clear the rope, and bring the rope over fast so you don't have time for that extra hop. Start out at the easiest pace you can without having to add the hop.

Pedal your feet. For variation, try jogging from foot to foot as you jump. The motion is more like pedaling a bike or light jogging than jumping up and down. You control the intensity by how fast you "jog" through your rope.

Keep your posture as erect as possible.

Keep your elbows in and wrists relaxed. With your elbows tucked close by your sides, your arms should barely move while you're skipping rope. Swing the rope with a relaxed motion of your forearms and wrists.

Stick to the low-jump. "There's no need to lift more than one inch off the ground," says Sottovia. You should rise just high enough so that the rope can clear the space between your feet and the mat.

Stop when you want to. If you're tired after a minute or two of jumping, just take a break—then try again when you feel like it.

Power Walking

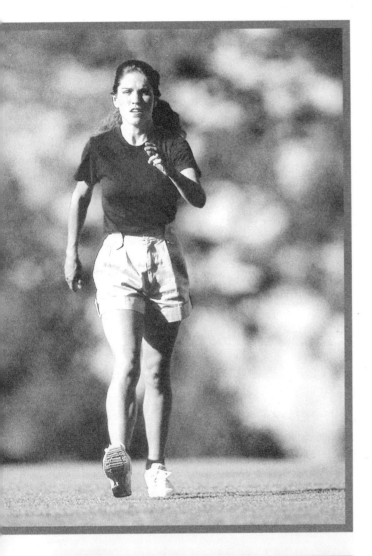

If you're like a lot of women who walk to lose weight and get in shape, you've probably been walking around your neighborhood religiously for months. You know every kid, every cat, and every dog within two miles of your house. You're out there, rain or shine. There's just one problem: You're getting a little bored. You don't want to jog, but you would like to somehow take your walks to the next level—burn a few more calories, or get slimmer, sooner.

Power walking is the sport for you. While the average walker usually covers about three miles in an hour-long walk, a power walker strives to do at least four miles in the same time period. Serious power walkers can eventually do about six miles in an hour, but that's going pretty darn fast. In fact, it's faster than some people run.

Most women will simply strive to bump up their 20-minute per mile stroll to a 15-minute mile power hike. Power walking is any walking done as exercise, rather than just recreation, according to Jeff Salvage, a Medford, New Jersey, junior national coordinator of U.S. Track and Field, a governing body of the U.S. Track Team.

"Power walking is the obvious next step for women who've made walking a habit," says Salvage, who is also a racewalking coach and author of *Walk Like an Athlete*.

Power Walking Stats

Calories Burned*	Body-Shaping Potential
Between 198 and 250 per mile	Tones hips, thighs, buttocks, and abdominals

*Based on a 150-pound woman. If you weigh more, you'll burn more calories; if you weigh less, you'll burn fewer.

Body-Shaping Benefits

Here's what you can expect when you power walk regularly.

- If you are a regular walker, but find that you have to walk long periods of time in order to burn as much fat as you want, then power walking will help you burn calories in less time.

- You will tone all the muscles in your lower body, including the gluteus (the large muscle in your buttocks), hamstrings (along the backs of your thighs), and quadriceps (in the fronts of your thighs).

The Right Footwear

"Try on as many walking shoes as possible before you buy a pair," recommends Carol Espel, a Walk Reebok master trainer and the executive fitness director of Equinox Fitness Clubs of New York. "You want to look for shoes that are lightweight and that breathe. (Look for mesh on the top or sides of the shoe.) The forefoot of the shoe should be flexible, so it bends fairly easily.

"A slanted, or beveled, heel makes it easier to walk with a heel-to-toe motion, which is one of the techniques of power walking. It puts less strain on your shin muscles, thus avoiding shin splints," adds Espel. "Ultimately, though, you have to find the shoe that's most comfortable for you."

What Else You'll Need

While walking is the easiest form of exercise, power walking requires some technique. "It's not just a matter of walking faster," says Espel.

"The difference between a 17-minute-per-

She Did It!

Ruth Power Walks into Her Class Reunion 32 Pounds Thinner

New Year's Day 1993 was one of celebration for homemaker and mother Ruth Artz. Her second child, a son, was born, and she made a resolution. "I had a school reunion to go to in May," she says. "I was determined that, by the time the party rolled around, I would lose the 32 extra pounds left after my pregnancy."

At five feet one inch, Ruth weighed 113 pounds before her pregnancy. At high risk for pregnancy-related complications, she had to give up her twice-a-week aerobics. By the time she gave birth, she weighed over 160 pounds; afterward, she weighed about 145.

"I went to see my aerobics teacher, Rosemary, and it turned out she had given up teaching," Ruth says. "Because her knees were bothering her, she was concentrating on the walking that she had been doing for 20 years, and she asked me to come along."

Ruth didn't think walking would be enough to get rid of the extra weight, but she tried it anyway. "Rosemary blew me away!" Ruth says. "She wasn't strolling. I couldn't even keep up with her at first. In fact, it took a while before I could reach her speed of four miles an hour."

Ruth noticed a difference in her body. "In about five months, I got down to about 115 pounds. I also made a real effort to watch what I ate and to drink a lot of water, and I used an abs workout video to flatten my abdominal muscles."

The next year, Ruth and Rosemary, who have remained walking partners until this day, began to compete in marathons. "Our normal walks are now 4.5 miles per hour (a little over a 13-minute-per-mile pace), but because they have time limits, we try to walk 12-minute to 11½-minute miles when we do marathons," says Ruth. In fact, Ruth and Rosemary always aim to complete the 26.2-mile course in six hours or under.

"Having Rosemary to walk with really helped—I don't know what I would have done without her," says Ruth. Together, they walk 30 miles each week, and they joined the Loma Linda Lopers, a running, walking, and fitness club in Loma Linda, California. "Half are runners, and half are walkers."

At 35, Ruth walked the Walt Disney World Marathon, and her figure reflects her accomplishments. "I'm 103 pounds now and I feel great," she says. "I'm in better shape now than I was in my early twenties."

Take It to the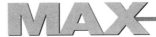

Ready to Race?

Proud that you're finally taking your walking seriously enough to call yourself a power walker? Here's even more reason to pat yourself on your back: Pick up the speed enough and perfect your technique into racewalking, and you have yourself an Olympic sport.

The women's world record for racewalking is just under 42 minutes for a 10-K walk (6.2 miles). That's a walking speed of 10.3 miles per hour.

"It's impressive, but speed is not the only point," says Jeff Salvage, a Medford, New Jersey, junior national coordinator of U.S. Track and Field, a governing body of the U.S. Track Team. "Racewalking has rules about technique. Rule number one: 'No loss of contact with the ground that's visible to the eye can occur.' In other words, one foot is always on the ground at all times. Rule number two: 'The advancing leg must be straightened (no bend at the knee) from the moment of first contact with the ground until in the vertical position (when it's starting to move back behind the body).'"

Sound complicated? It is. So here's what you'll need to racewalk.

Coaching. To make sure that you're racewalking correctly, you need someone with a keen eye and knowledge of the rules. So if you want to start racing, you should at least have a few sessions of coaching. Contact a local high school or college with a good track and field program, and ask them to put you in touch with someone who knows the regulations and techniques of racewalking.

Consider a running shoe. At racewalking paces, a well-designed running shoe might be a better option than a walking shoe, says Salvage. "There's a difference in flexibility and the position in which you place your foot down on the ground," he adds. "Racewalkers usually prefer a running shoe." He suggests you look for one with a low heel, flexible toe, stable heel counter, and plenty of room in the toebox.

Think about walking a marathon. Ever wish you could take part in all those 5-Ks, 10-Ks, and marathons held in your community? You can. Most events allow racewalkers to compete. You might start earlier than the runners, but you'll begin and finish the event in the same places. Believe it or not, professional racewalkers walk at a clip that isn't too far behind those of marathon runners. Most marathons are based on time, not gait, so you should ask what the time limit of the race is and decide whether it is reasonable for you, says Salvage.

mile 'health walker' and a 13-minute-per-mile 'power walker' is technique," notes Salvage, who coaches many women of all levels and ages.

Here's what you'll need for your metamorphosis.

A trail or a treadmill. While there's nothing wrong with simply walking around your neighborhood, if you want to power walk, you'll want to know exactly how long your training ground is. To do that, you can map out a course that's four to five miles long, do laps on a high school track, or walk on a treadmill that records your pace and distance automatically. Each of these choices has its own benefits.

"Getting started can be as easy as walking through a park or your neighborhood, which is wonderful because of the scenery and varying terrain," says Espel. "Tracks are good because you can concentrate on technique and don't have to worry about traffic."

Breathing in the fresh air and letting the wind pass over your body is healthy, says Salvage. Treadmills, on the other hand, allow you to pinpoint your pace and distance, which is also very helpful in the beginning. Keep in mind, however, that you aren't getting the benefit of the fresh air, points out Salvage.

Start with a warmup, advises Espel. Walk at a comfortable pace for about five minutes or until you break out in a light sweat. Then stretch your quadriceps, hips, hamstrings, and shins.

Water. If you're accustomed to waiting until you get home from your stroll to rehydrate, it's time to change. "You must carry a water bottle with you," says Espel. "Your power walks will be more intense than your old walks, so it's important to have water before, during, and after your workout." Drink at least a cup of water before starting out, a cup or more while you're walking, and still more water afterward, she recommends.

If you don't want to carry the water in your hand, invest in a fanny pack or waist pack that's big enough to hold a bottle of water, or buy one that has a strap in which to place the bottle. It's a must.

A progress log. Metamorphosing from a walker to a power walker means keeping track of your progress. "Your log doesn't have to be fancy or formal," says Espel. "Just write down when you walked, how far you went, how it felt, and how long it took you."

Getting Started

To hone your power-walking technique, you'll need to focus on your feet, your hips, and your arms. Espel offers these tips.

Feet: Think heel-toe. Take quick, short steps, not long, extended strides. "Your goal is to pick up your feet faster," says Espel. "To do that, you have to focus on rolling your foot from heel to toe. Come down on your heel, with your toes up, then roll through your foot, pushing off on your toes when that leg is behind you." It should almost feel as if you're rolling forward.

Hips: Think steady and straight. Lots of people think power walkers look as if they're waddling, assuming walkers are rocking their hips from side to side. Not so. Instead, your hips are used as an extension of your legs, so each hip moves forward and back (but stays level) as its accompanying leg moves forward. You're not pushing your hips, says Espel, but you're utilizing their power.

Arms: Think propulsion. Your arms play a big role in how fast you walk. Keep them stationary, and your stroll will never turn into a power walk. "The faster you pump your arms, the faster your body will move," says Espel. "That doesn't mean, though, that you want your arms to swing wildly without control." Instead, your arms should be bent at a 90-degree angle and move steadily forward and back, but your fists should never go back farther than your hips or higher than your sternum.

Eyes: Look ahead. Use your eyes to aim for a landmark far ahead of you, Espel suggests. "You should be looking at the horizon or focused on a spot down the block. That focus will add to your momentum as well as make sure that your posture is correct."

Posture: Lean forward from the ankles. "Imagine yourself looking like a ski jumper in midair," says Espel. "That's almost the angle at which you want your body." In other words, there should be no bend in your waist.

Here are some equations.

- If you're just beginning to change your walk into a power walk, then you might need music with 110 beats per minute, which is a 19-minute-per-mile pace—just a tad faster than the usual 3-mile-an-hour pace you may be accustomed to for exercise.

- If you're doing a solid power walk, pick music with 130 beats per minute, which translates to a 15-minute-per-mile pace.

- If you're going full throttle at the breakneck speed of a 13-minute-per-mile pace, pick music with 150 beats per minute.

Whole body: Stretch afterward. Power walking is harder on many lower-body parts than slow walking is, so you'll need to make sure that you stretch properly afterward, just as a professional athlete does after she works out or competes.

Specific areas to stretch? Again, the hips, quadriceps, hamstrings, and shins. "Shin pain is probably the number one complaint of fitness walkers," says Espel. "Ideally, your shins should adjust to a walk within the first five minutes. If they hurt or ache, you're going too fast." She suggests you slow your pace or try walking backward—retro-walking, it's called. This takes all the pressure off the shins. Once your shins feel better, resume walking forward.

Power Walking Workouts

Beginner

Using power-walking techniques, start to change the way you move during your walk. Bend your arms at a 90-degree angle, pump them, and try to walk heel-to-toe. Do this once or twice during your regular walks for a few weeks before moving on to the next level.

Intermediate

Start working intervals into your routine, using landmarks as your goals. For example, during your workout and using your new techniques, walk as fast as you can to a stop sign up ahead. Then give yourself plenty of time to recover (using a slower walk) before you start another speed interval. You've recovered when you are back to breathing a little harder than normal. Do this 3 to 5 times during each walk for 20 to 30 seconds each for at least 4 or 5 weeks, but don't do it every day. It's an every-other-day workout.

Experienced

Start timing yourself and measuring your heart rate during your walks. Subtract your age from 220—that's your maximum heart rate. You should never work out at that rate; rather, aim for 60 to 90 percent of that number.

You might want to purchase a heart rate monitor, available at sporting goods stores, suggests Carol Espel, a Walk Reebok master trainer and the executive fitness director of Equinox Fitness Clubs of New York. The monitors, which range in price from about $70 to $250, give a much more accurate reading than you would get from taking your own pulse manually.

You should only attempt to move through the three intensity workouts detailed on the left if you're already an experienced walker, cautions Espel. That means you are already walking at least three, and possibly more, days per week. Each of your walks should include a 5-minute walking warmup, 25 minutes of moderate-intensity walking, and then a 5-minute walking cooldown, plus some stretching.

"Then focus on technique and speed," says Espel, who leads many groups through Reebok's progressive walking program. "Technique should always be the most important part of your workout. Once you feel comfortable with your form, increase your speed gradually. Then, when your speed feels right, start to work on increasing the distance you go at that intensity.

"When exercising at high intensity, your goal is to work at 80 to 90 percent of your maximum heart rate for the longest portion of your workout, while always, of course, keeping your technique as flawless as possible," explains Espel.

Rowing

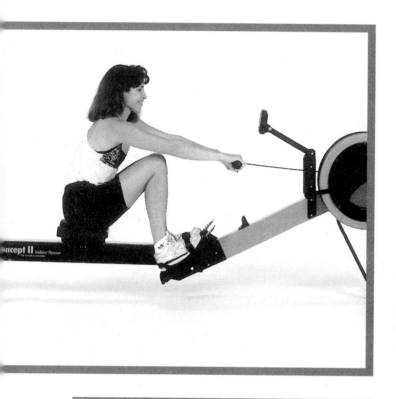

A rowing machine is nothing more than a stripped-down contraption designed to simulate the action of pulling yourself and a small watercraft along the surface of flat water—all in the comfort of your own home. Outdoor rowing burns nearly as many calories as weight-bearing exercises such as cross-country skiing. Rowing indoors, on your own terms, is a great way to whip your belly, butt, and thighs into top-notch shape.

Further, if your upper body yearns for something to do while you're working your belly, butt, and thighs, then rowing is for you, says J. Zack Barksdale, an exercise physiologist at the Cooper Aerobics Center in Dallas. It's a great high-intensity workout that uses virtually all of your muscles in a flowing sequence. Because rowing is not weight-bearing, it's also a great way for women with troublesome knees or weak ankles to work out, since rowing doesn't stress the leg joints.

"Rowing is a great workout for someone who wants to lose weight," notes Barksdale. "It really builds up your aerobic power, which means you'll burn a lot of calories when you do it."

Rowing Stats

Calories Burned*	Body-Shaping Potential
240 to 360 per half-hour	Tones the entire body, especially the muscles of the thighs, buttocks, abdominals, back, and arms

*Based on a 150-pound woman. If you weigh more, you'll burn more calories; if you weigh less, you'll burn fewer.

Body-Shaping Benefits

Here's what you can expect when you row regularly.

- You'll burn calories galore, because you're using all four limbs while your heart works—which uses up more calories than lower-body exercise alone, says Barksdale.
- You'll develop strong, toned abdominals, because you'll contract your abdominal muscles when you're rowing. When you contract your abdominal muscles consistently, they get stronger. When a woman's muscles get stronger, they get toned and develop more shape, even though they don't get bigger. Your legs and butt do a tremendous amount of work, so they also grow lean and strong.

■ As a bonus, you'll tone and strengthen your upper arms, an added trouble spot for many women as they reach midlife.

Psychological Benefits

Rowing leaves you with more energy and generates good-mood endorphins (brain chemicals that cause relaxation and euphoria). If you're a loner and don't care for aerobics classes or other forms of group exercise, rowing lets you work out on your own time, at your own pace, at home or in a gym.

If you love to be around other people—and crave competition—take an indoor rowing class (where everyone in the class rows her own machine, but the instructor plays group leader), suggests Holly Metcalf, president and founder of Row as One Institute, a rowing school and camp for women lo-

cated in South Hadley, Massachusetts. Call your local gym and ask if they conduct rowing classes. You'll get good rowing instruction and improve your skills and endurance while breaking up the monotony.

The Right Footwear

For all practical purposes, most women who want to row for exercise just buy rowing machines and put them to work in their living rooms, basements, or other workout space. That doesn't mean you should row in just any footwear. Wear low-cut sneakers to allow range of motion in your ankles, says Metcalf. She also recommends wearing tights and an exercise top. "Loose clothes, such as shorts and T-shirts, can get caught in the machine and won't allow you to move as smoothly."

Take It to the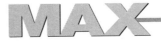

The Ultimate Rowing Workout

Most women who row to lose weight are content to scull at a gym or at home. Holly Metcalf isn't one of them. Metcalf rowed on Olympic and national teams from 1981 to 1987 and was part of a gold-medal winning team in 1984. For women who want to take rowing to the max, team rowing on the water is the ultimate workout.

"Women rowers love how their whole bodies feel strong, and that feeling is multiplied when you're on a rowing team," says Metcalf. "You feel everyone's strength working together. It's the sum of your power that makes the difference."

Join a women's rowing team. If rowing inspires you to take to the water, Metcalf suggests that you call a local college or high school to see if they have a rowing coach. He or she will probably know of a women's masters team (geared toward women in their forties or older) in your area—assuming you live near a major lake or river. This is a major commit-

ment: Most teams practice either during the early morning or early evening. How often depends on their training and racing schedule. But it's practically guaranteed to help you get in shape.

"An eight-person boat weighs about 250 pounds, while smaller boats weigh considerably less," says Metcalf. "So teamwork is involved not just in the rowing, but in carrying and caring for the boat." Hauling a heavy boat from the boathouse to the water not only adds to the teamwork involved but also acts as an added strength-training workout.

Learn the lingo. If you join a rowing team, you'll need to learn the words familiar to the other rowers. For example, *coxswain*, which is pronounced "cox-in." She's the leader of the team who sits on the front of the boat and doesn't row, but shouts orders to the rest of the team. You'll get to understand terms such as *back it down* (row backward) and *let it run* (stop rowing).

What Else You'll Need

If you're like a lot of women, chances are you—or someone in your family—already have an indoor rower stashed somewhere in the garage or basement. If it's more than a couple of years old, you may want to consider buying new equipment or using a rower at a gym or fitness club, says Barksdale. Check to make sure that your older rower has not become creaky or damaged over the years. If so, it may need a little oil to return to working order, he adds.

Unless your shoulders are very strong, you may be better off not using an older rower at all. Many rowers made in the 1980s feature two "oars" that move independently of one another (rather than a pulley), along with piston-driven resistance. Both features can make rowing potentially stressful on the shoulders and rotator cuffs, Barksdale cautions.

Here's what to look for.

Sturdy equipment with an ample seat and adjustable foot pads. The only parts of your body that touch the rower are your hands, feet, and backside. The foot pads should be easy to adjust for foot size. And when you row, the equipment should remain steady and secure on the floor.

If you're big-bottomed, pay special attention to how you fit in the saddle. Your backside must fit comfortably in the seat. Also, a big tummy may interfere with your range of motion and force you to hold your legs out to your sides, causing stress on the ligaments of your knees. Or you may round your back while rowing, which could potentially lead to back problems. If you have quite a bit of weight to lose, you may have to wait until your tummy and backside shrink to work rowing into your shape-up program, says Barksdale. If you're very overweight, you could also consider starting on a recumbent, he says.

Air or water resistance. Both air and water resistance give a smoother ride than the older piston-resistance machines, and they more closely simulate the outdoor rowing experience. The WaterRower actually uses a water flywheel for resistance, so it very closely simulates outdoor rowing on water. The water level can be adjusted to increase or decrease the resistance. The rhythm and adjustable wind resistance of the Concept II (found in most gyms) also mimic the feeling of river rowing. Both models are available through mail order.

Space. Indoor rowers are long—at least six feet. So if you're buying equipment, you'll need to make sure that you have enough room for it at home.

Getting Started

Done properly, rowing is a fluid, full-body motion. Your hands grasp the bar with an overhand grip while your feet are in foot pads and your butt is in a seat. The seat glides along a track as your legs flex and extend. Your arms rhythmically straighten and bend as you propel yourself through the rowing motion.

That said, rowing looks easier than it is, notes Barksdale. Even with the seat properly adjusted, rowing requires good posture and a lot of flexibility. To avoid any possible stress to your muscles or knees, warm up for a few minutes before starting to row, and make sure that your knees do not bend to an angle less than 90 degrees, he adds. Stretch your leg muscles, especially your hamstrings, before you get on your rowing machine.

As you begin to row, move backward. Your arms should be at a 90-degree angle with your body, and your shoulder blades should move backward and toward each other. As you glide forward, your arms should straighten as far as the rope or chain will allow. Take time to row properly. And if you're prone to lower-back problems, be sure to have someone teach you proper form on a rower before you begin your exercise program.

Here's a step-by-step guide.

The catch. This is the first movement of the series and begins with you sitting close to the front of the rower. Your hands hold the bar, your arms are straight, and you are leaning slightly forward. Your knees should be bent at a 90-degree angle, and your shins are perpendicular to the floor.

The drive. With this motion, you begin to go backward. Your legs straighten, and as your hands pass above your knees, your torso begins to move back and your arms begin to bend.

The finish. Bend your elbows and bring the bar toward your abdomen. (Straighten your legs without locking your knees.)

The recovery and preparation. To return to the catch and resume the pattern, stretch and straighten your arms and pivot on your hips. Now, let your knees slowly come up and bend to a 90-degree angle as you glide back toward the front of the rower.

What Not to Do

With rowing, what you shouldn't do is as important as what you should do.

Don't lock your knees or your elbows when you're at either end of the stroke, says Barksdale.

Although your legs and arms will be "straight," you can protect your joints by keeping them loose, relaxed, and slightly flexed.

Use your back and legs equally, rather than focusing on the pulling motion of your upper body. "Your arms and legs should move in a rhythmic, flowing motion as part of the equipment," Barksdale explains.

Finally, don't give up. Learning how to row properly takes a long time, says Metcalf. "Rowing appeals to people who like both mental and physical challenge," she notes. "In the beginning, you'll push yourself mentally because you have to learn proper form and technique. The physical challenge of a tough workout will come later on."

Rowing Workouts

Beginner

Row for 20 minutes at least twice a week. Keep the resistance light, but not so light that momentum moves you.

Intermediate

Row hard for 30 seconds, then easy for 30 seconds. Try to do 20 to 40 minutes at least 3 times a week.

Experienced

If you are rowing at this advanced level, warm up for 5 to 10 minutes, then keep a steady, high-intensity pace going for 40 to 60 minutes. Do not bend your knees past a 90-degree angle. Cool down. Repeat 4 or 5 days a week.

Many rowing machines come complete with a digital readout of distance traveled, time elapsed, and calories used so that you can track your progress and intensity level. Heart rate monitors are also available with some models. Machines can also be programmed to time your rest and work time if you want to do interval training.

"When you first start rowing, don't try to go as fast as possible," says J. Zack Barksdale, an exercise physiologist at the Cooper Aerobics Center in Dallas. "You'll tire out too quickly and not burn as much fat as you probably want to. Instead, warm up on a stationary cycle, then come over to the rowing machine and go at a moderate pace for 20 minutes, if you can." Going longer, rather than fast, will burn more fat.

Once you get used to the rower, try to increase your intensity for 30 seconds at a time, then back off for 30 seconds. At first, you'll be able to repeat this for only 20 minutes (if that), says Barksdale. But eventually, you can try to work your way up to a longer workout of 40 minutes or so. Be sure to warm up for 5 minutes and stretch your hamstrings and lower back before you row. Cool down for 5 to 10 minutes after rowing. Once your heart rate drops below 90 beats per minute, it is safe for you to stop completely. Barksdale suggests using a treadmill or stationary cycle for your warmup.

Finally, you'll be ready to keep the pace going longer. Aim for a high-intensity workout of 40 to 60 minutes. Again, make sure that you warm up and cool down at either end of the workout.

Spinning

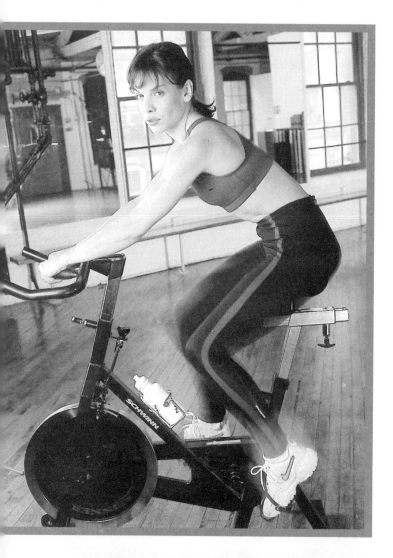

Also known as studio cycling, Spinning is basically road cycling brought indoors. It's done on a specially designed workout bike and is set to music or a series of visualizations.

Even if you tried stationary cycling and hated it, you'll love Spinning. For one thing, it simulates riding a bike more than stationary cycling does. A Spinning bike has a weighted wheel, called a flywheel, which picks up speed when you pedal, so you feel as if you're actually going down (or up) hills, or just riding along a country road. You can also stand on a Spin bike in order to climb the "hills" with more power (and thus change the muscles you're working in your legs). Finally, Spinning is a group activity. A certified Spinning instructor leads your ride—sometimes using visualization, sometimes utilizing speedwork, and sometimes combining every move you can do, making for some of the most intense—and addictive—workouts most women have ever experienced, says Ron Crawford, a certified Spinning instructor from Niles, Ohio, and president of World of Fitness, which operates two fitness facilities.

Body-Shaping Benefits

Here's what you can expect when you spin regularly.

- You'll burn 600 to 800 calories an hour—about as much as rowing on a machine at race pace.
- You'll tone your entire lower body, especially your butt and the front of your thighs.
- If you do a lot of standing and sitting intervals (known as jumps), you'll strengthen your abdominal muscles.

Psychological Benefits

Spinning is a true mind-body experience. The instructor will choose from a variety of "rides," each of which will add to your mental pleasure in

Spinning Stats

Calories Burned*	Body-Shaping Potential
About 535 per 45-minute class	Trims your butt and thighs, tones your abdominal muscles

*Based on a 150-pound woman. If you weigh more, you'll burn more calories; if you weigh less, you'll burn fewer.

a specific way. For example, some Spinning instructors lead their students through imaginary trips through the south of France or down the coast of California. Others lead you through intervals that simulate a road race. And others simply have you close your eyes and stay in touch with the way your body feels as you pedal through a variety of intensities and positions.

"It's almost a Zen experience," says Deborah Gallagher, a certified personal trainer and certified Spinning instructor in Vacaville, California. "You're moving in a repetitive fashion along with the music, but you don't have to worry about coordination. When I look at my students, I see joy on their faces."

The Right Footwear

Like the pedals on traditional racing bikes, Spinning bike pedals consist of a "cage," which holds your sneakered foot steady, and a "lock" for bike shoes. "Locking your foot into the pedal helps you move your legs more smoothly," explains Crawford. "But not everyone likes the feel of bike shoes." Most bike pedal manufacturers have a universal lock, which means that most bike shoes will fit into any bike pedal, Spinning or otherwise.

What Else You'll Need

Very few people purchase their own Spinning bikes because so much of the sport's appeal is its group atmosphere. So chances are you'll join a class. If you do, here's what Gallagher suggests you bring along.

Water. Spinning bikes include built-in water-bottle holders for a very good reason—you're going to need to stay hydrated during the class. Most of the holders will fit a small bottle of water—preferably one with a pop-up spout, so you don't have to interrupt your ride to open up your bottle.

A towel. You'll need a small hand towel, not only to sop up the sweat from your forehead, but also to wipe down your bike before someone else gets ready to use it.

Bike shorts (maybe). Like riding any bike, Spinning can irritate a tender tush (or other sensitive spots). "Bike shorts have extra padding in the butt to cushion you," says Gallagher. "They're available at most sporting goods stores."

A gel seat. Some gyms provide bike seats filled with gel, while others expect you to bring your own. "Available at sporting goods stores, gel seats have a lot more give than a traditional bike seat," notes Gallagher. "Some people prefer gel seats to bike shorts—especially if you don't look great in close-fitting shorts or can't find them in your size."

Getting Started

Yes, Spinning is a tough aerobic and lower-body workout. But as with all exercises, you have to start slowly and progress gradually.

Take a beginner class. "Most gyms offer a 'Begin to Spin' class for rookies," says Crawford. "The instructor will show you how to adjust your bike so that you're safe and comfortable as you ride." The bike needs to be adjusted for your height. If the seat is too low or the pedal tension is too high, for example, you may experience knee pain.

Begin to Spin classes are not as intense as intermediate or advanced Spinning workouts, and the instructors will explain directives used in class, such as "continue cadence" and "lighten up." They'll also check on your form, either by walking around or as they Spin. Most gyms have mirrored walls, so you can check out your form as you go, too.

The five basic Spinning moves include:

Seated flat. This is the basic sitting position on the bike. You'll use this for warmup, cooldown, and speedwork.

Seated hill. This is pretty much the same position as the seated flat, but when you increase the resistance of the flywheel, your butt will slide back a little bit in order to give your legs more power to pedal. Try to keep your upper body relaxed and, most important, don't jam the pedals on the downstroke. Your leg motion should remain fluid even though you're working hard.

Standing hill. Once the resistance forces you to incorporate more leg power, you'll naturally want to stand up. Your pedaling will slow down, but your legs will work very hard and you'll feel the resistance of the bike. Not only will this burn lots of calories, but it will really work the muscles of your legs and butt.

Running. It's not really running, but your legs will be moving quickly. In a standing position, you'll decrease the resistance on the flywheel, move your legs and torso slightly ahead of the seat, and with less resistance than you use when on a standing hill, push the pedals as quickly as possible, without losing control of the bike. Spinners usually "run" after a good warmup to increase their heart rates and get to the next level of exertion.

Jumping. This is not really jumping, but it is a very high intensity move. Keeping the bike at a fairly high and consistent resistance level, you'll do some interval work. Without changing your pedaling rhythm, or cadence, you'll stand up for a measured amount of time, then sit down for the same amount of time. You have to make sure that you're not throwing your weight forward or pushing your legs down hard; the motion should be smooth and fluid. Some instructors change the length of the intervals from four counts to another number.

Vary your hand positions. Since Spinning simulates actual road riding, your hand positions will also vary, depending on the ride, says Gallagher.

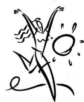

She Did It!

Spinning Classes Helped Denise Get Back into a Size 8

Denise Carissimo, director of admissions at Trumbull Business College in Warren, Ohio, was starting to feel stagnant in her life. At just 34 years old, the single mother of a nine-year-old son felt as if she had peaked. Plus, she was gaining weight—and getting bottom heavy.

"I normally wore a size 8," says Denise. "But I was stuffing myself into my size 10 clothes. I really should have been wearing a 12. And I just felt like it was time to make a change."

Denise headed over to the gym with the best of intentions. "I spent 30 minutes at a time on the stairclimber and treadmill, but it was boring and nothing was changing," she says.

Then she tried her first Spin class.

"I was addicted immediately," Denise says. "I began Spinning three times a week for 40 minutes each. The intensity level was great. It made me feel so alive and excited. Having a variety of instructors

with different personalities and tastes in music helped me to stay motivated. And even though I didn't change the way I was eating, I was dropping inches like crazy!"

Denise noticed the difference within two to three months. "My bottom half is trimmed down and I feel better. My waist is tiny. Even my calves look slimmer."

Those inches made all the difference in the way Denise's clothes fit. She began to comfortably wear her old size 8 clothing again. "I still weigh the same amount, but you would never know it from the way I look.

"I feel all of Spinning's benefits not only in my body, but in my personality, too," Denise says. Instead of going out on the town, she prefers Spinning. "Spinning is a social activity," she notes. Denise has made lots of new friends in her classes, including two women who have each lost more than 100 pounds.

Close together. Used when you're seated, your hands are next to each other, not grasping the handlebars too tightly. Your elbows and shoulders are always relaxed, with your knuckles slightly higher than your wrists. Your elbows should flare out a little bit.

Wider apart. Used for seated climbing and jumping, your hands are slightly separated and relaxed. Don't hold the handlebars too tightly.

On the ends of the handlebars. Used only for standing climbing, your hands are at the outermost edges of the handlebars, with your knuckles facing out and your fingers wrapped around the bar. "This is the position used when you're out riding your bike with others and you're trying to catch up with them," says Gallagher.

Aim for balance between speed (how fast you pedal) and resistance (how hard it is to pedal). You want to keep some resistance on the flywheel; otherwise, it will feel as if your legs are moving out of control.

Ride for yourself. Although Spinning is a group activity, there is absolutely no competition. "No one can tell at what resistance level you're riding," says Crawford. "And no one will force you to stand when everyone else is standing or to jump if everyone else is jumping." Tune in to the experience of how the ride feels for you, he says, not how you're doing in relation to anyone else in the class.

Spinning Workouts

Beginner

Take Begin to Spin classes twice a week, with no jumping allowed. Keep this schedule consistent for 4 to 6 weeks.

Intermediate

Move on to 3 classes per week. To work your legs, work out at a slightly higher pedaling speed.

Experienced

After 2 to 3 months of steady riding (3 times a week), you're ready for the big time: Include jumping and other intense moves like sprinting (high speed pedaling at light to moderate resistance, as though you're hurrying to finish a race).

Even beginner Spinning is intense. You need to take it slow in order to build up your speed, stamina, and endurance carefully, notes Deborah Gallagher, a certified personal trainer and certified Spinning instructor in Vacaville, California. "It takes three to four weeks before you begin to notice a buildup in the muscles and connective tissues in your legs. While you can do all kinds of rides, it's important to take it slow and not rush through all your different positions."

You can't necessarily anticipate what kind of rides an instructor will offer, says Gallagher. But in general, a beginner should stay at low levels of resistance and take the time to get used to the variety of instructors and rides available—seated flat, seated hills, standing hills, running, and jumping.

And remember—no competition!

Stationary Cycling

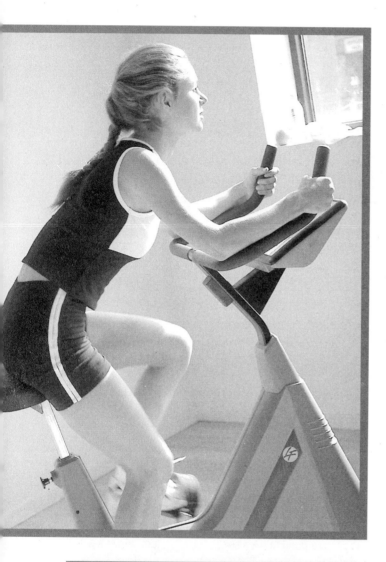

Stationary Cycling Stats

Calories Burned*	Body-Shaping Potential
130 to 330 per half-hour	Tones your leg and butt muscles

*Based on a 150-pound woman. If you weigh more, you'll burn more calories; if you weigh less, you'll burn fewer.

Look under the laundry piled up in the corners of 35 million American bedrooms, and you'll find a stationary cycle. This "used once, then forgotten" machine may make it seem as if exercise bikes have some inherent flaw. But that's not true. People just expect too much, psychologically, from their home workouts, says Edmund Burke, Ph.D., professor of exercise science at the University of Colorado in Colorado Springs and author of the *Complete Home Fitness Handbook.*

"Indoor exercise can lead to boredom," Dr. Burke says. "Either you have to plan to do other things while you're exercising, such as watching TV or listening to music, or you have to use your stationary cycle as an adjunct to another activity."

In other words, don't rely on stationary cycling as your sole means of slimming down and shaping up. Rather, think of your bike as an accessory in the wardrobe of your exercise plan—a once or twice a week "easy workout" to complement walking or doing aerobics regularly. Then your exercise bike is less likely to end up as a clothing rack.

Body-Shaping Benefits

Here's what you can expect when you use a stationary cycle regularly.

- You'll burn about five calories every minute while you exercise. That's a lot more than the usual one calorie per minute that you burn when you're doing other daily activities.

- You'll develop and strengthen the gluteal muscles in your buttocks, the quadriceps at the front of your thighs, and the hamstrings in the back of your thighs.

- There's no impact from your upper-body weight, so you can tone your butt and thigh muscles without putting any stress on your leg joints.

Psychological Benefits

Oblivion is one of the pleasures of stationary bicycling. It's absolutely safe—no wild drivers winging past as you pedal in the quiet of your home, and no risk of hitting a stone and flying head over heels into the gravelly road. So what you choose or don't choose to do with your consciousness while you're pedaling is entirely up to you.

Among your options: Set the bike in front of the TV, and you can lose yourself in a scenic video or, for that matter, watch your favorite movie. Switch on CNN and catch up with the news or lose yourself in a soap opera while your feet spin. Whether you watch fast sports or slow drama, you can be burning the calories and toning your muscles at a steady rate. And, of course, you always

She Did It!

Nancy Discovered the Permanent Route to Weight Loss

Nancy Allen's father died when she was 37. The loss hurt—as she knew it would. So much, in fact, that it seemed as though she stopped doing anything for a while.

"My dad died around Christmas 1995, and I just became a lump for about four months," she says. "Because I was getting older, this change of pace led to a pretty fast weight gain. I'm only five feet three inches tall, and I ended up being somewhere around a size 12."

After four months of inactivity, Nancy, of Chickamauga, Georgia, decided she'd had enough with languishing on the couch. On April 4, 1996—she remembers the exact date—she started exercising on the recumbent stationary bike that had been sitting in the corner of her living room for some time.

The months of inactivity had taken their toll, however. "I could only do about three minutes," she recalls. But when she got off, the impact of that little spurt of exercise surprised her. "I felt so much better!"

Within about a week, Nancy was pedaling up to 5 minutes every day. From there, she advanced rapidly until she could do about 15 minutes daily. Four years later, at the age of 41, Nancy was still doing a steady routine of 30 to 45 minutes daily.

"My target heart rate is 23 beats per 10 seconds. I'm usually puffing pretty hard," she says.

And the payoff was visible. Nancy went from a size 12 to a size 5. "My waist was somewhere around 33 to 34 inches, and now it is 26 inches," she says. "I have no saddlebags anymore, and my butt is gravity-defying."

Despite the heavy breathing, Nancy is able to do other things while she's on the bike. "I read or watch TV," she says. "Sometimes I even knit or crochet, but I have to stop when my hands get sweaty."

The stationary bike wasn't an end in itself. Once she felt comfortable with regular cycling, Nancy moved on to another important body-shaping exercise—weight lifting. After lifting at home for a while, she and her husband decided to join the Y. Now, two or three times a week, they attend 30-minute weight-lifting sessions there. "This, coupled with the recumbent cycling I do at home on alternate days, helps me to maintain those goals I have achieved," explains Nancy.

She credits the almost-forgotten stationary cycle and the human spirit that just wouldn't quit with starting it all. "All the equipment in the world won't help without the determination to use it," she adds.

Take It to the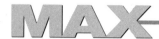

Bring Power to Your Pedal

With a little imagination, you can crank up your stationary cycling experience and keep from succumbing to boredom, says Cyndi Ford, an exercise physiologist at the Cooper Institute for Aerobics Research in Dallas. Here are two ways.

Ride the Tour de France in your living room. A number of companies sell bike ride videos that you can watch while you are exercising. You can tour the south of France or national parks while you pedal or even take part in famous road races. These tapes are often available wherever exercise videos are sold.

Count your miles. While novice riders simply let their bikes tell them how many revolutions per minute (rpm) they are doing, you can also track the total number of miles you ride. To chart your progress, time yourself over a "distance" of 10 miles. Keeping the resistance at the same level, ride those 10 miles again the next time you work out—and see if you can beat your previous time.

have the option of placing a book or magazine on the front of the cycle if you prefer to read.

"I've found that most people use stationary cycles as a mental break from other forms of exercise, because you get a good workout, but it doesn't put a lot of physical strain on your body, and you don't need a lot of skill to do it," says Dr. Burke.

What You'll Need

A good, new home bike costs a minimum of $350. But if that's more than you would like to pay, post a notice or ad for used bikes and see what kind of response you get. You may be able to get a used bike for much less than a similar new model.

Whatever you do, be sure to sit on the bike and pedal for a while to see how comfortable it is for you. "Wear your gym clothes, including your sneakers," Dr. Burke says. "If it doesn't feel right, try another model."

Whether you're buying new or used, here's what to consider.

Upright or recumbent. Traditional upright bikes aren't designed for women and overweight people, in general, because the seats aren't wide enough. And an upright can spell torture if you have lower-back pain. Before you write a check, be sure to try out a recumbent bike, which has a bucket-shaped seat that supports your back. Or you might like something in-between the upright and fully laid-back model, called a semirecumbent.

The right fit. First of all, you should be able to sit up straight on the bike even when you are pedaling full speed. This isn't a bike for the Tour de France, where you have to crouch over the handlebars and look like a flying bullet. If you need to hunch over to reach the handlebars, then the bike isn't the right size for you.

Adjustability. No bike is made-to-order, so you need to be able to make adjustments, says Cyndi Ford, an exercise physiologist at the Cooper Institute for Aerobics Research in Dallas. When you're trying out the bike, make sure that you can move the seat up or down to the right position. When you're seated on an upright bike, your hips should be square on the saddle. At the bottom of the downstroke, with your foot rested firmly on the lower pedal, the extended leg should be slightly bent at the knee. Also, look straight down and see whether you can see the toes of your foot below the knee. If you cannot see your toes, then you are too far forward. Sitting too far forward puts enormous stress on the kneecap. After you have made all the necessary seat adjustments, then see whether the handlebars are still at a comfortable level. If not, adjust them, too.

The same criteria apply to a recumbent bike. You should be able to move the seat forward or back, up or down. When it is in the correct position, your extended leg should be slightly bent at the knee.

A gel seat. Though you may think your hips and butt are well-padded, an ordinary bicycle seat can feel like an abrasive torture device after many miles of spinning. If you're getting a brand-new bike, ask the salesperson if you can have a softer gel seat instead of the standard-issue seat. If you're getting a used bike, you can still find a gel seat at most bicycle or exercise equipment stores.

Upper-body exercise handles. Rather than having normal stationary handlebars, some bikes have handles that you can push and pull, so you'll get some upper-body exercise while your lower limbs are also going full steam ahead. You might enjoy the extra upper-body flex, but movable han-

Stationary Cycling Workouts

Beginner

Progressive intervals. Over a 22-minute period, intersperse slow-paced, low-intensity riding with short, higher-intensity spurts. Ride at a slow pace and low intensity for 5 minutes, then pedal for 30 seconds at higher intensity. Keep alternating, but end up with some slow pedaling to cool down.

Intermediate

Pyramid workout. Ride for 10 minutes at high intensity, then follow with 2 minutes of low-intensity riding. Then do 8 minutes at a level of intensity that's even higher than the first 10 minutes—followed by another 2-minute, low-intensity interlude. Each increasingly harder interval should be 2 minutes shorter than the one before, but keep on increasing the intensity—and always insert a 2-minute interval to cool down. The whole routine should take about 40 minutes. Then give yourself some slow pedaling at the end to finish off.

Experienced

Hill training. If you want to test your maximum capacity, plan on riding for a certain amount of time—say, 40 minutes—and use progressively higher resistance throughout the ride. Increase the resistance every 3 to 4 minutes to increase the intensity of your workout. When you are halfway through the session, decrease the resistance at regular intervals over the same amount of time.

If your electronic bike has an electronic-display program, you have the option of sticking to the program that is displayed. But as an alternative, you might design your own program instead, focusing on resistance (or intensity), heart rate, speed, duration, or cadence (the rhythm at which you pedal).

"Once you have a base workout and you're riding two or three days a week, then you can begin to play around with the intensity and the amount of time you stay on the bike," says Cyndi Ford, an exercise physiologist at the Cooper Institute for Aerobics Research in Dallas. She says the best plan—for both calorie burning and body shaping—is a blend of sprint work with strength work.

These two types of workouts actually help you hone different muscle fibers. The sprint work—going fast at a low intensity—helps you work on what are called fast-twitch muscle fibers. The strength work—going slow at a high intensity—builds the slow-twitch fibers. If you mix and match the type of workout and the intensity, you will use a greater number of muscle fibers in different ways, which is more effective than doing the same exercises over and over again.

dles don't increase calorie burning very much. And they are an extra expense. So if you don't think you'll use that feature, skip it and stick to the pedal-only version.

Resistance. On some stationary bikes, resistance is created by a brake pad applying steady pressure. Others use electromagnetic resistance or a flywheel. The type of resistance might affect the feel of the bike, but otherwise, there is no particular advantage to any of them. You do want to be able to adjust the resistance so that you can vary the intensity of your workouts.

Electronics. Some bikes have elaborate programs—along with heart-rate monitors and other devices—to help you measure many different variables. With some, you can race against a computerized competitor. If you like these features and they keep you more challenged, you might want to opt for them. But they don't affect the operation of the bike or the slimming and trimming benefits you get from it.

Some other useful hints:

Padded bike shorts. The shorts worn by bicyclists have a built-in chafing-prevention device. It's called extra padding. Strategically sewn into the crotch and inner-thigh region, the padding can make indoor as well as outdoor riding more comfortable.

Repairs. Find out how, and where, you can get the bike fixed if something goes wrong. When equipment breaks, workouts come to a standstill.

Getting Started

On a stationary bike, there are a number of variables—speed, time, intensity, and resistance.

Here's how to get them to balance out and keep the challenges reasonable rather than reckless, says Ford.

Think tempo. Your workout pedaling speed will be affected by the resistance. When the bike is set to the right resistance, you should be able to keep a cadence, or rhythm, that is smooth and measured. If the resistance is too great, you'll find yourself pumping your legs to gather momentum for the next turn. If it's set too lightly, you'll find yourself pushing and pulling the handlebars, probably with an uneven cadence. The way you pedal should mimic the way you walk when you're striding along at a good pace—a measured and consistent tempo.

Stretch the time, not the heart. When you're starting out on an exercise bike, you need to let your legs and heart get used to the pace of exercise. At this stage, it is better to work out for a longer period of time at a low intensity for a few weeks rather than a short period at a high intensity. This will give your heart time to get used to your workouts.

Try some bursts. When you're able to cycle for 20 to 30 minutes at low to moderate intensity, you can try some short bursts at a higher intensity. But don't lose the cadence when you do that. You need to make increases that don't force you to pump too hard or spin too fast.

Vary the resistance. When your feet are spinning and your heart is pumping, your legs may actually be the first to cry "uncle!" In general, most people's leg muscles are weaker than their hearts. If your legs start to feel heavy or sore but you aren't breathing hard, decrease the resistance.

Step Aerobics

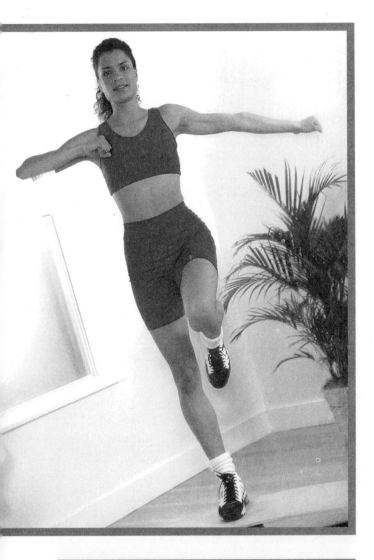

A high-intensity, low-impact movement choreographed on and around an adjustable platform, step aerobics was born in the late 1980s. During a step aerobic workout, you'll step on, over, and around a bench, all in time to heart-pumping music. It's one of the few exercise fads that has become a fitness staple.

You don't have to be highly coordinated to do step aerobics (although the more proficient you become, the easier the choreography is), says Gin Miller, the inventor of step aerobics, creator of Step Reebok, and star of Reebok Step Training videos, in Canton, Georgia. And you don't have to perform step aerobics at a gym. You can buy a step bench and various step videos in sporting goods stores and catalogs, making step aerobics one of the least expensive—and most effective—at-home workouts you can try.

Body-Shaping Benefits

Here's what you can expect when you do step aerobics regularly.

- You will burn lots of fat, since step aerobics is a high-intensity exercise.
- You'll tone and shape the muscles in your lower body, especially your butt, thighs, and calves.
- If you concentrate on keeping your abdominals contracted while you step, you'll tone and strengthen your abdominal muscles.

Psychological Benefits

Like other aerobic exercise, step aerobics will improve your mood as well as your ability to think creatively.

"As a bonus, step aerobics can also help women who feel klutzy get over their fears of choreography or footwork," says Miller. "It doesn't require as much coordination as dancing, yet you're still exercising to music and using some low-impact dance moves."

Step Aerobics Stats

Calories Burned*	Body-Shaping Potential
Approximately 300 per half-hour using a six-inch step	Works the entire lower body—hips, thighs, and buttocks

*Based on a 150-pound woman. If you weigh more, you'll burn more calories; if you weigh less, you'll burn fewer.

The Right Footwear

You'll want support while you do your step aerobics routine, so a good pair of aerobic shoes is your best bet. Look for flexible shoes that have plenty of cushioning and arch support on the bottom, recommends Tamilee Webb, the choreographer of numerous step videos and author of *The Step Up Fitness Workout*, who lives in San Diego, California. Some women prefer higher-cut shoes that give their ankles extra support.

What Else You'll Need

Once you've laced up your shoes, you'll need a step bench, a low and wide platform with grad-uated risers, so you can increase step height as you become more experienced at step aerobics. Some risers are attached to the step and simply fold under it when you want to change the step height.

Here's what to look for in a step bench, according to Webb.

Sturdy construction. Because you'll be stepping up and down on the bench, it should feel as solid as any step you would climb in your house. Likewise, any risers that come with the step should also be solid and not wobble at all as you go up and down the bench.

A step that is wide and long enough. You need plenty of room for both of your feet on the

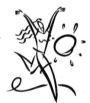

She Did It!

Beth Burned Off 25 Pounds with Step Aerobics

Beth Mendelson, age 41, loves her three boys—she would do anything for them. What she doesn't like is *looking* like somebody's mom. Step aerobics changed all that.

The turning point was when Beth, a homemaker from Silver Spring, Maryland, went to a restaurant with some friends. As they passed through the bar, "none of the men looked at me at all," she says. "I was 35 at the time, but I looked a lot older."

At five feet one inch and 140 pounds, Beth decided to do something for herself. "I had always been intimidated by traditional aerobics classes because I felt klutzy," she says. "But I figured I'd be okay exercising in my own home. So I went to the library and rented some regular aerobics tapes. But I still didn't like aerobics."

Then someone loaned Beth a step bench and step aerobics tape. "I loved it!" she says. "It was easy for me to build my confidence. For some reason—because the music is slower—my feet and brain work better with step than with aerobics."

Beth started with a beginner tape by Kathy Smith and then went on to Gin Miller's Reebok series. She loves tapes by Cathe Friedrich, one of the toughest instructors around. "I've found that I'm always able to pick up the choreography after using one tape just a few times," Beth says. "When I get a new tape, I really have to concentrate when I first use it; as I become more comfortable with it, I'm able to focus more on giving my body a tough workout instead of memorizing the new moves. I do some of my best thinking when I'm using some of the tapes I'm most comfortable with."

Step aerobics has really paid off for Beth. She now weighs about 115 pounds. "My thighs are slimmer, firmer, and much more muscular," she notes. "But, more than that, I feel like I look good now. I absolutely don't think I look my age."

Take It to the 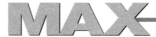 MAX

Basic Step Is Just the Beginning

Thanks to enthusiastic and creative instructors, step aerobics has become wildly popular among women. Once you become comfortable using beginner tapes at home and start to get in shape, you may want to consider stepping into an aerobics class or ratcheting up your home routine.

Instructors Gin Miller, the inventor of step aerobics, creator of Step Reebok, and star of Reebok Step Training videos in Canton, Georgia, and Tamilee Webb, the choreographer of numerous step videos and author of *The Step Up Fitness Workout*, who lives in San Diego, California, offer these suggestions.

Add some weight training. Some step instructors use both free weights and tubing after they have finished the step segment to work resistance training into their workout routines. These extra resistance workouts not only help you burn more calories but also allow you to target the areas you want to tone the most, including your upper body.

Create your own workout. Think you have all the step possibilities down pat? Then crank up your stereo and choreograph your own workout, using a combination of low-, moderate-, and high-intensity moves.

Low-intensity moves include the basic step (up-up, down-down), knee lift (up-knee, down-down/up-knee, down-down), and over-the-top (where you travel over the top of the step to the other side). *Moderate-intensity* moves are traveling movements (moving from side to side on the bench) and repeaters (standing with one foot on the bench and repeatedly bringing the other knee up). *High-intensity* moves may include lunges or any move that includes propulsion, such as leaps, hops, runs, and jumps. Make sure you perform the airborne movements on the up accent only, cautions Miller.

Pick the right music. While it's fine to use your favorite tunes to work out, you don't want to try to move to music that is too fast. Step aerobic music is not as fast as traditional aerobic music. Ideally, you're looking for a song with about 2 beats per second, or 120 beats per minute. But if you don't want to count beats, simply notice how you're feeling and moving during your workout. If you're tripping while you exercise, the music is simply too fast for stepping.

bench. Some choreography won't work with a narrow step, so if the step bench is too narrow, it's not a good buy. You should also be able to take at least one step out to the side while you're on the bench. The ideal step is two feet wide and three feet long. You can buy shorter (and cheaper) step benches, but the longer and wider the bench is, the more intense you'll be able to make your workouts.

Getting Started

Step aerobics is a high-intensity exercise, so you'll want to begin your workout routine slowly. Experts recommend videotapes specifically geared toward beginners (such as those offered by instructors such as Gin Miller, Tamilee Webb, or Kathy Smith, for example).

Once you select a tape, here's how to use it.

Take baby steps. The basic step pattern goes "up-up, down-down," up with the right foot, up with the left foot, down with the right foot, down with the left foot. "It's just like the way a child first learns to climb a staircase," says Webb. "The most important thing to remember is that you have to place your whole foot on the step, not just your toes and not just the ball of your foot."

At first, you'll have to look to make sure your foot is in proper position. Eventually, you'll get a feel for where you're stepping, and you can look ahead, not down, and follow the tape or instructor.

First, master the legs, then add your arms. When you're first learning to perform step aerobics, don't worry about moving your arms, even if the instructor on the workout tape is mixing her arms into the patterns. Instead, concentrate on getting the foot patterns down and feeling comfortable using the platform, says Miller. When you're ready, begin to incorporate the arm movements into your routine. Continuous arm movements increase your heart rate, and thus the number of calories you burn, by up to 10 percent.

Forget the hand weights. Hand weights can limit movement, and they can also cause pain and fatigue in your shoulders when used for long periods of time, cautions Webb.

Limit yourself to no more than four step workouts a week. Studies have shown that doing step aerobics more than four times a week markedly increases the chance of injury. So be happy that it's a high-intensity workout that will burn tons of calories in a very short amount of time.

Increase step height very gradually. The Reebok stepping platform—considered a "benchmark"-size step by experts—is 6 inches high. You can adjust the height by 2 inches at a time to make the advanced step bench a total height of up to 10 inches.

When you feel comfortable doing your step routine at the lowest height, add height 2 inches at a time, until your leg reaches a 60-degree angle or a comfortable step height. Only very tall or extremely advanced exercisers should use a step bench that's higher than 10 inches, says Miller. Step height (combined with your body weight) is the biggest variable in terms of how many calories you'll burn.

Step Aerobics Workouts

Beginner

Perform a 30-minute workout that begins with an 8-minute warmup and ends with a 5-minute cooldown. Start by doing this twice a week for 3 weeks to 1 month.

Intermediate

Increase one of 3 things: intensity (use harder moves and/or more arm combinations), duration (work out for a total of 40 to 50 minutes), or the number of times you exercise (try 3 or 4 times a week). Don't increase all 3 at once, and keep switching things around for a month to 6 weeks.

Experienced

Add the hard moves, like lunges. Don't work out for longer than 60 minutes, or more often than 4 times per week.

You may want to start out by simply stepping up and down on the first step of a staircase in your house in time to moderate tempo music, says Gin Miller, the inventor of step aerobics, creator of Step Reebok, and star of Reebok Step Training videos in Canton, Georgia. It won't hold your attention for very long, but once you can keep the stepping going for 10 minutes at a time, you're ready to move on to a beginner video.

"Once you've started using a beginner video, stick with it for two or three times a week for about four to six weeks," says Miller. "If you've been consistent with your workouts, it's time to reward yourself with a new tape—something intermediate."

Stick with your new tape for a month or so, increasing your workouts to a steady three times per week. Judge how hard you're working on a scale of 1 to 10, with 1 being a stroll and 10 being a sprint, says Miller. If you are between 4 and 6, you may want to wait until you feel around 3 (moderate) to tackle an advanced tape.

Stepping and Stairclimbing Machines

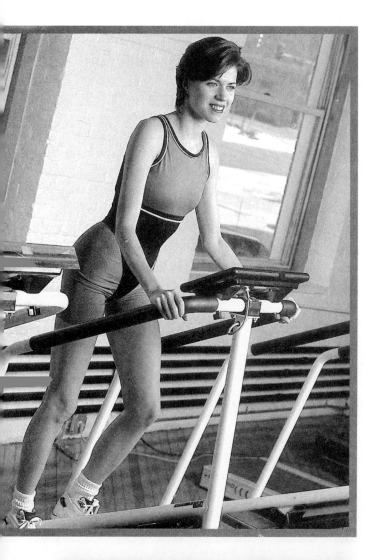

Are you intimidated by—yet envious of—those slender women moving up and down on the long line of stairclimbing machines at the gym? Well, there's a good reason these women are so svelte. Few workouts trim and tone your butt and thighs as efficiently as stepping.

"Like stairclimbing, using a step machine accomplishes two important jobs," says exercise physiologist Carla Sottovia, assistant fitness director at the Fitness Cooper Center in Dallas. It burns off overall fat, and it gives definition to the muscles of your lower body, including the gluteals (in your buttocks), hamstrings and quadriceps (in your thighs), and gastrocnemius (in your calves). As the excess fat melts away, the long, lean muscles underneath are revealed.

Although the terms *stepper* and *stairclimber* are used interchangeably, they are two different machines. Steppers work only your lower body. You balance on the handlebars, pushing with one foot at a time, alternately. Climbers work the whole body.

"The key to being consistent with your stepping workouts is finding an effective form of distraction," says Cedric X. Bryant, Ph.D., senior vice president of research and development/sports medicine at the StairMaster Corporation in Kirkland, Washington. "On a step machine, you can read, watch television, listen to music, or program the machine to vary your workouts. You can't very easily do that on stairs."

Body-Shaping Benefits

Repeatedly raising and lowering your body with either a stepper or stairclimber uses all of the large muscles in your hips, butt, thighs, and lower legs. As a result, stepping combines calorie burning (which uses fat as energy, so it comes off your body) with lower-body sculpting.

Stepping and Stairclimbing Stats

Calories Burned*	Body-Shaping Potential
250 to 350 calories per half-hour	Tones butt, thighs, hips, and calves

*Based on a 150-pound woman. If you weigh more, you'll burn more calories; if you weigh less, you'll burn fewer.

Here's what you can expect when you use a stepper regularly.

- You'll tone and strengthen your butt and thigh muscles, leaving you with a smaller butt and leaner thighs.
- You'll develop shapelier calf muscles.

What You'll Need

Any type of athletic shoe or comfortable sneaker will work on a step machine, so you don't have to go out and buy elaborate footwear.

You'll find steppers or stairclimbers in most gyms, so you don't necessarily have to buy one—unless you want to. Like other forms of exercise equipment, such as treadmills and weight machines, step machines are convenient, but the good ones can run you some money.

Here are some questions to ask and features to think about when you're considering a step machine at a gym or shopping for a home model.

Is it sturdy? The equipment should be able to support your weight easily and remain steady even while you're in motion, says Sottovia. The more expensive machines are usually sturdier and a better buy for people who have a significant amount of weight to lose.

Is it the right size? Every step machine has a prescribed range of distance that the foot pad can travel as you step. Some ranges are wider than others. It should be easy for you to stay in the midrange, or "sweet spot," of the step length. Likewise, the foot pads should be big enough to hold your entire foot with room to spare. Try each machine to see which one feels most comfortable to you, suggests Sottovia.

How does it work? There are two different kinds of step machine designs, dependent and independent. If you push down on one step of a de-

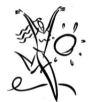

She Did It!

Glenda Stepped Away from 40 Pounds

At one point, Glenda Holmes was at her highest weight ever—293 pounds. A 46-year-old kindergarten teacher from Fresno, California, Glenda talked to her cousin Jim, who wanted to help her find a way to exercise. He suggested a step machine and offered to buy one for her.

They didn't talk about it again until just before Christmas, when Jim called to tell her someone would be calling to make delivery arrangements. "I had a cold around the holidays, so I didn't get on the machine until after the New Year," says Glenda. "The first time I got on it, I could only do two minutes with the machine set at the lowest intensity.

"I put the step machine in my dining room, so I'd have to walk past it every day," says Glenda. "I also decided that I would work out in the morning while listening to National Public Radio. That way, I knew I'd get it done early in the day before other responsibilities would get in my way."

This level-headed and realistic approach worked. Glenda lost over 40 pounds the first year and dropped two dress sizes. "My legs firmed up and my butt, I must say, developed a perkier, more lifted look," she adds.

Glenda worked up to 25 minutes at a time at a higher intensity on her step machine. "I do 20 minutes on the manual program, then I do the last 5 minutes on a higher-intensity program, before finishing with a thorough cooldown lasting 5 to 6 minutes," she says. "And I continue to get better and better at it."

Take It to the 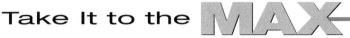MAX

Beat the Monotony of Endless Climbing

Once you've been slogging up and down on a step machine for a while, you probably will want a change in routine. To supplement your workout—or step up the effort—consider these suggestions.

Take the stairs—any stairs. You've heard it a thousand times: Use the steps and not the elevator in your office building. That's a good way to work stairclimbing into your busy day. But you can also use the stairs for 10 minutes of exercise a few times a day, says exercise physiologist Carla Sottovia, assistant fitness director at the Fitness Cooper Center in Dallas.

Don't bound up and down the stairs in dress pumps or heels, though. "Not only do heels throw you off balance, but they also take a toll on your knees, especially when you're going down the stairs," says Sottovia. "Wear sneakers, or at least flats."

Be Sisyphus. Sisyphus was the Greek king condemned to rolling a huge boulder up a hill, only to have it roll down again, forcing him to start all over. You could choose to mimic him by using the Stepmill, a tough, but effective, machine that looks like a flight of stairs and requires complete stairclimbing motion on full eight-inch steps, according to Cedric

X. Bryant, Ph.D., senior vice president of research and development/sports medicine at the Stair-Master Corporation in Kirkland, Washington. The stairs keep revolving (sort of like an escalator) so that you can climb them over and over (and over) again. What a workout!

Add your upper body. If you like the feel of using a stepper, but wish your upper body could get a workout, too, look into using a vertical climbing machine, such as the VersaClimber, by Heart Rate. It's a lot like climbing a stationary ladder, and because you work your arms and legs in full range of motion, you'll burn lots of calories, according to Dr. Bryant.

Visualize the Statue of Liberty. Need a visual goal to keep your workout exciting? Imagine you're climbing famous steps, like the Spanish Steps in Rome, Mayan ruins in the Yucatan Peninsula of Mexico, Telegraph Hill in San Francisco, or the stairs to the top of the Statue of Liberty. Or set a long-range goal—like the equivalent of climbing Mt. Everest. Find out how many steps it would take to reach your goal, then post it near your step machine or in your exercise log and chart your daily progress. Now that's a serious workout!

---

pendent machine, the other step will rise, creating greater stress on the knee joint. Independent steps aren't connected by anything and involve more natural and less stressful movement, says Dr. Bryant.

Most brands of step machines offer display monitors with manual or programmed features that set and measure the time and intensity of your effort. The programs also help you check your progress and guide you through a variety of workouts. You don't need an elaborately programmed unit to get a good workout, though, says Dr. Bryant. Choose a machine based on how the equipment moves as you exercise, not the display features, he says.

What type of resistance does it use? Experts recommend buying either hydraulic, cable, or chain steppers. Be careful, though, since hydraulic machines (which are less expensive) use oil, which can leak onto home carpeting. Leading brands of steppers include StairMaster, Tunturi, VersaClimber, and Tectrix.

Getting Started

Stepping might look as easy as marching, but stepping improperly can cost you 75 calories per workout. Bad form can also contribute to uncomfortable aches and pains during and after your workout. After all, you're not just bounding up the steps to answer the phone—you're stepping non-stop for half an hour. To step safely and effectively, you have to do it right. Here's how.

Warm up. As with any exercise, a good rule for stepping is "start slow, stop gradually," says Sottovia. "Warm up for five minutes with smaller steps on a low resistance level, then move into your workout with longer steps at a higher resistance. Slow down again at the end, and make sure you stretch your leg muscles afterward."

Don't lean on the rails. "When people lean, they tend to do about 20 to 25 percent less work than the machine credits them for, because they aren't using their full body weight when they step," says Dr. Bryant. "If you're working so hard that you have to lean on the machine, lower the stepping speed. Your hands should rest lightly, if at all, on the handlebars."

Slow down. Stepping quickly doesn't mean you'll burn more calories. It's the force of your leg working against the step, not how fast you step, that determines the value of the workout. Your steps should cover the middle range of the whole length of the step, and your speed should be steady, not fast or choppy, according to Dr. Bryant.

Stepping Workouts

Beginner

5 minutes at the lowest level you feel comfortable with, every day, if possible. Work your way up to 20 minutes at this intensity.

Intermediate

Once you can do 20 minutes of exercise every day, cut down on frequency, but increase intensity. Exercise for 2 days on and 1 day off, raising the intensity level every few workouts. Aim for 20 minutes, 3 or 4 times per week.

Experienced

Alternate between high and moderate intensity: For every minute of high-intensity exercise, do 2 minutes of moderate-intensity work. Continue for 20 minutes, 3 or 4 times a week.

Don't try to go all out when you first mount a stepping machine, say experts.

"If you start small and go slow, you'll eventually be able to light up the display monitor on your machine for relatively long, intense workouts," says Cedric X. Bryant, Ph.D., senior vice president of research and development/sports medicine at the StairMaster Corporation in Kirkland, Washington. "The key is to begin with short workouts that are within your capabilities."

Once you're comfortable working out for 20 minutes at a low to moderate intensity, try to begin high-intensity training. To do this, once again, you'll have to start slow. Cut down on the number of times per week that you exercise, but increase the level at which you exercise.

Swimming

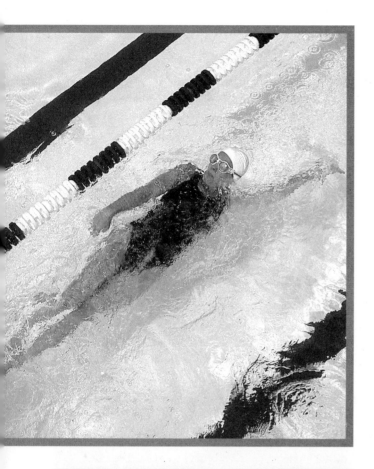

Few activities are as sensual and relaxing as swimming. And swimming may be the perfect way for a woman who needs to lose a few pounds to begin an exercise program, because extra fat helps keep you buoyant, making it easier to swim better and faster. If you have a lot of weight to lose—50 pounds or more—swimming is a good way to get started.

"Swimming isn't weight-bearing—it doesn't subject your joints and bones to a lot of added impact," says Jane Katz, Ed.D., professor of health and physical education at the John Jay College of Criminal Justice of City University of New York and author of *The All-American Aquatic Handbook* and *Swimming for Total Fitness.* "You're expending a lot of energy, which burns calories, but you don't have to support the weight of your whole body while you do it."

If you start to swim and stick with it, you could wind up as sleek, slender, and elegant as a mermaid.

Body-Shaping Benefits

Here's what you can expect when you swim regularly.

- You'll burn as many calories as running, without stressing your knees or bones.
- You'll tone your abdomen and hips.
- You'll tone and strengthen your legs. As a bonus, you'll also firm up your chest and upper arms.

Psychological Benefits

Despite the anxiety many women feel about getting into a bathing suit, most women feel light and beautiful once they're actually in the water.

"In the water, your body feels as though it weighs one-tenth your actual weight," says Dr. Katz. "So many women feel graceful, sensuous, and feminine when they swim."

If you're substantially overweight, having the weight of your body off your bones and joints for

Swimming Stats

Calories Burned*	Body-Shaping Potential
249 to 351 per half-hour, depending on what stroke you do and how fast you swim	High-calorie burning; tones the legs, hips, torso, arms, back, and chest

*Based on a 150-pound woman. If you weigh more, you'll burn more calories; if you weigh less, you'll burn fewer.

She Did It!

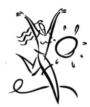

Gigi Lost 160 Pounds in the Pool

One phone call really can change a woman's life. "I remember the nurse at my doctor's office called to tell me that my cholesterol was slightly elevated," says Gigi Carnes, 39, a curator at Muscoot Farm in Katonah, New York. "When I asked her what that meant, she actually started to yell at me. 'You need to eat better!' she said. 'You need to lose weight!'"

Gigi says she couldn't deny that she had a problem: She weighed 310 pounds and wore a size 28.

"Ironically, when she called, I was in the middle of eating fried chicken thighs, cole slaw, and a huge box of french fries, with a bowl of rich, creamy, vanilla ice cream waiting on the side," says Gigi. "I just stopped eating and thought, 'Oh, my God—she's right.'" Gigi walked out the door and headed straight to a bookstore to find out how to eat well. Soon afterward, she started a low-fat, low-cal way of eating. "I didn't starve myself. I still ate three whole meals daily, which totaled about 1,200 calories."

At just about the same time that Gigi started to eat better, a nearby swim club opened up in May for the season. "I had loved to swim as a kid," she says. "And once, in 1979 when I lost 30 pounds, I did a lot of swimming. But otherwise, whenever I was in a pool, all I did was splash around. You couldn't really call it exercising."

This time, Gigi got into her bathing suit and started swimming. She swam five days a week and sometimes six in the hot days of summer. "The weight just rolled off me," she says. "By July, I needed to tie a cord around my shorts to keep them up. Swimming was obviously making a difference."

Less than a year after starting to swim regularly, Gigi was 160 pounds lighter.

So how did Gigi manage to get her bathing suit on and step into the pool at 310 pounds when so many thinner women feel too self-conscious to swim? "I focus on my swimming goals, not on my weight," she says. (Gigi is proud to say she can swim one mile in just 44 minutes.) "Plus, it's not as intimidating as you might think from the ads on TV—most people at gyms and swim clubs don't really look that great. In a pool, you see what real women look like, and that makes it easier to not feel self-conscious about how you look."

In fact, Gigi takes delight in wearing a swimsuit. "I own 29 bathing suits!" she says. "I'm a sucker for suits that are on sale." She pairs her suits with five different goggles and 14 different bathing caps that match her suits.

Gigi believes that two key things have led to her successful weight loss. First, she chose an activity she loves. "Whenever I make plans, my first priority is to figure out when I can get my swim in," she says.

Second, says Gigi, "I was willing to let go of my old habits in order to make way for new, healthier ones. I was open to different foods and a new way of life. When you start seeing results and your plan comes together, it makes everything worthwhile."

an hour or so may also be a physical relief. "Many women find they have extra energy when they're in the water," notes Dr. Katz.

The Right Footwear

You could swim barefoot. But if you're swimming to shape up, experts recommend the following footwear.

Swim fins. Available at scuba diving shops and sporting goods stores that sell gear for water sports, swim fins help you swim faster—and give your legs a better workout. "Because fins create more resistance against the water for your muscles, you kick faster," says Dr. Katz. "Look for medium-length fins, not the extra-short ones. The length is what's helping you go fast."

Shower sandals. To protect yourself against athlete's foot, a nasty skin infection that is picked up from fungus in and around public pools and showers, you'll want to wear rubber flip-flops, sandals, or water shoes to walk to the pool and also to take a shower, says Dr. Katz. For flip-flops and sandals, the kind sold in discount stores is fine, she says. Water shoes can be found in sporting goods stores that sell water sports gear.

What Else You'll Need

Let's start with the big item.

A pool. Maybe you'll be swimming in a lake or the ocean. But most women who swim regularly are probably doing laps at their local pool or YWCA.

Take It to the 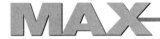 MAX

Power Up in the Pool

If swimming is your aerobic exercise of choice, you'll burn more calories if you go beyond the basic crawl and add other strokes to your repertoire, says Jane Katz, Ed.D., professor of health and physical education at the John Jay College of Criminal Justice of City University of New York and author of *The All-American Aquatic Handbook* and *Swimming for Total Fitness.* "The best way to learn more strokes is to take a fitness swimming class," she says. "The instructor will help you swim more efficiently and correct any mistakes you're making."

Here are some of the strokes that will make swimming more challenging—and interesting.

Flip onto your back. A major calorie burner (345 calories per half-hour if you weigh 150 pounds), the backstroke is a wonderful complement to the crawl. If you don't like to keep your face in the water, you'll like this stroke.

Stay on your side. The side stroke doesn't burn the most calories (249 per half-hour if you weigh 150 pounds), but it is a relaxing way to cool down and work the oblique muscles located along your torso. Toned obliques mean a toned waistline.

Fly like a butterfly. One of the toughest strokes to master, the butterfly pays off in terms of calories burned (351 per half-hour if you weigh 150 pounds). Not all instructors introduce beginning swimmers to this stroke, but if you can master it, you'll feel like a powerhouse in the pool.

Learn the new breast stroke. The breast stroke has been reinvented since you were in the guppy swimming group at summer camp. It calls for more whip in the kick and a more efficient, faster, narrower arm motion that doesn't strain your muscles as much as the old method, which required a complete extension of the arms. The breast stroke is also harder than it used to be. But it's still a great way to strengthen your pectoral muscles in your chest (and thus lift your breasts). You'll burn 330 calories per half-hour if you weigh 150 pounds.

A bathing suit. If you're like a lot of women, the thought of wearing a swimsuit in public makes you cringe. "It's just a matter of getting from the edge of the pool into the water," says Dr. Katz. "Once you're in there, no one can see what you look like."

That said, Dr. Katz advises women who swim for exercise to buy a racing suit designed and produced by sportswear companies. "Shop at a sporting goods store first, rather than a department store," she says. "You're not looking for something to lounge in, but rather something that will hold your body in place and keep you streamlined in the water." For exercise swimming, she advises women to stay away from suits with skirts or other added layers of fabric.

Fortunately, the traditional racer-back suit, which is available in almost all sizes, is flattering to almost every figure, since it covers your backside and upper thighs more adequately than fashion swimsuits that are cut high on the thigh. For large-breasted women, Dr. Katz recommends fitness swimsuits with support. "You can purchase these at specialty fitness stores where swimsuits are geared to accommodate your form."

Finally, Dr. Katz has one other piece of advice for the bathing-suit shy: "Swim at a facility that's not too high-brow. More expensive clubs tend to be more looks-oriented, but your local Y caters to every type of body."

Goggles. To minimize levels of harmful bacteria, pool water must contain a certain amount of chlorine and other disinfecting chemicals that can irritate your eyes, so you need goggles. They're a must for swimming laps, says Dr. Katz, because they allow you to see the lane markers along the bottom of the pool. Goggles aren't expensive; pick up a pair at a specialty fitness store where someone can help you choose the best-fitting ones. For beginning swimmers, Dr. Katz recommends goggles with good peripheral vision and padding around the rim of the eye piece. You should feel light suction around the eyes—just enough to keep water out.

A bathing cap. Public pools sometimes require women (and sometimes men) to wear a bathing cap. Wearing a cap also helps to protect your hair from chemicals in the pool water, which can dry or discolor your hair. And if your hair is long, a cap keeps it from becoming tangled while you swim. Look for something sleek and simple at a specialty fitness store. A silicone bathing cap is best because it doesn't pull your hair as much as other materials do, explains Dr. Katz.

Soap and a scrubbie. Pool chemicals can dry and irritate your skin if you don't shower with soap and moisturize after you get out of the pool, says Dr. Katz. You can use bar soap and a washcloth, but Dr. Katz says that liquid soap is often easier to carry in your gym bag. Just squirt some on a scrubbie (those balls of nylon that are sold in drugstores), lather up, rinse well, and moisturize when you get out of the shower. Your skin will thank you.

Shampoo and conditioner. Shampoo and condition as soon as possible after each swim, advises Dr. Katz. "Try a shampoo and conditioner formulated to help remove chlorine; these are available at hair salons."

A T-shirt or robe. If you feel self-conscious walking from the shower or locker to the pool, Dr. Katz recommends bringing some sort of cover-up to the pool.

Getting Started

"Swimming for exercise is not the same as taking a dip when you're hot and want to cool off after a day in the sun," points out Dr. Katz. "You have to swim at a consistent pace for at least 20 minutes in order to get your heart pumping and your fat burning."

Crawl first. Unless you're proficient in another stroke (breast, back, side, or butterfly), you'll probably want to do the crawl, which is sometimes called freestyle swimming. Before you attempt to learn several strokes, simply work on being able to consistently do a crawl for 10 minutes at a time, says Dr. Katz.

Learn to roll. Sure, swimming looks as if your arms and legs are providing all the power. But the real source of a swimmer's power comes from—

surprise—the hips and trunk. "Efficient swimmers are always in a rolling motion," says Dr. Katz. "They're never still in the water." The key is to move from your hips, turning your head to one side to breathe as the opposite arm comes out of the water, then starting to roll toward the other side for your next breath and its matching stroke.

Turn your head and inhale. If you haven't swum laps for a long time, you may feel awkward trying to pace your breaths. When you breathe, turn your whole head along with your body toward one side. Your mouth will lift slightly out of the water for an inhalation. As your body rolls back into a straight line, you'll slowly blow bubbles as you exhale into the water. Continue your body roll to the other side, turning your mouth out of the water on the other side for your next inhalation. Alternating breathing in this way helps to balance your stroke, says Dr. Katz. When you become a proficient swimmer, alternate breathing sides every third pull.

Lead with your head, not your chin. Your head, not your chin, should lead the way down the lane, says Dr. Katz. You want your body in one streamlined position so that you're looking toward the floor of the pool. Don't worry about hitting the wall—when you see the end of the black line in your lane, start to make your turn, and swim back down the lane.

Watch out for other swimmers. If you've joined an aquatic facility, YWCA, or gym, chances are you'll be sharing the pool with others, so you have to learn the etiquette of sharing lanes. In some clubs, swimmers do circle-swims, swimming to the right-hand side of the lane and turning counterclockwise at the end of each lap. At other pools, each swimmer has one side of a lane—that is, you stay on one side of the black line that goes down the middle of a lane.

Swimming Workouts

Beginner

Swim freestyle laps for a total of about 100 to 300 yards every other day or at least 3 times a week for 1 to 2 months. If you have to stop in between laps at first, that's okay. Work up to swimming nonstop for 10 minutes. If you use fins, you'll burn more calories.

Intermediate

Swim 350 to 550 yards in about 15 minutes without stopping, at least 3 times a week for 2 months.

Experienced

Swim 600 yards (24 laps in a 25-yard pool) to 880 yards at a time without stopping, 3 times a week. Mix and match your strokes, if you want. This should take about 30 minutes.

"This beginner program is designed for someone who knows how to swim but hasn't been doing laps regularly," says Jane Katz, Ed.D., professor of health and physical education at the John Jay College of Criminal Justice of City University of New York and author of *The All-American Aquatic Handbook* and *Swimming for Total Fitness*. "Wearing swim fins, you'll start out swimming slowly and gradually increase your speed over the course of a few months."

Don't forget to warm up before swimming and cool down afterward, says Dr. Katz. "You need to do at least five minutes of water exercise and stretching before you begin to swim your laps. To warm up, walk in the shallow part of the pool or tread water in place."

To cool down, do the stretches in Stretch into Shape on page 180. Stay in the shallow end of the pool and use the steps or edge of the pool if you need to hold on to something. Or you can stretch in the locker room before and after your swim, says Dr. Katz.

Tennis

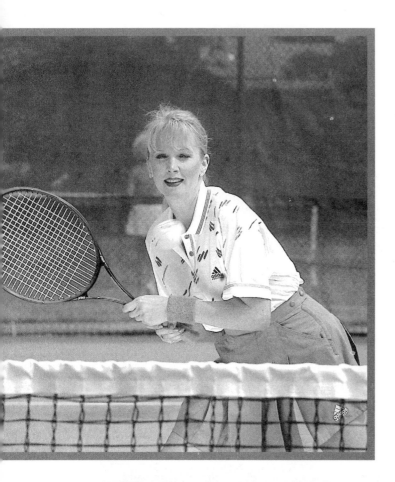

Tennis. Now here's a woman's sport. Chris Evert, Martina Navratilova, Billie Jean King, Martina Hingis—great players, all. You don't have to play like a pro, however, to develop a body about which you can crow.

"When I look at the women who play tennis consistently at our club, they're all in pretty good shape," says Jim Coyne, director of tennis at the Claremont Resort in Berkeley, California.

If you haven't played tennis since you retired your old wooden racket after college, you'll find that the equipment has improved. But you still play on a rectangular court with a net. And the rules and score-keeping are the same. You may need some lessons to brush up on your technique, but if you're looking for a fun way to work more exercise into your life, this centuries-old sport is worth a second look. Or if you've never picked up a racket, it's definitely worth a try. (You don't even have to wear a little white skirt and socks with pom-poms on the heels—unless you want to.)

Body-Shaping Benefits

Whichever arm you use primarily to play tennis will become stronger and shapelier as a result of playing the game, but this sport primarily provides a lower-body workout. If you play regularly:

- Your gluteus (in your backside), quadricep (along the front of your thighs), hamstring (back of your thighs), and calf muscles will all get a good workout from the quick starts and stops and lateral movements required in tennis.

The Right Footwear

Wearing the right shoes is important in tennis. Running shoes and cross-trainers are not designed for the game's constant lateral movement, says Paul van der Sommen, owner and tennis instructor at the Oneonta Tennis Club in Oneonta, New York.

Tennis Stats

Calories Burned*	Body-Shaping Potential
Burns 475 calories an hour in a highly competitive match	Tones the gluteus, quadricep, hamstring, and calf muscles

*Based on a 150-pound woman. If you weigh more, you'll burn more calories; if you weigh less, you'll burn fewer.

"If you wear tennis shoes, you'll have less risk of ankle injury when playing."

Here's what to look for, according to Barrett Bugg, exercise science specialist for the U.S. Tennis Association, based in Key Biscayne, Florida.

Good arch support. A shoe that's well-designed for racket sports will have good support for the arch and be well-padded at the ball of the foot, where you exert the most pressure. If the arch supports feel too high, try another style.

Toe room. There should be enough room in the toebox to move your toes and avoid blisters. That means no more than one-quarter inch between the toes and the toebox or front of the shoe. The toebox is subject to the most wear and tear during tennis, so make sure it's made of leather or rubber, not fabric, which will wear out faster.

Wide soles. The outsole, or bottom, of the shoe should be wider than the upper—the part of the shoe above the sole. Otherwise, you won't be getting enough lateral support as you move from side to side on the court. Look for a midsole made of ethyl vinyl acetate (EVA) or polyurethane. Some shoes have air or gel within the midsole. Press the

shoe. The midsole should give a bit. The insole, or interior, of the shoe should be made of fabric that will breathe and control moisture.

The right size. Buy tennis shoes that are one-half size larger than your regular shoe size, so they can accommodate heavy tennis socks.

Thick socks. Look for thick socks in moisture-wicking fabric or synthetic/cotton blends that provide extra cushioning to absorb shocks and prevent blisters. Ankle-length socks are best— even with pom-poms at the heel, low-cut socks tend to creep back into tennis shoes. Some players wear two pairs of socks to minimize blisters and maximize moisture absorption and cushioning, Bugg adds.

What Else You'll Need

Tennis doesn't require much equipment. Here's what you'll need.

The right racket. Beginners should buy a lightweight, oversize racket, which will improve their chances of making contact with the ball, Coyne says. If your racket's too heavy, your arm

She Did It!

Ronda Lost Weight—And Mellowed Out

When Ronda Sorensen took up tennis, it wasn't exercise she craved. It was adult conversation. Ronda had quit her job to stay home with her two young children, and she missed talking to other grown-ups during the day.

Playing tennis solved the problem, and it offered Ronda an added benefit. After playing regularly, she lost about 10 pounds. "People always say I look leaner," says Sorensen, 38, of Alameda, California. "And I think I'm stronger, too."

Ronda also believes in the mental magic of

tennis. "If you've had a bad day, like with your kids, it's much better to be batting around a bunch of balls than getting angry with your children. When I come home from playing tennis, I'm Mellow Mom."

Ronda plays three sets of tennis three or four days a week, typically spending 1½ to 2 hours each day on the court. She even competed in an amateur tournament in Florida, which further helped to keep her in shape.

"I've seen myself improve, and I want to get better," Sorensen says. "I just love the game."

Take It to the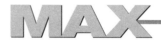

Get the Most out of Every Game

In 1996, at the Australian Open, Brenda Shultz-McCarthy delivered the fastest tennis serve ever clocked by a woman—121.8 miles per hour. You don't have to blast balls into the next county, though, to crank up your tennis game and maximize your workout. Once you've learned the basics, take the following steps to get the most out of the game.

Play singles. You have to cover more court and hit more shots when you play singles, so you get a better workout, says Jim Coyne, director of tennis at the Claremont Resort in Berkeley, California.

Play with someone who's good—but not too good. If your opponent's skills are similar to your own, you are more apt to have longer rallies and get a good workout, says Barrett Bugg, exercise science specialist for the U.S. Tennis Association, based in Key Biscayne, Florida. A partner who plays

better than you can improve your game and your workout if she makes you work hard with her shots, but not so hard you can't return them.

In tennis lingo, for example, an ace is a serve so powerful or artfully placed that the player on the receiving end can't return it. If you play opponents who hit the ball so hard that you seldom return it, you won't get much of a workout, explains Paul van der Sommen, owner and tennis instructor at Oneonta Tennis Club in Oneonta, New York.

Go solo. Even if you can't find an opponent to play some days, you can still work on your game. Find a wall to hit balls against. Or rent a ball machine to send balls whizzing at you on the court. "Ball machines are wonderful," van der Sommen says. "They don't make errors, and they don't whine or complain."

---

will get tired. But if it's too light, you'll be waving it like a wand, not learning proper strokes.

Look for a racket with midlevel string tension, to absorb impact but provide power. As for grip, a finger's width should separate the tip of your middle finger from the crease at the base of your thumb as you grasp the handle.

If you plan to play at a club, ask at the pro shop if you can rent or borrow a racket for the day and see if it feels like a model you might want to buy.

Fresh balls. All tennis balls are created equal, van der Sommen says. So if you can buy a can cheaper at a discount store, do so. Balls last longer in warmer climates. If it's summer or you live someplace like Florida where the weather is warm year-round, you can use the same balls two or three times, he says. If it's cold outside, they lose their bounce after play—use the balls only once.

Tennis attire. Some tennis clubs have a dress code requiring women to wear a skirt or a dress

when playing tennis and men to wear a collared shirt. Others permit you to wear shorts. Some allow only all white attire, or light colors. Of course, if you're playing on a public court—say, at a local community park or high school—you can wear what you please.

Whatever you wear should be comfortable, but not baggy or too snug. It you wear clothing that's too large, the excess fabric may slow you down. Clothing that's too tight can restrict your movements and not allow your skin to breathe. If you wear shorts instead of a tennis skirt, look for wide legs and side vents, to give you freedom of movement. Wear a sports bra to control bounce and support your breasts comfortably during play.

Cotton fabric is traditional for tennis, but it's best when blended with synthetics like Lycra or Supplex, which help clothing keep its shape longer and resist wrinkling.

Getting Started

You needn't be rich or competitive to enjoy tennis. "It's a wonderful sport to learn if the emphasis is not on winning," notes van der Sommen. Here are some tips on getting started.

Take lessons. Private tennis lessons can easily cost $60 an hour, van der Sommen says. A more affordable option is to take a clinic or class with no more than four students. Check out your local community college for tennis clinics and workshops.

Don't let yourself be pressured into committing to a whole series of lessons (or a club membership) until you've taken at least one lesson, van der Sommen says. That way, you can see if you like the tennis pro and the game itself.

Notice if the tennis instructor comes in with one bucket half-full or four buckets or a shopping cart full of balls, says van der Sommen. It's a good indication of how much practice and instruction you can expect. "The more you hit the ball, the better you're going to get," he says. And make sure there are no stray balls on the court while you're practicing. If you accidentally step on one during play, you could twist an ankle.

Choose your court. Grass is the worst surface on which to learn tennis; clay is the best, according to van der Sommen. But if you're just starting out, look for an indoor court, he says. There will be no sun to blind you, no wind to skew your shots, and a less distracting background that enables you to better see the ball.

Warm up. You're not going to get a tennis workout if you have to sit on the sidelines with a pulled muscle, so warm up before you play. Start with brisk walking or easy jogging, then stretch for several minutes, Coyne suggests.

Calf muscles, in particular, can get tight, so stretch your quadriceps and hamstrings (in your thighs) before, between, and after matches, van der Sommen says.

Tennis Workouts

Beginner

Enjoy noncompetitive play for at least a half-hour against someone of equal or greater ability than yourself.

Intermediate

Play competitively for 45 minutes to an hour.

Experienced

Engage in an hour to 90 minutes of tournament-type play.

A traditional women's tennis match is made up of a group of sets. Each set varies in length, but ends when one of the players wins 6 games, says Barrett Bugg, exercise science specialist for the U.S. Tennis Association, based in Key Biscayne, Florida. Not many people can win in a competitive environment without a lot of effort, he adds. Opponents play to win the best of three sets. If the score becomes tied at 6-6, a 12-point tie breaker is played. When that happens, the first player to hit 7 points wins, Bugg explains.

The intensity of any workout depends, of course, on whether the games have much rallying, says Bugg. So if you or your opponent is scoring lots of quick points, you may want to extend the amount of time you play, he explains.

Conversely, if you plan to play for, say, an hour, but your racket feels like a lead weight after 45 minutes, listen to your body. "If your muscles start to feel so tight and fatigued that you can't even hold the racket, call it a day. Otherwise, you're going to be sore the next day," says Bugg.

Walking

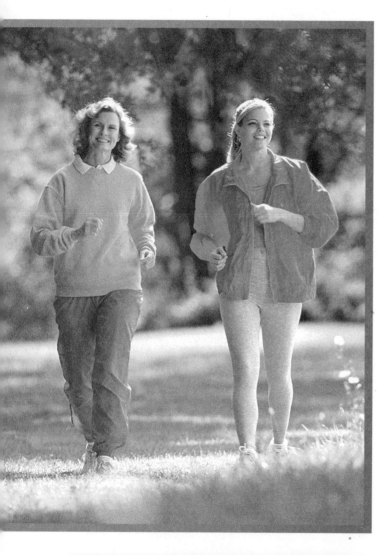

What could be simpler than putting one foot in front of the other? That's all there is to walking. You don't need fancy equipment, a health club membership, or even good weather. Indoors, you can walk on a treadmill or stride around a mall. Outside, the sky's the limit.

Best of all, walking can give you all the rewards of aerobic exercise, but it puts less stress on your knees, hips, and back. A walking routine can help lower your risk of heart disease, reduce your cholesterol and blood pressure, speed up fat loss, and increase muscle tone, says Rosemary Agostini, M.D., clinical associate professor of orthopedics at the University of Washington and staff physician at the Virginia Mason Sports Medicine Center, both in Seattle.

Body-Shaping Benefits

Here's what you can expect when you walk regularly.

- Your body will burn more calories and more fat all day long because you've revved up your metabolism.
- You'll help tone your abdominals, hips, thighs, and buttocks.
- You'll use all the major muscles—glutes, quads, hamstrings, back, biceps, and triceps.

Psychological Benefits

Walking makes you feel better. If you want proof, just ask the women who take walking classes from nationally known racewalking instructor and coach Bonnie Stein in Redington Shores, Florida. Cynthia Gates Baber, a licensed social worker and psychotherapist at the Scottish Rite Children's Medical Center in Atlanta, conducted a study of 25 women in one of Stein's walking classes. At the start of the eight-week program, Baber discovered that 48 percent of the women

Walking Stats

Calories Burned*	Body-Shaping Potential
100 per mile	Tones abdominals, hips, thighs, and buttocks

*Based on a 150-pound woman. If you weigh more, you'll burn more calories; if you weigh less, you'll burn fewer.

showed signs of stress, and almost half had been in therapy for depression. By the end of eight weeks, only 32 percent of the women showed signs of stress.

The Right Footwear

Priority one for all walkers is good shoes. Here is what Stein recommends that you look for when you shop for shoes.

Flexibility. The shoe should bend where your foot bends—at the ball of your foot, not in the middle of the shoe.

An ample toebox. When you walk, you bend and push off with your toes. There should be a thumb's width from the end of your longest toe to the front end of the shoe, says Stein. If the toebox isn't big enough, your toes will be tingling 20 minutes into your walk.

Light, thin materials. Look for shoes that are lightweight, with a thin heel and a flexible sole. Running and walking shoes with soles that are extremely thick and cushioned are not good for walking. Also stay away from aerobics, tennis, and basketball shoes, Stein says. Cross-trainers are too stiff and inflexible for walking and don't offer the proper support.

What Else You'll Need

If you venture outdoors on your walks, you'll want to be prepared for any conditions.

Water. Drink two cups (16 ounces) of water about two hours prior to your workout, then 5 to

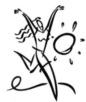

She Did It!

Karen Whittled Her Weight by Walking

Barely five feet tall, 47-year-old Karen Primerano wore size 14 jeans. She had tried to lose weight by consuming diet foods and liquid diet drinks, but she always managed to regain any weight that she lost. After several years of unsuccessful dieting, she had finally had enough.

"One day," says Karen, "I said to my husband, 'That's it. I've spent my last nickel on anything diet.' So we went out and bought a treadmill.

"I was so out of shape that it took me months to work up to walking 20 minutes. In the beginning, I couldn't walk for even 5 minutes at a slow pace without being totally out of breath," she recalls. But she stuck with it.

Every week, she increased her treadmill time by 1 minute, until she was up to 20 minutes at a time. She used the treadmill every night during the week, and on weekends, she walked two to three miles around her neighborhood.

As the weeks went by, the pounds started easing off. Karen lost 40 pounds, and she was able to trade in her size 14 jeans for a slim size 6.

"I noticed the inches coming off right from the start," says Karen. "That encouraged me. So I began to make improvements in my diet. It had finally dawned on me that there is no fast way to lose weight. You have to change your lifestyle and the way you think."

Karen still walks, and now, more than two years after she started, she has kept off those 40 pounds.

"Walking is the exercise of choice for me," she says. "You can walk no matter where you are—on vacation, visiting friends, on business trips. I wouldn't trade walking for anything."

Take It to the 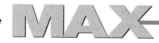 MAX

Customize Your Walking Technique

To maximize the body-shaping benefits of walking, follow these tips from Kate Larsen, a walking instructor and certified group fitness instructor in Minneapolis.

Take short, quick steps instead of long strides. You'll work your glute muscles (in your buttocks) as you log miles.

Practice the heel-toe roll. Push off from your heel, roll through the outside of your foot, then push through your big toe. Think of your big toe as the Go button and push off with propulsion. Keep your other toes relaxed. (This takes practice.)

Squeeze your glutes. Imagine squeezing and lifting your glutes up and back, as if you were holding a $50 bill between them. This will strengthen and tone your glute muscles. Developing the ability to maintain this deep contraction throughout your walk will take a while.

"Zip up" your abs. During your walk, imagine that you're zipping up a tight pair of jeans. Stand tall and pull your abdominal muscles up and in. You can practice this even when you're not walking. This will also strengthen your lower-back muscles.

Pump your arms. Imagine that you're holding the rubber grips of ski poles in your hands. Stand straight, drop your shoulders, squeeze your shoulder blades behind you, and push your elbows back with each step. Keep your arm movements smooth and strong, moving past the outside of your hips.

Keep your chest up and shoulders back. Use your walk as an opportunity to practice perfect posture. Imagine that someone dumped ice down your back. That's the feeling you want to have as you hold your chest up and shoulders back.

Hold your head up. Look about 10 feet ahead of you. Imagine that you're wearing a baseball cap with the bill of the visor level to the horizon, so that you have to look up just enough to see the road. This keeps your neck aligned properly.

Smile and have fun. Learning these techniques takes time and concentration. Be patient and enjoy your workouts. Dress comfortably; find a partner or wear a headset (if you're walking indoors only) and listen to music you love; and if you're walking outdoors, vary your route.

Practice mental fitness. Don't replay the problems of the day while you walk. Try to maintain a state of relaxed awareness by paying attention to your breathing and noticing how your body feels. Visualize and tell yourself you're getting healthier, stronger, and leaner.

---

10 ounces every 15 to 20 minutes during exercise, says Dr. Agostini. After you're done, drink 16 ounces for each pound of weight lost during the workout.

Sun protection. Wear sunscreen and a floppy, wide-brimmed hat or baseball cap, sunglasses with 100 percent UV protection, or a visor to shade your eyes and protect your face from sunburn. A visor is best for really hot weather because it doesn't hold the heat in.

Wet-weather gear. There's plenty of rain gear available to make wet-weather walking enjoyable.

You can also find wet-weather activewear in mail-order catalogs such as L. L. Bean and Eddie Bauer.

Cold-weather gear. When it's cold outside, you want clothing made with a fabric that pulls the moisture away from your skin. Look for T-shirts, turtlenecks, and other attire made with CoolMax or other synthetic fibers designed for activewear. You can dress in layers, but don't wear cotton next to your skin, because it won't wick away the sweat. Cover your ears with a headband or a hat. Just be aware that even at a cool 35° or 40°F, a hat may make your head perspire, so a headband is a better choice. When the temperatures dip below freezing, however, wear a hat. When the weather is cool, you may want to wear gloves. When it gets really cold, switch to mittens. Stein likes polar fleece for headbands and mittens because it doesn't trap moisture.

Getting Started

With your walking shoes firmly on your feet, it is time to hit the road. Here are some pointers from Stein.

Take it slow. If you need to lose 50 or more pounds or you are relatively inactive, don't overdo it at first. Aim for a daily 20-minute walk at a pace that makes your breathing just a bit labored but doesn't leave you out of breath. "At the end of 20 minutes, you'll probably feel great, as though you could do more—but don't," says Stein. "In the first two to three weeks of walking, don't go more than 20 minutes per session."

Keep going. If you can, walk the entire 20 minutes without stopping. But even if you can walk only 10 minutes at a time, you'll get some benefits. Slow down and rest for a few minutes, then begin again.

Listen to your heart. "The best indicator of whether you're walking briskly enough to gain health benefits is your target heart rate," says Dr. Agostini.

Plan to walk every day. "Even on days when you don't feel like doing it, just get out and walk a few blocks," says Stein. You'd be surprised at how, once you get going, those few blocks can turn into a mile or more.

If you're an indoor walker, consider buying a treadmill. Stein recommends a motorized version. Set it at a speed that lets you walk comfortably without holding on. When you feel balanced and are used to it, you can increase the speed. Walk on a treadmill for the same amount of time that you would if you were walking outside.

For more information on walking for weight loss, visit our Web site at www.banishbbt.com.

Walking Workouts

Beginner

20 minutes, 6 or 7 days a week for 2 weeks

Intermediate

25 minutes, 6 or 7 days a week; increase walking time by 10 percent increments each week until you reach 40 minutes

---

Experienced

Continue to increase walking time by 10 percent until you reach 45 to 60 minutes, 6 or 7 days a week. If you don't need to lose body fat, you can walk 20 to 30 minutes, 3 days a week to stay fit.

Beginners should aim for a level of exertion equivalent to a 6 or 7 on a scale of 1 to 10, advises Bonnie Stein, a nationally known racewalking instructor and coach in Redington Shores, Florida. You should be able to carry on a conversation without being short of breath.

Another way to measure exertion is to monitor your heart rate. To calculate your target heart rate, subtract your age from 220, then multiply by the level of exertion at which you want to exercise (60 percent of your maximum is good for beginners). For example, if you are 50 years old and want to start out at 60 percent exertion, the math would work like this: $220 - 50 = 170$; $170 \times 0.60 = 102$.

Thus, your heart rate should be 102 beats per minute when you walk. As you develop endurance and lose weight, increase your walking time and the intensity by recalculating your target heart rate at a higher percentage or by aiming for an exertion level of 7 or 8.

Water Aerobics

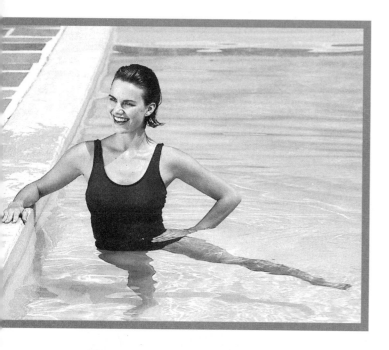

You don't have to know how to swim to do water aerobics. As long as you're comfortable in water up to your chest, you are a candidate for this extraordinarily effective form of exercise, says Marti Boutin, a training specialist for the Aquatic Exercise Association headquartered in Nokomis, Florida. Also known as aquatics, water aerobics are gaining popularity among professional sports stars, Olympic athletes, and regular people.

What do they know that you should? Three things: Water aerobics is easy on your joints and still provides a great aerobic workout. The resistance provided by moving through water, which is 12 to 14 times greater than traveling over land, gives your muscles continuous resistance training. Finally, because of the reduced impact in the water, you can execute moves that you might not be able to do on land.

Water Aerobics Stats

Calories Burned*	Body-Shaping Potential
200 to 250 per half-hour	Tones abdominals, hips, thighs, buttocks, calves, arms, and more

*Based on a 150-pound woman. If you weigh more, you'll burn more calories; if you weigh less, you'll burn fewer.

Body-Shaping Benefits

Water workouts on a regular basis can bring you a steady stream of rewards.

- By engaging in an energetic water aerobics workout, you'll burn calories just as well as if you did an aerobic workout on land, without the added stress on your joints.

- The three-dimensional effects of water provide resistance in all directions, toning your muscles from head to toe. Water exercise creates a beautifully shaped and balanced body.

- You'll work your abdominal and back muscles, along with your legs, extra hard in the water to maintain erect body alignment and balance, resulting in strong, defined abdominals and legs.

Psychological Benefits

Water aerobics gives you a wonderful sense of well-being during and after a workout, says

Boutin. Exercise releases endorphins, naturally sedating compounds in your brain that reduce stress. The water offers a comfortable environment, and its massaging effects soothe tired muscles, she says. The moment you become immersed in water, you enter a new environment of sensation and perception.

The Right Footwear

Water fitness shoes are soft, flexible shoes that are specifically designed for walking in water. They add comfort, provide a nonskid base, and help protect your feet, says Boutin. Water fitness sneakers, which provide more support than the shoes, are also a good choice, she adds. But if you like, you can do water aerobics in your bare feet.

What Else You'll Need

Water aerobics requires minimal equipment. A bathing suit and a pool will do the trick. For added efficiency and safety, you can opt for additional water aerobics equipment.

Water. A backyard pool or the one at the local Y are both perfect. The water should be approximately chest deep, and you should have enough space to move through a full range of motion without bumping into the side of the pool or the person next to you, says Boutin. Water temperature is important: The Aquatic Exercise Association says it should be between 80° to 85°F for water fitness classes. As your body temperature rises from the vigorous parts of the routine, this temperature keeps you cool, Boutin explains.

She Did It!

Linda Gets Hip to Water Aerobics

"I love to be active," says Linda Grable, a 50-plus office manager in Redondo Beach, California. Despite having been born with a dislocated hip that made her vulnerable to injury, she was a runner and worked out at a gym. Over the years, however, she developed arthritis in both hips. Her doctor recommended two hip replacements.

"Since the surgery, I haven't been able to do any exercises that may put stress on my hips," Linda says. "I can no longer run, use the step machine, or take aerobics classes. I had to explore different activities.

"One day, I got a flyer for a water aerobics class in the mail," Linda recalls. "I read the class description and thought about it for a few days. Then I decided, 'Hey, I'm going to do this!'" And she's thrilled that she did.

"Water aerobics finally allows me to do the things I used to be able to do on land," she says. "I felt so limited after surgery. Now, for the first time, I was able to do jogging and jumping jacks, lunges and kicks. I am so tickled!"

The one-hour class is "a really, really good workout," Linda says. "It's almost constant movement, so I know I'm giving my heart a good workout." The class also incorporates resistance training for more focused muscle toning.

"I'm back in great shape again," she says. "Sometimes after class I practically crawl out of the pool, but it's fun. I used to feel so deprived, not being able to exercise. Now I can do everything in the water that I can't do on land."

Take It to the MAX

Tips for Longer, Harder Water Workouts

Water workout experts offer these tips for keeping motivation high.

Join a class. The leadership and motivation provided by a good instructor can be an inspiration, says Marti Boutin, a training specialist for the Aquatic Exercise Association headquartered in Nokomis, Florida. The companionship and camaraderie you develop with your classmates also helps you to stay motivated.

Add variety. Don't just do water walking and leave it at that, says Boutin. "There's a huge range of things you can do in the water, from lap swimming to water yoga. By experimenting with new things, you sustain your interest."

Partner up. Working out with someone else keeps you committed to showing up and, once you're there, staying in the water longer and working out harder, notes Boutin.

Keep a workout journal. A written record of what you've accomplished heightens your motivation to do even more, Boutin explains. Include the day of your workout, how long you stayed in the water, the type of workout, any resistance training equipment you used, and the number of repetitions you did. Also jot down how you felt before, during, and after your workout.

Watch a video before you work out. Watching even a few minutes of a water aerobics video before you work out, whether you're working out on your own or in a class, teaches you something new about form or motivates you to exercise that much better, says Boutin.

Add music. If you're working out on your own, add music to boost your energy level and make the workout more fun.

Swimsuit. Comfort is the key here. Wear a suit that you can move well in. If wearing a swimsuit makes you feel embarrassed because you're out of shape, just pull a T-shirt over your suit.

Resistance-training aids. Working out in the water tones your abs and helps to flatten your stomach. Adding other equipment, such as water dumbbells, Styrofoam noodles, and webbed gloves, helps tone other muscles groups—notably, your thighs, buttocks, and arms—while increasing the intensity of your workout, Boutin says.

Flotation belt. For deep-water workouts (where your feet don't touch the bottom), a flotation belt is essential for safety and also provides good back support.

Getting Started

Here's what experts advise to launch yourself into a water aerobics program.

Get a book or video. Books such as *Fitness Aquatics* by Lee Anne Case can introduce you to some of the main moves. So can videos such as *Your Backyard Swimming Pool Is Your Home Fitness Center*, from the U.S. Water Fitness Association.

Sign up for a class. Your local YMCA and other health facilities offer a wide range of classes. Make sure the instructor is nationally certified in aquatic fitness and trained in both general and water safety precautions. According to the American Council on Exercise, a good class should include a warmup, a gradually intensifying aerobics portion, muscle conditioning exercises, and a cooldown consisting of flexibility exercises.

Warm up. Experts recommend that you perform a three- to five-minute warmup in the water before a water aerobics workout. Start with knee lifts and then use straight leg kicks to warm your muscles. You may also want to stretch for three to five minutes at the side of the pool before you get into the water.

Get your heart pumping. The aerobic portion of your workout can include anything from water walking to lap swimming. Experts recommend that you gradually work up to your target heart rate and stay at that level for at least 20 minutes.

Cool down. Use the last three to five minutes of the aerobics segment of your workout to cool down, says Boutin. Gradually decrease the intensity, so your heart rate drops and you breathe more slowly.

Monitor your intensity. In order to get the most out of your workout and ensure that you are working at a safe level, keep track of how hard you're exerting yourself, says Boutin. Check to make sure your pulse is in your target heart rate zone, described on page 198. Or you can take the talk test: If you cannot comfortably hold a conversation with the person next to you, you're working too hard, she says.

Keep yourself nimble. You should conclude the class with the same kinds of stretches you did to warm up, says Boutin. This will help keep you flexible and prevent muscle soreness.

Get into the swim at least three to five times a week. "If you're consistent, you'll reach your goals," notes Boutin. Perform your water aerobics workout for at least 20 minutes, preferably on alternating days to allow for rest and recovery, she says.

Water Aerobics Workouts

Beginner

Target heart rate 60 to 65 percent of maximum, 2 to 3 days a week

Intermediate

Target heart rate 65 to 75 percent of maximum, 3 to 4 days a week

Experienced

Target heart rate 75 to 90 percent of maximum, 4 to 6 days a week

Intensity makes all the difference in water aerobics. "Don't be fooled into thinking that water aerobics is a 'no sweat' workout," says Marti Boutin, a training specialist for the Aquatic Exercise Association headquartered in Nokomis, Florida. Your heart rate may be lower in the water, but that doesn't mean you aren't working hard. The cooling and compression effects of the water, the decreased gravitational pull, and other factors may act to lower your heart rate.

Try these techniques to add to the intensity.

- Lift your knees higher while water walking and take longer strides.

- Jog or run instead of walking.

- Cup your hands and push or pull the water away from you.

- Add equipment that increases intensity, such as drag, buoyant, or weighted equipment.

Yard Work

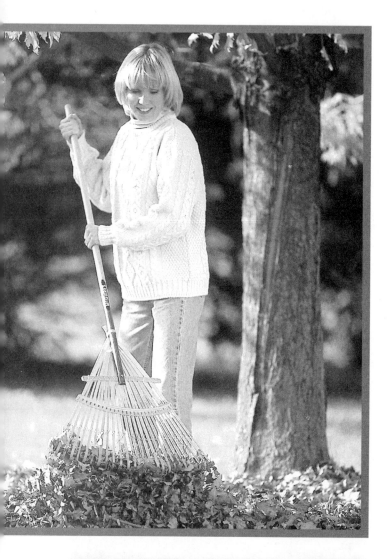

If you've ever maintained a lawn in the summer or raked and bagged an autumn's worth of leaves in October, you would probably claim that yard work makes for one good workout. You'll be happy to hear that exercise experts agree.

"Anyone who doesn't think that yard work leads to an enormous sense of fitness has never had to spread a truckload of topsoil over her lawn," says exercise physiologist Richard Cotton, chief exercise physiologist for the American Council on Exercise in San Diego. Yard work can also improve your aerobic fitness at the same time that it tones your muscles.

Body-Shaping Benefits

The walking, bending, heaving, and hoeing of yard work engages almost all of your torso, leg, and arm muscles, says Barbara Ainsworth, Ph.D., associate professor of exercise science and director of the Prevention Research Center at the University of South Carolina in Columbia.

- You'll get a challenging, calorie-burning aerobic workout from mowing, raking, and other rigorous, rhythmic tasks.
- You'll work your back, chest, abdomen, buttocks, legs, arms, and shoulders by pushing a lawn mower or pulling a rake or hoe. Trimming bushes and trees gives your arms and back an even greater workout.

The Right Footwear

Any activity that involves working with sharp tools on uneven terrain calls for protective footwear. Don't even think of tackling chores in a pair of flimsy loafers or canvas sneakers. Instead, lace up the sturdiest shoes you own—ones with hard soles and sturdy uppers. If you must, press your walking shoes or hiking boots into service for yard chores.

Yard Work Stats

Calories Burned*	Body-Shaping Potential
Mowing: 76 per 10 minutes	Tones arms, shoulders, chest, back, buttocks, abdomen, and legs
Raking: 37 per 10 minutes	
Hedging: 52 per 10 minutes	

*Based on a 150-pound woman. If you weigh more, you'll burn more calories; if you weigh less, you'll burn fewer.

What Else You'll Need

If you have a yard, you probably have at least a rake or two on hand, some kind of grass mower, and hand tools of some kind. Using the proper tools in the correct way can go a long way toward maximizing your yard "workout."

The right tools. Manual tools you have to push or pull with your own strength will build strong legs while you firm your abdomen and buttocks. A push lawn mower instead of a riding mower or an old-fashioned rake instead of a motorized leaf-blower will help give you the workout you're looking for.

When buying tools like clippers or edgers, choose manual versions. Pay particular attention to your ergonomic comfort: Look for comfortable handles and angles that require effort yet don't put undue strain on your back or other parts of your body. If possible, opt for a manual mower or a self-propelled push mower.

The right clothes. What you wear can make all the difference between a good experience and a not-so-good one, even in your own backyard. In warmer weather, wear loose-fitting lightweight clothes that will breathe when you perspire. In cooler weather, dress in layers

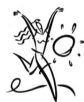

She Did It!

Suzanne Trimmed Her Waist by Trimming Her Trees

When Suzanne DeJohn, 38, moved from Boston to rural Vermont 10 years ago, she couldn't wait to get outside and begin working in her new yard.

"I love being out in the fresh air, listening to the trees rustle," she says. "I thrive on it."

So fond is Suzanne of the outdoors that she took a job as a landscaper. For five years she dug vegetable and flower beds, mowed and watered lawns, raked leaves, and hauled dirt, mulch, and rocks. At the same time, she took to tending a garden of her own at home. It's hard work, she says, but it's fun. What's more, it's the best physical fitness regimen she has ever engaged in.

"Yard work is a great form of exercise," she says. "I feel my fitness level increase each year, and friends have even commented on my strong muscles and good health." No longer a landscaper, she now works on staff for the National Gardening Association, teaching courses and answering the public's questions via the Internet. You can still find her out in her three-acre yard

every weekend, however, and often on weekdays after work.

"There's so much to do," Suzanne says. "My husband does most of the mowing, but I do the rest. We have quite a few maple trees, so there's a lot of raking, and there are trees and bushes to trim. I also spend a lot of time piling mulch and compost and manure into a wheelbarrow and spreading it around.

"I'm not a big person," Suzanne says. "I'm five feet six inches tall and of average build. I'm Italian, so I do love to eat, but I'm able to burn off those calories with yard and garden work.

"I'd much rather work in the yard and garden than go to a gym. The fresh air is wonderful, and I find a certain peace of mind outdoors. When I'm finished, I have a sense of accomplishment. I have something to show for all my work, whether it's a new perennial bed, a big pile of leaves, or a stone walkway. I can work all day and be so busy I hardly know I'm exercising."

Take It to the MAX

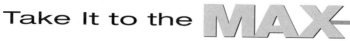

Turn Yard Maintenance into Self-Maintenance

Experts offer these tips for turning yard work into healthy and rewarding exercise.

Do it one day at a time. Don't overwhelm yourself with an entire list of yard work chores to finish right now, cautions Barbara Ainsworth, Ph.D., associate professor of exercise science and director of the Prevention Research Center at the University of South Carolina in Columbia. "Instead, think of one manageable task for each day. Maybe today you can edge the yard for 30 minutes, tomorrow you can spend a half-hour mowing, and the next day you can rake and bag the grass clippings. The day after that, you can trim the bushes. Don't expect to do everything in the first couple of hours."

Warm up mentally. There's a psychological warmup period for yard work, just as there is for other forms of exercise. "Sometimes I find it hard to get started on a difficult job like hauling mulch to my flowerbeds, but once I get through the first 10 to 15 minutes, I'm usually into it altogether," says Suzanne DeJohn, horticulture staff coordinator at the National Gardening Association in Burlington, Vermont. "It helps to remind myself how much I enjoy being in the fresh air. I also tell myself that this is a good way to get exercise, and that when I'm finished, I'll have something to show for all my hard work."

Do it with friends. DeJohn and her friends enjoy helping each other out with yard work. "I'll help someone clear brush one Saturday, and the next Saturday, she'll come help me fix a fence," she says. People she knows from another group rotate working at each other's homes one day a month. "Each person gets a workday every three or four months. They spend Saturday morning working, and the host provides lunch. It's great!"

Create new challenges. As you grow stronger, you can come up with new ways to make yard work even more of a workout, suggests Richard Cotton, chief exercise physiologist for the American Council on Exercise in San Diego. "Try walking a little faster behind your mower," he suggests. "Or switch from a power saw to a manual pruner for a great forearm and hand workout."

that you can easily take off or put back on as necessary.

Sun sense. Always wear a hat and sunscreen to protect against ultraviolet rays.

Getting Started

The grass is growing, the leaves are falling, and those dandelions are taking over the lawn. There's lots to be done and no time like the present. Here are some suggestions to help you tackle your yard.

Do a little at a time. If until now you've been paying the kid down the block to maintain your two-acre spread, don't hand him a pink slip quite yet. Start out by taking over only small portions of yard work and counting them as big accomplishments, Dr. Ainsworth suggests. "Just walking around watering your lawn burns more calories and is a lot better for you than sitting on the couch," she notes.

Warm up. Ease into light activity first, Dr. Ainsworth advises. "Don't immediately take the mower out and pull the crank on the engine. That's a huge strain on your back." Instead, do a few minutes of raking or some other activity that makes you gently move and stretch your whole body, she suggests.

Vary your activities. Don't lean over the rake all weekend. In fact, don't engage in any single yard work activity for hours on end, says Dr.

Ainsworth, or you'll risk stressing particular muscle groups and end up aching. Instead, break big tasks into smaller chunks of about 10 minutes each. "For example, rake a section of leaves into one pile," she says. "Trim bushes for 10 minutes, then bag the leaves you raked. Now mow a section of lawn."

Get close to your tools. Tools such as trimmers and hedgers can be heavy, awkward, and dangerous. "These tools put a strain on your hand, arm, and back as they work to support the weight of the implement," Dr. Ainsworth explains. To reduce the strain, pull the tool in closer toward your body as you work with it.

Watch your back. Whether you're picking up the hose or leaning over the mower, the frequent bending involved in yard work can really put pressure on your back. Practice proper bending and lifting techniques, suggests Dr. Ainsworth. Instead of bending at the waist, squat down with your legs, and lift back up with your legs instead of your back. When you're bagging leaves, a task that can be a real strain on your back, the best position is to kneel with one leg.

Switch sides. Give the muscles on both sides of your body a good workout. "Do your raking from the left, then switch to the right, and keep alternating periodically," says Dr. Ainsworth. "Otherwise, you'll end up out of balance, with one side of your body noticeably stronger than the other. There's also more risk of muscle strain if you stick to one side."

Drink a lot of water. Don't just water the grass. Water yourself frequently with a swig from a water bottle. If you don't, you'll risk dehydration, which can cause fatigue and muscle cramps. And don't wait to drink until you're thirsty. By then you're already dehydrated, explains Dr. Ainsworth.

Stop when you're tired. Don't be a weekend warrior, working in your yard from dawn till dark Saturday and aching from head to toe on Sunday. Instead, spread your yard work over the entire weekend, Ainsworth advises. Better yet, spread it out over several days throughout the week.

Yard Work Workouts

Beginner

Watering and seeding a lawn for 10 minutes, 2 or 3 times a week

Intermediate

Mowing with a self-propelled push mower, raking, or trimming shrubs or trees for 30 minutes at a time, 3 times a week

Experienced

Digging, spreading fertilizer, or mowing with a manual mower or doing other chores for 35 to 45 minutes, 4 or 5 times a week

"These levels are based on research that shows that it takes just as much energy to do some yard work tasks as it does to perform conventional exercises," says Barbara Ainsworth, Ph.D., associate professor of exercise science and director of the Prevention Research Center at the University of South Carolina in Columbia. "For instance, raking a lawn is comparable to bicycling at 10 miles per hour, and mowing a lawn with a manual mower can be as challenging as taking an aerobics class."

Ease into yard work at lower intensity levels for 10 minutes at a time, suggests Dr. Ainsworth. "Gradually increase your sessions to 30 minutes each at least three times a week for maximum health and fitness benefits," she says. You can add more high-intensity activities as you're able to handle them. To burn calories big time, work in your yard for 35 to 45 minutes at least five times a week, she adds.

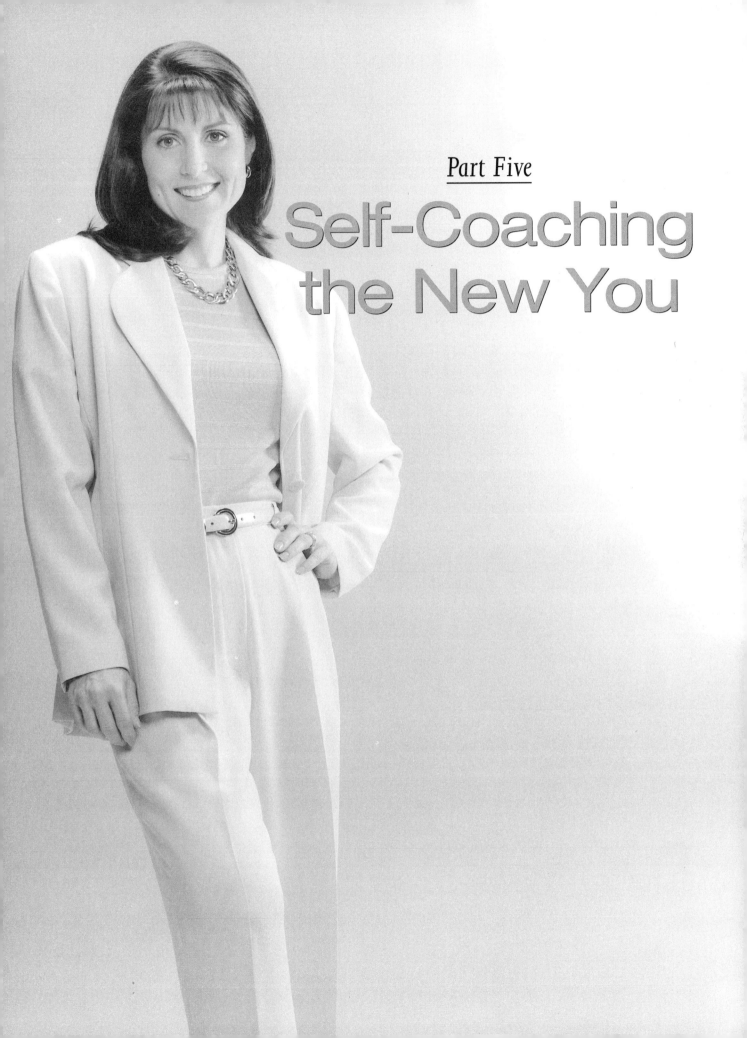

Part Five

Self-Coaching the New You

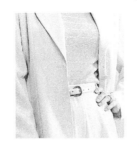

Your New Food Attitude

The average woman trying to lose weight has lost 100 pounds, gained 125, and been on 15 diets, says Debra Waterhouse, R.D., a registered dietitian in Oakland, California, and author of *Outsmarting the Midlife Fat Cell.* So chances are, you've tried to lose weight before, only to gain it back again.

The truth is, most people who do lose weight and keep it off haven't done so by finding the perfect crash diet or sipping a magical powder drink that melts away their fat cells, says Waterhouse. Lifelong weight control focuses not on your belly, butt, or thighs, but on your brain.

Women who lose weight and keep it off succeed because they change their eating habits and the way they regard food, says Waterhouse. They regard their bodies and attitudes not as obstacles, but as vehicles to success. Further, they don't pin their hopes on a celebrity or other personality who will dictate an absolute path of what to eat and when. Instead, they rely on themselves.

How do you develop a new food attitude? By exploring outmoded attitudes that may have trapped you on a dizzying diet carousel and refocusing your energy on more effective strategies—new strategies that put you in control.

Restyle Your Eating Style

Here are some common yet self-defeating food mindsets, along with refocusing strategies from experts in weight control. Use their suggestions to make over your food attitude.

Old attitude: *All I have to do is tell myself not to eat so much.*

New attitude: *I'm going to make some changes in my food milieu: what I buy, where I store food, how I prepare meals, where I eat, what I do while I'm eating, and how I order at restaurants.*

Cultivating a new food attitude means making meaningful food decisions, not relying on willpower to avoid temptation, says Kelly Brownell, Ph.D., director of the Yale University Center for Eating and Weight Disorders, who developed the LEARN (Lifestyles, Exercise, Attitudes, Relationships, and Nutrition) Program for Weight Control at the LEARN Education Center in Dallas. In his program, Dr. Brownell tells people to plan their meals, shop from a list, and go to the store on a full stomach—time-honored strategies that work.

"If your refrigerator resembles a salad bar because you shopped wisely, you'll suffer only minor damage if your resolve weakens," Dr. Brownell points out.

Other suggestions from Dr. Brownell include:

- Do nothing else while you eat.
- Eat on schedule.
- Eat in one place.
- Do not clean your plate.

Old attitude: *The holidays are coming (or the office bash, a cousin's wedding, or other food fest), so there's no point in even trying to watch what I eat right now.*

New attitude: *I'm going to develop coping strategies for tempting situations.*

"Don't make excuses, take control!" urges Laurie L. Friedman, Ph.D., deputy director of the Johns Hopkins Weight Management Center in Baltimore. Going to a holiday get-together? Offer to bring a salad, a lower-calorie appetizer or dessert, or even an exotic fruit plate. That way, you won't binge on cheesecake because you had no choice, she says. If you choose to eat some cheesecake, eat a small portion and enjoy it. But never let yourself be at the mercy of food or the situation.

"At a buffet, I suggest that people walk through and really look at everything before choosing. Just select a few things that are most appealing," Dr. Friedman says.

Old attitude: *Starting today, I will never eat chocolate (or french fries, or cheeseburgers, or Bavarian cream pastries) again.*

New attitude: *I can still eat whatever I want—occasionally. I just need to set limits for myself and stick to them.*

Every indulgence doesn't have to turn into a binge, says Dr. Friedman. "Some women may have foods that they like a lot or that trigger a binge for them," she notes. "While they're trying to lose weight, I ask them to temporarily avoid certain foods that might undermine their efforts. But vowing to avoid french fries forever is an empty promise.

"The long-term goal is moderation," Dr. Friedman adds, noting that for many people, high-fat foods lose some of their appeal once they get used to eating healthier choices.

When the women Dr. Friedman counsels do crave bacon cheeseburgers, she urges them to pay extra attention to the taste and texture of each bite. "Sometimes the idea or the smell is better than how it actually tastes when you're eating it," she says. You may find that after a bite or two, the pleasure fades and you can stop.

Old attitude: *Well, of course I ate a carton of ice cream at the end of a perfectly healthy day of eating. I'm a slob, I have no self-control, and I deserve to look this way.*

New attitude: *No one is perfect. I'm going to think about why this happened, take steps to prevent it the next time, and give myself a break.*

Don't fall into what Dr. Brownell calls light-bulb thinking, telling yourself that you are either perfect, eating healthy foods in reasonable portions, or horrible, slipping up and eating a big piece of cake—in essence turning the light out on your whole effort.

Instead, put your slipup in perspective: Over the course of a month, one 2,000-calorie mistake will not make much difference.

The real danger lies in heaping guilt and despair on yourself because you're not perfect, says Dr. Brownell in his LEARN program. If that happens, most likely you'll react by eating even more.

Old attitude: *I'm just going to follow the high-protein, low-carbohydrate diet that worked for my boss. I know it's a fad, but she lost weight really fast.*

New attitude: *I need to identify my own food attitudes and plan strategies that work best for me.*

The theory behind high-protein diets is that if the body doesn't have carbohydrates available, it will turn to stored fat for energy. A high-protein diet relies heavily on meat, eggs, and other animal sources of protein, while minimizing bread, potatoes, and other carbohydrates.

This diet works in the short term because it controls calories, and you lose a lot of water weight. The problem is that you can't stay healthy on this diet for the long haul: Animal foods are usually high in fat, and they don't provide enough vitamins and minerals or fiber. Also, when you restrict carbohydrates, your body breaks down lean muscle mass—exactly what you *don't* want to do to tone your muscles. Worse, this diet launches your body into a state of carbohydrate starvation: Your body begins to break down stored fat, but it also lapses into a dangerous state called ketosis, causing diarrhea, headaches, weakness, low blood pressure, fatigue, and sleeplessness. What's more, eating too much protein is hard on your kidneys.

So forget the high-protein diet—or any fad diet. Experts emphasize that any diet that eliminates certain food groups and depends heavily on others is unwise from a nutritional standpoint. It also does nothing to help you foster realistic eating patterns.

To do that, says Dr. Brownell, "evaluate your strengths and weaknesses and choose foods and cooking techniques that help you the most."

Begin by keeping a food diary of everything you eat for a week. Tally the calories and divide by seven days. Take note of the time, what you are doing while you eat, and what you are feeling.

A food diary will help you identify "automatic" eating habits, such as munching mindlessly, even when you're not hungry and not really appreciating the food. By paying attention to your eating, you'll also be able to spot patterns that may be thwarting your efforts to lose weight. Do you skip meals, then overeat? Do you tend to eat higher-fat, higher-calorie foods after 10:00 P.M.?

"Once people know which situations are risky for them, they can either avoid them or plan in advance how to deal with them," says Dr. Friedman. They might pack rice cakes and a gelatin snack as an afternoon pick-me-up at work, or decide not to eat in front of the television, she says.

Keeping a consistent food diary can even help keep you on track during the toughest time of the year—the holidays, says Raymond C. Baker, Ph.D., a psychologist at the St. Francis Medical Center in Peoria, Illinois. He studied 38 dieters to see who gained and who lost weight from late November through the new year.

"Lo and behold, the people who monitored their diets most closely lost the most weight," Dr. Baker says. Those who monitored their diets the least actually gained weight, even though they were enrolled in a weight-loss program.

"Be your own scientist," urges Dr. Baker. "See what works for you." He noted that many people who maintain weight loss continue their monitoring over the long haul, for a year or more. That way, they see patterns over time, rather than dwelling on one bad day or one great week.

Old attitude: *I eat nothing but salads, but I still gain weight. My problem is in my genes.*

New attitude: *Weight control may be tougher for me than other women, but I'm going to be honest with myself about what I eat.*

Most people eat much more than they think they do, recalling a three-ounce steak when it was actually an eight-ounce steak, or forgetting the pastry they grabbed as they walked by the snack room at work. When you keep a food diary, everything counts—even the french fries you eat off your child's plate, says Felicia Busch, R.D., a registered dietitian in St. Paul, Minnesota.

Grazing on junk food does make a difference if you are snacking several times a day, Busch points out.

You also need to think about precisely what you're eating. A salad drenched in a rich, creamy, or oil-based salad dressing and topped with mayonnaise-based macaroni salad carries the same fat and calorie burden as a plate of pasta with cream sauce, adds Anne Dubner, R.D., a registered dietitian and nutritional consultant in Houston.

Finally, consider whether you really may have eaten an extremely low calorie diet for so long that you've slowed down your metabolism. Women who consistently eat less than 1,200 calories a day get themselves to a state where they burn fewer calories, so their attempts at losing weight go nowhere, says Dubner. You can get back to normal within a few months by eating at least 1,200 calories a day and exercising to readjust your metabolism, she says.

Old attitude: *I'm under a lot of stress now. I'll eat more sensibly when things calm down.*

New attitude: *Things may never calm down. I have to find other ways to cope besides food.*

Stress is really just a euphemism for what psychologists see as a whole Pandora's box of emotions. Dr. Baker encourages people enrolled in his weight-control program to stop to analyze the real emotion behind the stress. Are they bored when they eat? Angry? Overwhelmed? Sad?

Ask yourself the same questions. Once you decide what's bothering you, you'll be able to find better alternatives to munching the feeling away, says Dr. Baker. If you're overwhelmed, take time to get organized instead of racing for the doughnut box. If you're sad, think of nonfood ways to soothe yourself: You might run a hot, candlelit bath sprinkled with lavender while you listen to music. If you're angry, take a run or a brisk walk.

For handling ongoing or long-term stress, experts recommend learning meditation or deep-breathing techniques.

Old attitude: *I have no willpower. If the cookies are there, I'm going to eat the whole bag.*

New attitude: *I am an adult who can and will make rational choices about what I eat.*

Ask yourself, "Am I making a conscious decision to eat this, or am I getting carried away with my emotions? Am I trying to avoid working on this project, so I'm eating instead?"

Once you learn to differentiate between a "want" and a "choice," you'll begin to have a much more relaxed relationship with food, says Dubner. "A choice is something that's rational. A want is emotional," she explains.

To further analyze your "wants," think about what you crave and why, then substitute something satisfying but lower in fat and calories, recommends Dubner. For example, when you're about to dig into the double chocolate chip cookies, ask yourself if it's the crunchiness that appeals to you or the sweetness. Would a crunchy carrot dipped in fat-free Ranch dressing suffice? Or a cup of hot chocolate made with skim milk?

If you decide that you really want a cookie after all, decide if you can eat just one or two. If you can't, then eat more, says Dubner, but realize it is your choice. Your brain is not at the mercy of a rushing current of need that carries you helplessly downstream. Thinking through your choice prevents out-of-control bingeing.

Old attitude: *I tried counting calories and measuring out portions for a while. But then it seemed like I went over the deep end and ate more than ever. I don't think it's possible for me to eat in moderation, especially when it comes to something like Oreo cookies. They're meant to be eaten by the bag in front of the TV.*

New attitude: *I'm not going to force myself to go on a rigid diet. I'm going to learn healthier ways of eating for life.*

Give portion control another try, says Dubner. But this time, use it as a guideline or tool, not as an extreme restriction. Measure out foods you like once. Take a look at the fat and calorie content, so you'll have a general idea how much they add to your total food intake for the day. But you don't have to weigh and measure all your food on a daily basis. "That will just drive you crazy," she says.

Old attitude: *Part of food's appeal is the camaraderie. At my office, eating chocolate is a common bond among the women I work with. We talk about it, share it, give it to each other as gifts.*

New attitude: *I'm going to appreciate my friends for who they are and not what we eat together. I'm going to ask them to do the same.*

If you have trouble being assertive, you're not alone. Dr. Baker found that many men and women in his weight-control program have a difficult time stating their needs to others. He advises a take-charge approach. What would happen if you proposed to your chocolate-loving buddies that you all embark on a month of healthy eating?

"Sometimes other people in the group are struggling, too," Dr. Baker says. Under your plan, you could still share the cooking and eating elements of your friendship without having to sacrifice something important to you—getting in shape. Maybe you could have a potluck soup and salad night, or make healthy box lunches to trade on your break.

Also, give your friends some credit. Do they really only invite you to the party because you bring chocolate torte, or is it actually your company they enjoy? If they care about you, they'll want the best for you. Explain your reasons for wanting to make some changes and ask for their help. You may be surprised at their warm response.

Old attitude: *My mother and sister are health food nuts. I grew up having to hide the Twinkies. Even as an adult, I feel they're still pressuring me to lose weight—and now my husband has joined in. I was always a rebel, so my immediate reaction is to eat as much food as I can get my hands on.*

New attitude: *I'm going to take responsibility for my own well-being. I need to tune them out and go about losing weight slowly and patiently in my own way.*

Someone who eats Twinkies for revenge is thinking of food as a weapon, rather than as nourishment or pleasure, says Dubner. If you're eating to satisfy or annoy someone else, you have lost touch with your inner voice, the one that will guide you to foods you enjoy while you accomplish personal goals for your body and your life.

Explore your own motivations for changing your eating patterns, Waterhouse suggests. How do you personally feel when you overeat? On the other hand, how do you feel when you eat healthy meals all day and go for a walk? What are your personal goals for fitness and health?

Value yourself and let motivation for change come from within, says Waterhouse. You may be pleasantly surprised that healthy eating is a springboard for other changes in your life.

Old attitude: *I know women who stay slim because they exercise all the time and eat big plates of bulgur, tofu, and other beans and grains. But that's not for me. I refuse to abandon all fun in my life and eat strange foods.*

New attitude: *I'm not going to eat foods I hate, but I will try new things. Making healthy lifestyle choices is fun, and doing something good for myself is satisfying.*

Who says "strange" foods taste bad? Like the reluctant character in Dr. Seuss's well-known *Green Eggs and Ham*, you may want to recapture some of the risk-taking you probably excelled at when you first left your mother's table, says Busch. You just might discover that your friend eating the tabbouleh isn't doing it just to be good—she actually likes to eat it because it's delicious!

Visit alternative grocery stores on sampling days and try just a nibble of the week's free offerings, Busch suggests. People who might cringe at the thought of eating raw fish in the form of sushi—a low-calorie, low-fat food—might change their minds if they try a vegetarian version. Besides, eating raw fish isn't safe, she adds.

"One suggestion I give almost everybody is to buy one thing you haven't tried before every time you go to the grocery store," Busch says.

Beyond new choices, you may be underestimating the number of healthy foods you already like, says Dubner.

Every food group contains many, many choices. So if you hate bulgur and cottage cheese, eat whole-wheat bread and a low-fat pudding cup instead. For other suggestions, see the "New Foods to Try" sections throughout part 2.

Old attitude: *I see women who can eat anything they want and still stay skinny as a rail. I'm short, and I gain weight when I just think about food. It's not fair.*

New attitude: *I'm going to concentrate on looking and feeling my best and stop dwelling on things I can't change.*

Life, indeed, is unfair. Start by accepting that, say experts. Your genetic background, metabolism, skeletal structure, and body type all factor into the person you see when you look in the mirror, acknowledges Dubner.

"If you're destined to be a round person, you're never going to be a skinny-minny, Twiggy-type person," Dubner says. You can exercise and eat healthy foods, however, to make your figure proportionate and firm. As a bonus, you can also keep your heart healthy and your bones strong.

Don't compare yourself to the slender woman eating the overstuffed corned beef sandwich and fries, warns Dubner. "You don't know how much she exercises. Maybe that's the first meal she's eaten all day, and that's not very healthy."

Old attitude: *I lost 50 pounds. Now I can finally eat anything I want.*

New attitude: *My new food attitude is a healthy and productive one. Sure, I can indulge in a special dessert once in a while, but my switch to healthy eating is something I'll stick with for a lifetime.*

"If you gained weight in the first place, you're prone to gaining it back again," says Dubner. The "I'm fixed now" syndrome is the biggest reason people regain weight, no matter how thrilled they were to reach their goals.

Stick with your food diary and study it periodically to find your vulnerabilities. If you never really shook loose of that late-night snack, make sure you've stocked your kitchen with popcorn and pretzels. "Sometimes, it's much easier to change the food than it is to change the behavior," Dubner notes.

For more first-person stories of women who changed their attitudes toward food, visit our Web site at www.banishbbt.com.

Personal Food Diary

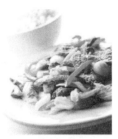

Experts say the best way to get an accurate picture of what you're eating is to keep a food diary for three days. Photocopy these pages and then continue to record what you eat—including snacks and beverages. That helps you to look at your overall diet, rather than focusing on "good" or "bad" foods at any one meal.

Date

Breakfast
Lunch
Dinner
Snacks
Beverages

Date

Breakfast
Lunch
Dinner
Snacks
Beverages

Date

Breakfast
Lunch
Dinner
Snacks
Beverages

Date

Breakfast

Lunch

Dinner

Snacks

Beverages

Date

Breakfast

Lunch

Dinner

Snacks

Beverages

Date

Breakfast

Lunch

Dinner

Snacks

Beverages

Date

Breakfast

Lunch

Dinner

Snacks

Beverages

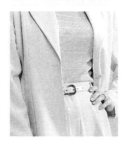

Action Tips for Exercisers

Okay, you're convinced: Getting some form of calorie-burning exercise a couple of times a week is the only way you're going to leave unwanted pounds behind. Doing crunches, leg raises, and other forms of resistance training for your tummy, backside, hips, and thighs is the only way you're going to trim and tone your belly, butt, and thighs. The question is, just *when* is all this exercise going to take place? Experts agree: Finding time—and staying motivated—isn't always easy.

"After a long day at work, it's easier to plop down in front of the TV than to go out for a run or walk," says Joyce Nash, Ph.D., a clinical psychologist in San Francisco and Menlo Park, California, and author of *The New Maximize Your Body Potential.* "To overcome the time trap, schedule exercise on your calendar and treat it like an important appointment," she suggests.

"Women I advise always ask me how to 'keep the music playing,' as I like to put it," says Lisa Hoffman, an exercise physiologist and personal trainer in New York City, and author of *Better Than Ever: The Four-Week Workout Program for Women over 40.* "At times, you'll be really motivated to exercise, and at others, you won't feel like doing anything. It happens even to me."

Life's hectic pace doesn't help.

"I don't know of any woman, whether she be a mother or a working woman or both, who isn't exceptionally busy, searching desperately for time for herself," notes Liz Neporent, an exercise physiologist and president of Plus One Health Management in New York City.

Competing obligations squash plans, too.

"Women are socialized to put other people first," says Dr. Nash. "Putting our needs first or even equal to others makes us feel terribly guilty. We're thinking, 'I can't go to the gym, I have to watch the kids tonight or work overtime at the office.'"

The key to success is to anticipate problems, says Judith Young, Ph.D., executive director of the National Association for Sports and Physical Education in Reston, Virginia. "Identify the things that can prevent you from following through on your plans and make plans for dealing with them," she says.

Here's a list from the experts of top exercise obstacles—with practical tips for countering each.

Problem: *You hate to exercise.*

Solution: *Choose activities that you really, truly enjoy.*

Just because your sister-in-law runs, your neighbor goes for marathon bike rides, and your pals at the office go to aerobics classes religiously doesn't mean you have to. Opt for belly dancing, elliptical training, inline skating—or just plain walking, if that's your pleasure, say experts.

Problem: *You've tried exercise before, but you dropped out after two or three sessions.*

Solution: *Announce your intentions to your family and friends. This makes it more likely that you'll stick to your program.*

Problem: *You exercise every day for the first week, then get distracted, and by week three, you've abandoned exercise altogether.*

Solution: *Start out exercising just twice a week. This leaves room for you to have a desire to do more, instead of setting yourself up for failure because you haven't fulfilled greater ambitions.*

Problem: *You have too much to do and too little time.*

Solution: *You have lots of company, says Neporent.* Surveys show that most people who want to exercise but don't blame lack of time. You can find the time, though. Here's how.

- Figure out your best time of day, says Dr. Young. Some women get up early to work out first thing in the morning, getting it over and done with before the world starts humming. Others can't function before two cups of coffee, so they save their workouts for later in the day.

- Make exercise appointments. Write them down in your daily planner or stick a reminder on your refrigerator door. This helps you create an exercise habit while also training your family to anticipate and respect your exercise regimen. Fit other appointments around your exercise session, rather than vice versa.

- Do it for 10 minutes. Studies have shown that accumulating 30 minutes of daily exercise in 10-minute chunks has positive calorie-burning and heart-strengthening effects, says Neporent.

- Try this: Walk 10 minutes before work, do another 10 at lunchtime, and finish the day with 10 minutes after dinner.

- Exercise with short videos. A number of exercise videos now incorporate a week's worth of short—no longer than 15 minutes—routines on the same tape. Do one routine a day and rewind at the end of the week.

- Walk around the block while dinner's cooking instead of waiting for the meat loaf to bake.

- Make phone calls on a speaker or portable phone while you're on a treadmill or bike or doing a stretch routine. In fact, this is a great time to take the "talk test" of exercise intensity: Your breathing should be such that you can hold up your end of a conversation.

Problem: *My family needs me. The kids whine when I'm not available, and my husband says I'm ignoring him.*

Solution: *Include your family in exercise.*

- Join a health club that offers baby-sitting services or kids' activities. You get your exercise while your child gets entertained.

- Do your workout during your child's soccer or softball practice, suggests Dr. Young. Instead of just daydreaming on the bench, walk, jog, or bike.

- Use your small ones as exercise aids, says Dr. Young. Plop your seated infant at your feet and do curl-ups toward her, saying "peek-a-boo" as you sit up. Or sit in a chair, balance your toddler astride your ankles and shins, hold her hands, and bounce her gently up and down, working your quadriceps, she suggests.

- Encourage your husband to exercise with you. This can be a big boost to your exercise routine while relieving the guilt that can arise from "abandoning" your spouse to do something for yourself, notes Hoffman.

If you still have problems, talk it over with your family, says Dr. Nash. Explain the changes you want to make, why they're important to you, and what help you'll need from them. For example, "I want to go for a walk three mornings a week, so you'll need to get up and eat breakfast by yourselves." If your plans will cause them difficulties, work out compromise solutions.

Problem: *My family doesn't seem to mind if I exercise, but I still feel guilty when I leave them to work out.*

Solution: *Tell yourself that you deserve some time to take care of your body, says Dr. Nash.*

- Consider yourself a positive role model for your children, Dr. Young says. Your routine will demonstrate the benefits of exercise, from having more energy to being in a better mood. Emphasize the concept further still by taking your child along on walks and bike rides.

Problem: *You work in an office all day and can't seem to fit in any exercise.*

Solution: *Be creative and flexible.*

- Work out flexible work hours, recommends Hoffman. Arrange for a later starting time so that you can hit the gym before work, or for an earlier starting time so you can exercise after work. Or extend your workday so you can take a long lunch break for exercise.

Quick Answers to Common Excuses

Some days, outside forces coax you to skip a workout. Should you tough it out, or ease off? Experts offer this advice.

"I have cramps." Laying off is definitely valid if you have bad menstrual cramps or heavy bleeding. But a little exercise may actually help relieve cramping, says Rosemary Agostini, M.D., clinical associate professor of orthopedics at the University of Washington and staff physician at the Virginia Mason Sports Medicine Center, both in Seattle. Coax yourself into exercising for just a few minutes and see how you feel.

"I have the flu." If you're sick, hang up your sneakers. Exercising now will probably only make you feel worse, especially if you have a fever, says Dr. Agostini. When your body is fighting a virus, it needs rest and lots of fluids to marshal its resources to fight the bug. Give yourself time—and permission—to sit it out, she says.

"It's rainy and cold outside." Carry a mini folding umbrella with you so you don't have to miss your walk during a rain shower, or wear a waterproof jogging outfit, suggests Liz Neporent, an exercise physiologist and president of Plus One Health Management in New York City. In cold weather, bundle up, starting with a sweat-permeable inner layer of moisture-wicking synthetic fabric, such as polypropylene or CoolMax. Add an insulating middle layer of fleece or wool to keep the cold out, and finish with a waterproof or windproof outer layer, such as Gore-Tex.

"It's too dark to exercise outside by the time I get home." Wear white clothing and reflective gear to protect yourself against traffic when you're out in the dark, advises Judith Young, Ph.D., executive director of the National Association for Sports and Physical Education in Reston, Virginia. If you exercise at a gym at night and are concerned about safety, go with a friend or at least ask someone at the gym to walk you to your car after your workout.

"Business travel and vacations mess up my routine." Sneak exercise into your travel plans, says Dr. Young. At airports, challenge yourself to walk along, but faster than, the moving sidewalks. At your destination, see the sights on foot. Stay at a hotel with exercise facilities, or take along a jump rope. Pack an exercise video and plug it into your hotel room's VCR. And consider an active vacation spent hiking, biking, or skiing.

- Exercise in your office. Close the door and do crunches or pushups, says Neporent. If you don't have privacy, do exercises in your chair like "writing the alphabet" with your toes, which works your shins and calves. Trace each letter from A to Z on the floor with the big toe of each foot. You can also strengthen your thighs by tightening and releasing your thigh muscles while sitting.

Problem: *You work the night shift.*

Solution: *There's no rule that says you can't exercise at odd hours, points out Dr. Young. As long as you're* getting enough sleep and have a safe place to exercise—say, on home exercise equipment—there's no reason you can't exercise at 1:00 A.M. after your midnight shift.

Problem: *You have trouble staying motivated when you exercise alone.*

Solution: *Make exercise time social time.*

- When a friend asks you to a movie or dinner, suggest that you go for a hike together instead.
- Tell your co-workers you plan to walk during your lunch hour, and ask them to join you if you'd enjoy company.

- Get an exercise buddy. Working out alone can be a welcome break, but sometimes making a commitment to work out with someone else makes it more likely you'll actually do it, says Dr. Young. Choose someone who is convenient, such as a neighbor down the block, and who has similar exercise interests and skill levels. Agree from the outset that you'll both be positive and supportive rather than critical of each other, she adds.

- Have an online buddy. If you have computer access to the Internet, send e-mail messages about your workouts to online exercise buddies.

Problem: *You can't afford a lot of expensive equipment, gym fees, or fancy workout clothes.*

Solution: *Keep it simple.*

- Take up something simple like walking, jogging, or using exercise videos, says Neporent.

- Amortize the fees at your health club: The cost per visit decreases with each visit, so the more you exercise, the cheaper it is. Say the annual fee is $500—pretty steep if you go only once. Go twice, and it's $250 per visit; four times, $125; and so forth. So if you go three times a week over the course of the year, it comes down to $3.20 per visit.

- Join a gym where you can pay per month or per session. Then go only when you need to—like when it's too cold to exercise outdoors.

- Ask for workout clothes instead of other gifts for your birthday, Christmas, Hanukkah, or other special occasions. The same goes for exercise gear like water aerobics aids, aerobic videos, bicycling gel seats, and so forth.

Problem: *You'd like to go to the gym, but it's just too much trouble to drive there, especially in bad weather, so you often end up skipping your workout.*

Solution: *Exercise at home.*

- A motorized treadmill, stationary bicycle, or exercise video will do just fine for aerobic exercise, says Hoffman. And you can do your workouts to trim your abdominals, hips, thighs, and buttocks at home on a mat.

- To create the feel of a health club and help you to keep an eye on your form, add a mirror to your workout space, suggests Neporent.

- Tell your family that you need some time for yourself, Neporent says. Unless they're going to work out with you, this is your time, not the time to help your kids write a book report.

Problem: *Your hair and makeup get messed up when you exercise, and you have to go back to work.*

Solution: *Dealing with perspiration will solve both problems, says Paula Begoun, makeup artist and author of* Don't Go Shopping for Hair Care Products without Me. *Perspiration makes frizzy hair frizzier and straight hair limp. It also can cause makeup to move and streak. Further, salt from sweat gets trapped under makeup, irritating your skin.*

- Pull your hair back to get it off your sweaty neck, says Begoun. This will keep you cooler, and your hair will be less likely to get wet, which can destroy just about any hairdo.

- Avoid wearing makeup during exercise, suggests Begoun. The combination of makeup and perspiration may irritate your skin. If you don't want to remove and reapply your makeup for a quick lunchtime workout, use a "stay-put" makeup, which doesn't drip or move. Then, to prevent streaks, gently dab perspiration with a soft cloth as you exercise.

Problem: *You mean to work out, but you forget your workout clothes half the time, or you're too rushed to get your exercise gear together before leaving for work.*

Solution: *Plan ahead. Pack your workout clothes a day in advance or have extra workout clothes stashed in your desk at work, says Hoffman.*

Problem: *You start out with enthusiasm, but you just can't seem to stay motivated.*

Solution: *Remind yourself why you're doing this.*

- Put your reasons down on paper. Write down both the benefits of exercising and getting in shape and the costs of not doing so, suggests Dr. Nash. For example, "Benefit of exercising: I look better in my clothes. Cost of not exercising: I feel fat, tired, and bad about myself." Display your list in a prominent place.

- Mentally rehearse doing exercise. What your mind believes, your body achieves, says Dr. Nash. When you wake up in the morning, spend a few moments in bed mentally picturing yourself exercising. Surround yourself with inspirational posters and pictures of women involved in various forms of exercise.

- Give yourself a gold star. Using a calendar that displays a month at a time, apply an adhesive gold star for every day that you exercise. Or use a variety of stickers to designate different activities, like happy faces for bike rides and stars for speed-walking.

- Note your progress. You'll feel more motivated if you check your progress against your initial goals every two months or so, says Neporent.

- Train for an ambitious goal. Once you're in the swing of regular exercise, pump up your motivation by aiming for an event, suggests Hoffman. For example, if you're a walker or runner, sign up for a local 5-K or 10-K race.

Problem: *Some days exercise feels easy, but sometimes, it's a real effort to get through.*

Solution: *Expect tough days and deal with them. It happens to even the most avid of exercisers, says Hoffman. One day you run around the block effortlessly and care-free, the next you count every minute and feel like you're carrying a bag of cement on your back. Expect the mentally tough days and just do your best to push yourself through them, knowing that tomorrow is another day. If you are slowed by a physical (rather than a mental) soreness, however, take it easy, she adds.*

Problem: *You react to any setback with frustration and give up.*

Solution: *Know that backsliding is normal. Maybe your old habits caught up to you or life got so hectic that you didn't exercise for a week or two. Just get back on track as quickly as possible and don't waste time beating yourself up over it, says Hoffman.*

Problem: *You've been exercising for months, but you're getting bored, and you can't get excited about activities you used to enjoy.*

Solution: *These are signs that your exercise regimen is getting stale, say experts. To renew your interest in exercise:*

- Change the scenery. If you usually work out indoors, logging miles on a treadmill or stationary bike, move your workout outside for a refreshing new environment, suggests Dr. Young. Or bring your running-around-the-block workout inside.

- Take up an entirely new activity. If you've always stuck to solitary pursuits, sign up for a team sport, such as volleyball, or a partner game, such as tennis. Or sign up for a class to train for running a marathon.

- Watch television or listen to music on headphones while you're walking on a treadmill or lifting weights. For your stationary bike and stairclimber at home, buy a plastic rack that fits onto the console and holds reading material—like motivating fitness magazines—and a water bottle, says Neporent. For safety, don't wear Walkman-type headphones when you're out on the roads, however: You won't be able to hear traffic or pay attention to your surroundings.

- Try an occasional "take it to the max" workout: If you always do 25 crunches, aim for as many as you can short of muscle cramps, says Dr. Young. If you jog, go to a local track and run a mile as fast as you can, timing yourself with a stopwatch.

- Try new exercise toys. Heart rate monitors, exercise tubes and rubber bands, exerballs, and aquatic exercise gear can make workouts more fun and challenging. Find out which new training gadgets are available for your favorite activity, or try something altogether new with them.

For more information on motivational tips, visit our Web site at www.banishbbt.com.

Personal Exercise Log

Date

The key to banishing your belly, butt, and thighs with exercise is consistency. Photocopy this exercise log and use it to record your aerobic efforts and body-shaping workouts every day. You should see results in as little as four weeks!

Aerobic Exercise

Activity	Duration

Workouts for Waist and Tummy

Exercise	Sets/reps
Curl-Ups 1	
Curl-Ups 2	
Curl-Ups 3	
Knee-Up Crunches	
Crunches with Knees Up, Spread	
Inclined Board Crunches	
Hip Raises	
Modified Knee Raises	
Pelvic Tilts	
Reverse Curls	
Single-Knee Lifts	
Diagonal Curl-Ups 1	
Diagonal Curl-Ups 2	
Diagonal Curl-Ups 3	
Side Crunches	
Side Bends	
Side Jackknives	

Workouts for Hips, Thighs, and Buttocks

Exercise	Sets/reps
Leg Extensions	
Lunges	
Squats	
Wall Squats	
Leg Curls	
Prone Single-Leg Raises	
Back Leg Extensions	
Bent-Leg Extensions	
Pelvic Lifts	
Bent-Knee Crossovers	
Side-Lying Straight-Leg Raises	
Standing Abductions	
Seated Abductions	
Side-Lying Bent-Leg Raises	
Fire Hydrants	
Inner Leg Raises	
Seated Inner Leg Raises	
Butterfly Leg Raises	
Single-Leg Pelvic Lifts	
Scissors	

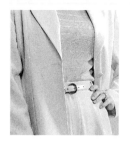

Instant Minimizers

You don't have to wait until you've banished your belly, butt, or thighs to find the right dress for a night on the town, the perfect jeans for casual wear, or a wonderful outfit for the office. You can find clothes that flatter your figure now, whether you've just started your shape-up program or you've been exercising diligently and still have a few inches to lose. With the right style, color, and details, you won't even notice your trouble spots—and no one else will, either.

Slimming Tips from Fashion Experts

Rest assured: You don't have to buy a closet full of new clothes to minimize the appearance of your belly, butt, and thighs (unless you want to). Start with a couple of key pieces: innovative shapewear (a modern version of the girdle), plus a go-everywhere jacket, crisp jeans, and a figure-flattering skirt or pair of pants. Then combine these pieces with wardrobe items you already own, to create "new" outfits that flatter your individual figure. But first, here are some general guidelines from industry experts.

Layer—for now. Once you've successfully slimmed down and shaped up, you may be able to wear dresses and separates that hug your figure. Until then, you can cheat with a jacket or loose blouse that eases the transition from top to bottom, says Liria Mersini, owner of the Cello clothing line in Santa Monica, California.

Up-to-date layering goes beyond the dowdy overblouses of yesteryear. Modern layering is still simple, but more sophisticated. A summer-weight wool duster jacket over a matching fitted dress, for example, is great for all shapes because it camouflages your trouble spots while giving a slim illu-

sion. Or try a short vest over a thigh-length oversize cotton blouse (a superb casual look for anyone with heavy upper thighs or a thick waist).

Don't assume more coverage is better. Sometimes, covering your lower body with lots of fabric draws attention to a trouble spot instead of camouflaging it, says Nancy Nix-Rice, an image consultant from St. Louis and author of *Looking Good: A Comprehensive Guide to Wardrobe Planning and Personal Style Development*. The right style will use just the right amount of fabric—not too much, not too little for your figure type.

Be bold. An interesting top or jacket can divert attention away from the tummy, derriere, and thighs, says Nix-Rice. Wear tops embellished with bright colors, beads, or textured fabric.

Make black work to your advantage. Anyone who has ever felt self-conscious about her weight has relied on the slimming effects of wearing dark colors, especially black. But black alone can get boring and depressing. So can all navy and all brown, which in some fashion seasons stand in for black. So Nix-Rice takes this concept one step further. She suggests wearing a dark or muted solid color on bottom and a printed or light-colored top. This tactic will make your body look more proportional while giving your wardrobe some life, she says.

Select fabric that works with you, not against you. Certain materials create a slim silhouette, but stretch when you sit. Slinky knit fabric is popular for its good recovery and swing, says Peggy Lutz, designer and owner of Peggy Lutz Plus in Sebastopol, California. Other fabrics are suitable when cut on the bias (diagonal to the vertical and horizontal weave or knit stitch). The fabric is cut "on-grain," and when joined, the finished garment hangs perfectly up and down and across the body. Bias-cut garments are more expensive, but they have more stretch and drape—the effect is wonderful. The garment hugs your body's contours without clinging and stretching.

Test for ease. Try moving in the clothes. Sit, walk—the more comfortable you are, the less you'll draw attention to your trouble spots by fussing over them.

Look for details with vertical lines. Even a subtle seam in a jacket or pleats in a pair of pants can make a difference, says Katie Arons, of Hollywood, California, a well-known plus-size model and author of *Sexy at Any Age*.

Go for a tailored look. If you're heavy, don't fall into the trap of thinking you should wear loose, baggy clothes. Not so. Tailored clothes—fitted and semifitted suits and classic dresses, skirts, and pants—are more flattering (and more appropriate in the office). In many cases, company policy requires a tailored look—most often a suit. Professionals also need suits for work. But to look her best, a heavier woman must choose tailored clothes carefully, say experts.

Wear what fits. Although it may be tough to admit that you no longer fit into a smaller size you once wore, it's important to be honest with yourself and realistic. Wearing a garment that pulls down in back when you sit, has wrinkles at the side seams, or cups under your buttocks will only draw attention to your trouble spots.

Consider plus-size clothing. Designers and manufacturers who offer plus-size clothing (starting as low as size 14) specialize in creating garments and outfits designed to minimize your tummy, derriere, and thighs.

Jeans That Fit and Look Sharp

Women of all ages wear jeans. And with so many styles from which to choose, you can get comfort and flattering fit without compromising style, even if you can't wear slim, tapered styles marketed to teens.

To determine the best jeans for your shape, check out the following tips on styles that minimize the appearance of your belly, butt, or thighs, from

experts Norma Willis, pattern manager for the Lee and Riders labels in Merriam, Kansas, and Sarah Schwennsen, design manager of women's wear bottoms for Levi Strauss and Company in San Francisco.

Relaxed-Fit

You want: Jeans that disguise your thighs or allow room for an ample derriere. If your thighs are the problem, you need a silhouette that pulls the viewer's eyes away from the thighs. If you have an ample derriere, you need a cut that provides enough ease to wear the jeans comfortably and doesn't wrinkle at the top of your thighs or cup under your buttocks.

Look for: Jeans with more fabric in the seat and upper legs, and a flat front. You can wear waistline pleats that carry through to fuller legs, but you don't want your thighs swaddled in yards of fabric. Schwennsen recommends Levi's 519 Low-Cut Relaxed Flare for a relaxed fit through the hips and thighs and a boot-cut leg and 555 Guy's Fit, which has a low rise and straight legs. (Both these jeans solve several other fit and appearance concerns as well.)

Boot-Cut Legs

You want: Jeans that won't emphasize your derriere or thighs.

Look for: Legs that extend straight to the knee, then widen slightly at the hem. Now called a boot cut, this isn't the same dramatic bell-bottoms style that women wore in the 1960s. This shape pulls attention away from your waist and down to your hemline.

If you aren't comfortable with the boot-cut shape, opt instead for legs that drop straight from the hips to the hem. Avoid a tapered leg because the narrow ankles and lower legs will only draw attention to your thighs, hips, and waist.

Low-Rise Waist

You want: Jeans that make your stomach look flat.

Look for: Jeans with a low-rise waist, which sits on or under your belly button. A full-rise front can ride over your tummy and settle at your waist, emphasizing a belly.

For a protruding derriere, experts disagree on which is better: jeans with an all-around low-rise waist, or a low rise only in front. Schwennsen says a low-rise all around is better because there's less fabric across your rear, making it look less prominent. Willis, on the other hand, prefers a low-rise front and full back so your back won't be exposed when you sit. Jeans cut with more fabric in the crotch or loose, full-cut fronts are less likely to pull down when you sit. Try both and decide what works for you.

Full-Span Pocket

You want: Support to hold in your tummy bulge, and a streamlined style that fits comfortably.

Look for: Jeans with a full-span pocket, which secretly holds your tummy in place. Made of two fabric pieces that extend from each side seam to the center front, this pocket gives you a firm fabric "girdle" that controls your tummy.

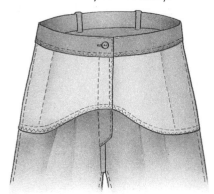

Pocket Details

You want: To minimize the appearance of your derriere.

Look for: Good fit plus patch pockets that aren't too big or too small, or that sit too low.

Outside pockets can also dramatically minimize your derriere because they break up the expanse of your rear—as long as the pockets are proportional and properly positioned. Avoid small patch pockets and keep in mind that if pockets are sewn on too low, it'll look like your derriere dropped.

Shopping for Shorts

Just because your hips, thighs, or backside need work doesn't mean you have to forgo shorts. Your first impulse might be to choose a garment that covers as much real estate as possible: baggy sweats or "elephant leg" shorts. Resist the urge. If you're apple-shaped—with a prominent tummy but slim hips—you can look particularly great in shorts, says Rita Farro in her book *Life Is Not a Dress Size*. Same goes if you're pear-shaped, with heavy hips and thighs that taper to slender knees, calves, and ankles. But whatever your shape, you can find shorts that offer comfort, fit, and style.

Pick the best features from among available styles—walking, boxer, or cargo—and stick with them. Take your cue from the following guidelines, offered by Gail Grigg Hazen, of Saratoga, California, and author of *Fantastic Fit for Every Body*, who has fitted many women with figures just like yours.

Elasticized Waist

You want: Easy fit and comfort while moving and sitting.

Look for: A waistband with elastic inserts at the sides or back.

If you carry a fair amount of weight in your belly, butt, or thighs, you need shorts that are roomy enough to accommodate your curves when you sit or bend. As you've no doubt discovered, tailored waistbands tend to stay put when you move. Elastic waistbands have plenty of give, but they create unflattering gathers at your waist and hips. The answer: elastic inserts at the sides of the waistband, or an elasticized back waistband.

Because women who carry their weight in their lower bodies often tend to be short-waisted,

Grigg Hazen also recommends narrow waistbands. A wide waistband further shortens the distance between the midriff and waist.

Full Legs

You want: To downplay the appearance of your tummy.

Look for: Shorts with loose upper legs.

If you carry your extra weight in your waist and abdomen but have a slim backside and hips, it's tempting to show off your attributes by choosing shorts that hug your legs. This strategy will backfire, since the same style that hugs those gams also fits snugly around your tummy, creating a roll at your waist. Your best bet is to wear shorts that are loose through the hips and legs. Or you can get a temporary tummy-tuck wearing shorts with full-span pockets (often used in jeans for this figure problem).

Not-So-Short Shorts

You want: To draw attention to your trim waist and away from a full bottom and heavy thighs.

Look for: Shorts that are slightly fuller in the leg, with a wide hem that falls mid-thigh.

The legs don't need to flare dramatically, but they should cover the heaviest areas and flatter your waist.

The exception would be bicycle shorts—streamlined black Lycra-blend tights that are sold in sporting goods stores that reach mid-thigh and don't ride up as you cycle. They're not really a fashion item, though, and should be worn only for cycling, not everyday wear.

Capri Pants

You want: To minimize the appearance of full thighs and avoid chafing (a common problem if you perspire and your thighs rub together as you walk).

Look for: Below-knee styling for warm weather, in loose moisture-wicking fabrics like ramie or silk.

Everyday Clothes That Flatter

Ever since work clothes went casual, the line between office wear and everyday clothes has blurred. Depending on your profession, khakis and a twin set (matching sweater and cardigan) will suffice on casual Friday. Or you can slip a stylish vest over a blouse and skirt and reserve the jacket for days you attend meetings.

If you carry most of your weight in your belly, butt, or thighs, combining separates is your best option. You can fit each piece to a specific part of your figure. Layering is especially helpful, says Arons. Toss a loose-fitting, long blouse, shirt, or jacket over a dress or fitted top and pants or skirt. Choose cotton or rayon in summer, chamois or flannel in fall, and wool in winter.

To further minimize your tummy, thighs, or derriere, look for these features.

Tapered Skirt

You want: A skirt that accommodates a protruding derriere or heavy thighs when worn with a straight, tailored jacket.

Look for: A skirt that's cut generously through the hips, with a tailored waistband, fitted front, flat front pleats, tapered hem, and back slit.

If a skirt falls straight from hips to hem, it can easily make your figure appear boxy, says Nix-Rice. To work well, a straight skirt needs to skim the body, never fit too tightly. She suggests a skirt that's tapered slightly from hip to hemline. The converging lines will narrow and elongate your figure. You'll look slimmer without compromising comfort.

To alter a garment you've purchased, start the taper just below the heaviest spot at the thighs.

To get a sleek look and comfortable fit off the rack, without hiring a professional seamstress, look for a waistband that's elasticized in the back or at the sides. And opt for a back slit.

"A slitted skirt looks wonderful on a woman with a round derriere," says Lutz.

Sculpted Hem

You want: A skirt that compensates for an ample derriere.

Look for: A skirt with a longer back or a scooped front. If you're wearing pants and your derriere needs more fabric, your backside "borrows" the fabric by pulling it from the front. But if you're wearing a dress or skirt, your fanny simply pulls up the skirt, leaving the hemline uneven. The solution: An intentionally uneven, asymmetrical hem. You may have to visit a shop that specializes in plus sizes, but the quest is worth your while. Ask for a hem that's shorter in the front, also known as an irregular hemline.

If you can't find a scoop-front skirt, buy skirts that fall mid-calf or longer. If your skirt is ankle length and the back rides up, no one will notice.

A-Line Top

You want: Tummy coverage, especially if you're wearing pants or a skirt that contrasts with your top or has a high waistband.

Look for: An A-line top to layer over a tapered skirt or straight-leg pants.

Try what designer Lutz calls a trapeze top, made in stretchy or gently flowing fabric and worn long, so if you stand with your arms at your sides, it falls somewhere between your fingertips and your knees. You can get a similar effect with less fabric by wearing a straight tunic top with side seam slits, creating an A line when you walk. Side slits also add more vertical lines to the outfit.

Flat-Front Pants

You want: Pants that minimize the appearance of your tummy, hips, and thighs.

Look for: Construction features and details that minimize bulges with as little fabric as possible.

Most of the guidelines for buying jeans (see page 315) also apply to pants and trousers. As a bonus, it's easier to find trousers that hold in the tummy—mainly because the linings are cut slightly smaller than the pants, functioning as internal support.

Quality garments often include extended pocket bags, which start at the side seam and attach at the center front seam or front opening. If you like to wear pants with pleats, look for either a quality lining or the extended pocket bags. These will prevent your tummy from pulling open the pleats.

To minimize both tummy and derriere, avoid fly fronts. For a smoother line, look for a back zipper or a button closure tucked into a side seam pocket instead. For similar reasons, avoid pants with a side zipper at the hip, says Nix-Rice. If you're heavy, it will invariably buckle, bulge, and stick out.

Sarong Skirt

You want: A skirt that diverts attention from your hips, thighs, and tummy.

Look for: Skirts with an additional panel of fabric that wraps around the front of your body and ties at one side. Called a sarong, this style is increasingly popular for both casual and office wear, especially when paired with a matching, fingertip-length jacket. The second front works by fooling the eye into thinking the extra fullness comes from your skirt, not your tummy. And the diagonal downward line contributes to the slimming effect. (Be careful that the fabric wrapped across your tummy isn't full of gathers or stretched completely flat. Unless the sarong is gently draped across your tummy, the second, wrapped front will draw attention to trouble spots.)

Watch the shape at the hemline, and make sure that the skirt tapers from knee to hem, rather than swinging out.

Office Wear That Suits Your Figure

Casual Fridays aside, tailored pants, skirts, and jackets are still the unofficial uniform for many working women. Experts agree that in order for you to look effective and professional, your office wear must fit perfectly. If your only trouble spot is your tummy, you'll have an easier time. But if your body is pear- or hourglass-shaped, it's difficult to find ready-to-wear suits that fit well.

A woman who has a prominent derriere and thighs needs garments with specific designs. The clothes should look great when you stand, yet they should be cut with the right shape and ease to spread as you sit. Unless a designer started with a model that had the classic pear- or hourglass-figure, the garment won't fit your shape. And buying a larger size won't help.

If you are pear-shaped and must wear a suit to work, consider hiring a dressmaker or tailor. An expert can cut garments to minimize your figure variations. If that's not an option, follow the guidelines for flat-front pants and tapered skirts, above. Then follow these tips when purchasing a jacket.

Cropped Jacket

You want: A style that diverts attention away from your lower body.

Look for: Waist-length jackets. While a cropped jacket does reveal all if you have a triangular figure, it will pull the viewer's eye up to your face, which is just where you want it, says Nix-Rice. To enhance this effect further, choose a jacket made from fabric with texture or one that has interesting embellishments, such as decorative stitching at the neckline or piping, for example.

Women who want to define their waists should try an even shorter jacket, known as a bolero, recommends Lutz. The bolero shape includes slightly extended shoulder seams that balance the upper body of a triangular figure. Lutz suggests combining the bolero with a camisole top and a six-gore, calf-length skirt. To pull the look together, add a three-inch-wide belt.

If you aren't comfortable drawing attention to your waist, consider wearing separates that have the same color or print.

Kimono Jacket

You want: A relaxed jacket that complements several dress and skirt styles, while minimizing your belly, butt, and thighs.

Look for: A loosely fitted jacket in soft fabric, that hangs straight or wraps and ties at the center front with a fabric belt, with three-quarter-length sleeves and a fingertip-length hem.

A fingertip-length hem is great for a slimming look, particularly when both side seams are slit from hem to waist. Combine the kimono jacket with a tee dress, which is "kicked out" at the hips and slit at one side seam, suggests designer Lutz. If you don't own a tee dress, try any dress that has a simple silhouette and neckline.

Swing Jacket

You want: A jacket that diverts attention from your tummy or obscures your derriere (or both).

Look for: A fluid jacket cut in an A-line shape that barely brushes your derriere and thighs. This swing styling adds instant panache to any dress or top and bottom. Avoid bulky fabric, which will

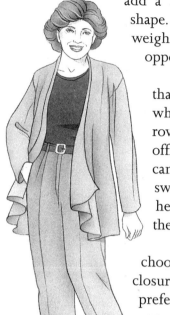

add a size or two to your shape. Slinky knits or light-weight gabardine have the opposite effect.

Choose a hemline that rests near the knee, where your leg is narrowest. In more creative office environments, you can wear a duster, a swing jacket with a hemline that drops to the ankle.

Whatever length you choose, don't worry about closures. A swing jacket is preferably worn open, so you have two very desirable long, vertical lines at the center front opening. Wear fitted garments underneath.

Shapewear for a Great Foundation

If you add only one item to your wardrobe this entire year, make it a piece of shapewear: combination bras and panties and other one-piece undergarments that hold you in—comfortably.

More and more women are replacing their underwear with these wonder undies. Nothing takes off as many pounds and firms up so many areas in just seconds. In fact, the undergarment company Bali calls one of its lines Inches Slimmer, and says the briefs "take off inches instantly." Plus-size model Katie Arons says shapewear helps her look her best at a photo shoot.

"It enables me to wear clothes I couldn't otherwise model," says Arons. "I can pull on a girdle and then pull on something that fits snugly through the hips." Her favorite shapewear? Pantyhose. Givenchy Ultimate Smoothers, says Arons, are comfortable, sturdy, and just as effective as a girdle. "I can wear them every day."

Tights, often used for a sportier look, are a great opportunity for color toning. Blend shoes and hosiery with the hemline for a continuous flow of color from waistline to floor, suggests Nix-Rice.

One for All

You want: Tummy support, derriere-firming hold, and torso-smoothing panels.

Look for: Hip slip, full-body slip, long- or high-leg briefs.

Regardless of the style or manufacturer, these items really hold in your belly, butt, and thighs. Unlike girdles of old, the new shapewear is comfortable. Choose light, medium, or firm control. Even if you need firm control, the fabric is soft and pliable, and hems often stay in place without thick, stiff elastic that impedes circulation. Look for all-over control, with panels at the thighs and tummy to smooth and flatten these areas.

While shapewear holds that jiggly stuff in place, not all shapewear targets the rear for extra support. The Playtex Sleek Shaper Longleg brief meets all the criteria.

Whatever you choose, look for comfort and quality. When trying on these garments, really move around: Sit, bend, and walk up and down the fitting room aisle several times. This is important because hems tend to creep up if the garment doesn't have grippers (elasticized areas that keep the garment in place) or they're low-quality. The grippers shouldn't creep out of place. Otherwise, you could find yourself surreptitiously yanking at the hem—which is now neatly curled around your waist—in the middle of a meeting or an evening out with your honey. Avoid grippers that look like opaque glue dribbled in squiggly lines along the hem. They don't hold very well, and as the garment ages, little wormlike pieces will fall off when you walk.

Swimwear Made for the Water

If you're planning to work your swimming workouts into your vacation schedule, you'll want

Go Easy on the Shoulder Pads

The football linebacker look of the 1980s is long gone—for now. But shoulder pads are still around, and they've always helped give shape to tailored jackets.

If you have heavy hips and thighs, shoulder pads can help balance a proportionately larger lower body, says Nancy Nix-Rice, an image consultant from St.

Louis and author of *Looking Good: A Comprehensive Guide to Wardrobe Planning and Personal Style Development*. But don't go overboard, or you'll end up looking larger all over. Her advice: If you have soft, sloping shoulders, you can wear thicker pads. If you already have square shoulders, use only thin pads—or forgo them completely.

---

swimwear that's up to the task. And you'll also want to look good. You can still find swimwear with frilly skirts—if that's your style. But skirted suits aren't the only way to camouflage figure flaws when you take to the water.

When you step into the dressing room to try on a new suit, don't eye yourself too critically. This can't be said enough. Others will be far less apt to notice your trouble spots if you accept yourself and have a confident attitude.

One piece or two? Some fashion experts say a one-piece suit is the only way to go. Others say either one can look great, as long as you choose the right style. You have to decide what works best for your physique.

"I'd just as soon see women in suits that they love, in colors that light them up, having a wonderful time in the water—alone or with others," says Alice Ansfield, the publisher of *Radiance: The Magazine for Large Women*. "Women of all sizes can enjoy the pools, lakes, and oceans of the world—and well they should."

She ought to know: Every year, *Radiance* publishes photos of its readers in swimsuits, showing many flattering styles on various body shapes. A woman with a triangular or pear-shaped figure, for example, looks good in a suit that draws the viewer's eye upward.

To find a suit that works with, not against, your body, follow these expert guidelines.

Dynamic Tops

You want: To divert attention away from your tummy, derriere, and thighs.

Look for: Anything with a stylish or pretty design above the waist.

Consider a ruffle, lace, or an interesting design at the bodice, says Ansfield. A diagonal design or pattern down the front also works well. So do wide shoulder straps or halter styling.

High-Cut Legs

You want: To reduce the appearance of your thighs.

Look for: A slightly higher leg opening.

This style "stretches" the leg so heavy thighs aren't as obvious. Keep in mind, though, that a very high cut leg means less fabric to cover a prominent derriere.

Consider, too, the shape of your thighs. If there's a bulge where your leg joins your body, a high-cut leg won't be very attractive. In this situation, look for long legs (called a boy cut) that cover and smooth your hips. For two-piece suits, choose bottoms with full-cut legs. In other words, the legs are cut to sit at the joint where your legs meet your hips.

Sarong Swimsuit Skirt

You want: Slimming coverage for your tummy and thighs.

Look for: A wrap that ties over the bottom of your one- or two-piece suit.

Almost any lightweight, washable fabric will do. A pareo, very similar to a sarong, is simply a large fabric rectangle that you creatively wrap or tie around your body to cover your bathing suit.

You can buy removable skirts to slip off before you take a dip. If you want to keep everything under wraps while in the water, look for a shorter version of the sarong, in mesh or other swimsuit material. Several manufacturers sell two-piece mix-and-match tops and bottoms as well as mesh sarongs.

Evening Wear

Whether your style is sophisticated, demure, sexy, or casually elegant, you can find dressy garments cut for your shape. If you're trying to tone your belly, butt, or thighs, you don't have to hide under ruffles (unless you want to). For example, for a publicity photo for her book, *Sexy at Any Size*, Katie Arons—a size 18—wore a knock-your-socks-off sexy two-piece outfit pulled together with a sheer, duster-length jacket. The tank-style top was fitted, and the slightly A-line skirt was ankle length with a daring slit up the center front. Arons, who has worn many types and styles of garments during her modeling career, says the key to wearing fitted garments is completing the outfit with a loose blouse or jacket. Even if it's sheer or worn open, no one will notice your tummy, derriere, or thighs.

If you prefer pants to dresses and skirts, even for evening wear, follow the basic advice on pages 318 to 320 to purchase dynamic velvet trousers and a matching satin jacket.

Fitted and Cropped

You want: A sleek look that diverts attention away from your hips and thighs.

Look for: A slim dress topped with a gorgeous cropped jacket.

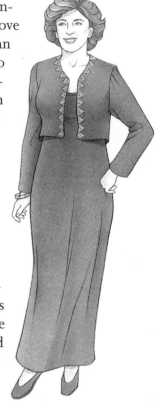

Ideally, the jacket hemline should stop just above or at your waist. With an open front to create two vertical lines, slightly extended shoulders, and an abbreviated jacket, you'll instantly have a gorgeous, shapely figure.

This look is particularly flattering when paired with a slim dress that swings into an A-line hem. But fabric choice is important. Choose a medium-weight fabric that moves gracefully and has some stretch. Crepe, when used for a fitted or semi-fitted garment, ripples over body bumps.

Basque Waistline

You want: A fitted look, but you also want to obscure your rear and thighs.

Look for: A basque dress with a hemline that is either floor-length or hits your lower calf and that shows off your upper body while camouflaging the lower portion. It should have a fitted bodice that explodes into a dramatic, full skirt from a dropped waist that starts at the top of the hips. The silhouette draws the eye down, away from trouble spots that are no longer visible under the gathered skirt.

A woman with a full derriere or hips can carry this style nicely. But don't abandon hope if the first few dresses you try on don't work. Not all women with pear-shaped figures carry their extra inches in the same place, so it's simply a matter of finding a compatible garment. The amount of fullness in a skirt and the position of the waistline will vary.

A-Line Dress or Jacket

You want: A flattering outfit that minimizes your tummy.

Look for: A-line dresses and skirts, or a semi-fitted dress with a matching swing coat. From full-coverage to revealing, the top of this swingy dress or skirt style can vary greatly. Even the hemline width can differ. What all have in common is a silhouette that moves outward as it travels down the bottom half of your body, creating an "A" shape. In a dress, the fabric skims the waist and flows out over the hips.

Even a slip-dress, thought to be very revealing, can look fabulous. Choose luscious fabrics, but keep in mind that if the fabric is light-colored and light-reflective, like pink satin, others will see your tummy.

The Classic Empire

You want: Sophisticated styling without holding in your tummy all night; a classic dress that you know flatters and slims.

Look for: An empire waist—it's fashionable and flattering for every body shape, says Barbara Pflaumer of Alfred Angelo, a wedding and evening wear manufacturer in Horsham, Pennsylvania. The trick is avoiding a stiff, full skirt. Crepe, satin, and other fabrics with beautiful drape will gently skim and camouflage your lower body.

For more information on apparel makers and designers who cater to women who wear larger sizes, visit our Web site at www.banishbbt.com.

Photography Credits

Cover by Mitch Mandel/Rodale Images 1999

All interior photos by Mitch Mandel except:

© Comstock, page 286

Courtesy of Concept II Ltd., page 256

Tim De Frisco/Rodale Images, pages 232, 238

John P. Hamel/Rodale Images, pages 264, 277, 294

Courtesy of ICON Health and Fitness, page 215

© John P. Kelly/The Image Bank, page 210

Ed Landrock/Rodale Images, pages 242, 260, 273

© Araldo de Luca/Corbis, page 1

© David Madison, page 205

© David Madison/The Image Bank, page 251

© Lori Adamski Peek/Tony Stone, page 201

Photo Courtesy of Precor, page 223

Rodale Images, page 246

Sally Ann Ullman/Rodale Images, pages 282, 290

Kurt Wilson/Rodale Images, pages 219, 269

© David Woods/The Stock Market, page 235

Index

Underscored page references indicate sidebars and tables.
Boldface references indicate photographs and illustrations.

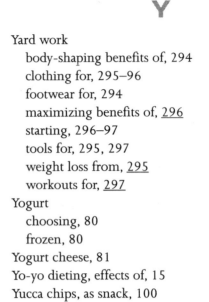